T0344761

# ANNALS *of* THE NEW YORK ACADEMY OF SCIENCES

**EDITOR-IN-CHIEF**
Douglas Braaten

**ASSOCIATE EDITOR**
Rebecca E. Cooney

**PROJECT MANAGER**
Steven E. Bohall

**EDITORIAL ADMINISTRATOR**
Daniel J. Becker

Artwork and design by Ash Ayman Shairzay

The New York Academy of Sciences
7 World Trade Center
250 Greenwich Street, 40th Floor
New York, NY 10007-2157

annals@nyas.org
www.nyas.org/annals

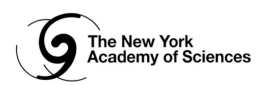

**The New York
Academy of Sciences**

Published by Blackwell Publishing
On behalf of the New York Academy of Sciences

Boston, Massachusetts
2012

# ANNALS *of* THE NEW YORK ACADEMY OF SCIENCES

VOLUME
1247

ISSUE
# The Year in Immunology

ISSUE EDITOR
## Noel R. Rose

The Johns Hopkins University

## TABLE OF CONTENTS

# Become a Member Today of the New York Academy of Sciences

The New York Academy of Sciences is dedicated to identifying the next frontiers in science and catalyzing key breakthroughs. As has been the case for 200 years, many of the leading scientific minds of our time rely on the Academy for key meetings and publications that serve as the crucial forum for a global community dedicated to scientific innovation.

 **Select one FREE *Annals* volume and up to five volumes for only $40 each.**

 **Network and exchange ideas with the leaders of academia and industry.**

 **Broaden your knowledge across many disciplines.**

 **Gain access to exclusive online content.**

## Join Online at **www.nyas.org**

Or by phone at **800.344.6902** (516.576.2270 if outside the U.S.).

Ann. N.Y. Acad. Sci. ISSN 0077-8923

## ANNALS OF THE NEW YORK ACADEMY OF SCIENCES

Issue: *The Year in Immunology*

# Preface for *The Year in Immunology*

## Homeostasis in innate and adaptive immunity

Each year the distinguished editorial advisory board of *The Year in Immunology* series suggests topics and authors that have contributed most to forward thinking in the year just passed. Although each review is entirely independent, the articles collectively often illustrate interlocking themes for the year. For 2011, it is likely that future historians of immunology will look back at a year emphasizing immunologic homeostasis.

The immune system is one of the most potent of our physiologic responses. Consequently, it can produce great harm as well as essential benefit. As Darwin taught us, evolution endeavors to provide a biologic constitution with the greatest likelihood of success in a particular environment. This concept is well illustrated in immunology. A life on earth free of infectious disease on one hand, and autoimmune and allergic disease on the other, requires a careful and dynamic balance of the many interacting components of the immune response. The goal of a healthy homeostasis is shown in both the innate and adaptive responses. It is seen as the adjustment of responses to exposure to microbial colonization, infection, aging, and the environment. Consequently, the most effective recent therapies restore homeostasis and thus alleviate the threat of ongoing disease.

Lane and colleagues introduce us to the relatively new arrivals on the monocyte terrain, the lymphoid tissue inducer (LTi cells), originally identified in neonatal lymph nodes as CD4$^+$CD3$^-$ lymphoid cells. Their function in maintaining homeostasis of both innate and adaptive immunity first became obvious when mice deficient in the orphan retinoic acid receptor gamma (ROR$\gamma$) demonstrated reduced formation of organized lymphoid follicles following bacterial colonization of the gut. Because of their broad phylogenetic distribution, LTi cells have had a long evolutionary history, and they are integrated into the regulation of several steps in the immune response, including both innate and adaptive. Another ancient seminal pathway, the Wnt signaling pathway, is also deeply involved in regulation of both innate and adaptive immune systems. Important in the regulation of peripheral T cell responses, Wnt's role in thymocyte development and T cell maturation is discussed by Xue and Zhao. Gamma delta T cells are another product of the ancient evolutionary background of the immune system. Korn and Petermann describe the role of gamma delta T cells in producing interleukin 17 (IL-17) during inflammatory responses, for protection against a variety of mycotic and bacterial infections, and in autoimmune diseases such as multiple sclerosis. The forkhead box O (FoxO) family of transcription factors—also with a long evolutionary history—has been found to be important in maintaining immunologic homeostasis, especially by controlling development of adaptive immunity. Thus, dysregulation of FoxO activity results in chronic inflammation and loss of self-tolerance. The controlling mechanisms of this family of transcription factors are described by Mashreghi and colleagues.

doi: 10.1111/j.1749-6632.2012.06458.x

For many years, helper T cell development was believed to follow two alternative pathways, Th1 and Th2. Then, additional alternatives came along with the description of regulatory T cells ($T_{reg}$ cells) and IL-17–producing T helper cells (Th17 cells). Bopp, *et al.* describe the newly recognized Th9 cell—T helper cells that produce IL-9 and other specific cytokines—differentiation pathway and distinguish it from the effects of Th2 responses. The role of IL-9 in allergic asthma, certain microbial infections, and autoimmunity and self-tolerance are all receiving renewed attention.

A remarkable property of the immune system is its ability to adapt to changing circumstances. During newborn and infant years immune responses may be restrained in order to protect from possible immune attack on still vulnerable developing organ systems. At the other end of life, the immune system compensates for the involution of the thymus. The immune system must contend, moreover, with additional stress caused by chronic infections by, for example, cytomegalovirus (CMV) and HIV. The consequences of stress on immune aging are discussed in an article by Goronzy, Weyand, and Le Saux. The ability of the intestine to harbor trillions of microbial passengers entails remarkable resiliency of the intestinal immune response at both adaptive and innate levels. Detailed study of the defining exposure to certain intestinal inhabitants, particularly helminthic worms, has revealed some of the most critical homeostatic mechanisms maintaining intestinal tolerance. The regulatory devices of the intestine are reviewed comprehensively by Elliott and Weinstock. Intestinal homeostasis also depends on the humoral immune response, especially secretory IgA. Bemark and colleagues analyze the relationship between IgA production and the gut microbiota, and outline some of the factors distinguishing an unwanted response in the form of allergy and autoimmunity from an effective response to mucosal vaccines.

Finally, a better understanding of the essential elements of immunologic homeostasis has helped in designing drugs to correct the immunologic imbalances that lead to inflammatory diseases. Calabresi and colleagues review the mechanism of action of several newly introduced disease-modifying drugs for the treatment of multiple sclerosis. Some of these recently approved agents provide fresh insight into regulatory steps in the immune response. For example, fingolimod, a structural analog of intracellular sphingnosine, exerts its effects by mimicking sphingnosine-1-phosphate (S1P) and binding to the S1P receptors. Without these signals, the egress of T and B cells from secondary lymphoid tissues is impaired and the level of circulating lymphocytes reduced. The effect is most pronounced on the trafficking of memory T lymphocytes, with less effect on important protective functions such as release of inflammatory cytokines. Lo and Tsokos have scrutinized the newer drugs approved for the treatment of systemic lupus erythematosus. Of special interest is belimumab, which inhibits the B cell growth factor BLyS (BAFF). Belimumab has proved to be effective in a subpopulation of SLE patients. The availability of these target drugs underlines the growing importance of looking at homeostatic deficiencies in individual patients. A drug that may be highly beneficial in individuals with one particular deficiency may be of little value or even harmful in others with a different mediator or cytokine profile.

The year's advances in immunology present a spectrum from molecular research to clinical application. They well exemplify how growing knowledge of the inner workings of the immune response can identify the critical steps for maintaining its homeostatic balance and can lead us to better and safer treatments for immune-mediated diseases.

As issue editor of *The Year in Immunology* series, I am pleased to acknowledge with gratitude the excellent support provided by the staff of *Annals of the New York Academy of Sciences*, and the general support of The New York Academy of Sciences, in producing this year's issue.

NOEL R. ROSE

*The Johns Hopkins University*
*Baltimore, Maryland*

Ann. N.Y. Acad. Sci. ISSN 0077-8923

ANNALS OF THE NEW YORK ACADEMY OF SCIENCES
Issue: *The Year in Immunology*

# Lymphoid tissue inducer cells: innate cells critical for CD4+ T cell memory responses?

Peter J.L. Lane,[1] Fabrina M. Gaspal,[1] Fiona M. McConnell,[1] Mi Yeon Kim,[2] Graham Anderson,[1] and David R. Withers[1]

[1]MRC Centre for Immune Regulation, College of Medical and Dental Sciences, University of Birmingham, UK. [2]Department of Bioinformatics and Life Science, Soongsil University, Seoul, Korea

Address for correspondence: Peter J.L. Lane, MRC Centre for Immune Regulation, College of Medical and Dental Sciences, University of Birmingham, UK. p.j.l.lane@bham.ac.uk

Lymphoid tissue inducer cells (LTi) are a relatively new arrival on the immunological cellular landscape, having first been characterized properly only 15 years ago. They are members of an emerging family of innate lymphoid cells (ILCs). Elucidation of their function reveals links not only with the ancient innate immune system, but also with adaptive immune responses, in particular the development of lymph nodes and CD4+ T cell memory immune responses, which on one hand underpin the success of vaccination strategies, and on the other hand drive many human immunologically mediated diseases. This perspective article is not an exhaustive account of the role of LTi in the development of lymphoid tissues, as there have been many excellent reviews published already. Instead, we combine current knowledge of genetic phylogeny and comparative immunology, together with classical mouse genetics, to suggest how LTi might have evolved from a primitive lymphocytic innate cell in the ancestral 500-million-year-old vertebrate immune system into a cell critical for adaptive CD4+ T cell immune responses in mammals.

Keywords: memory; effector; lymphoid tissue inducer cells; lymph nodes

## Introduction

Reina Mebius was the first to characterize murine lymphoid tissue inducer cells (LTi),[1] but they were initially identified as CD4+CD3− lineage negative lymphoid cells in neonatal lymph nodes by Kelly and Scollay.[2] Their function in the development of lymphoid tissues was revealed when it was found that mice deficient in the orphan retinoic acid receptor gamma (RORγ) lacked both this CD4+CD3− LTi population and lymph nodes.[3,4] Although RORγ is expressed in nonlymphoid tissues, it is selectively expressed in hemopoietic cells as the splice variant, RORγt; coexpression of green fluorescent protein (GFP) with RORγt showed LTi to be the only RORγt expressing hemopoietic cells in the developing embryo.[5] Mapping the fate of these LTi on the basis of their GFP positivity,[6] it was demonstrated that the CD4+ population present in gut cryptopatches,[7] originally thought to be sites of intestinal T cell generation,[8] were in fact LTi that in-

cluded a CD4− subset; furthermore, LTi were required for both the development of cryptopatches and their subsequent transformation into isolated lymphoid follicles (ILFs, focal follicular accumulations of LTi with dendritic cells [DCs] and B and T cells), postnatally, after bacterial colonization of the gut.[9]

These studies linked LTi unequivocally with the development of lymph nodes, cryptopatches, and ILFs through their expression of the tumor necrosis family superfamily members (TNFSF) for the lymphotoxin beta receptor (LTβR) ligands (LTα$_1$β$_2$)[10] and TRANCE,[11] but more recent studies have also shown that LTi are rich sources of the cytokine interleukin 22 (IL-22)[12] that is linked with the promotion of defenses at epithelial sites.[13–15] This would permit the LTi a function in the promotion of innate immunity that is distinct from the induction of lymphoid tissues. In addition, our work has shown that LTi persist in adult lymphoid tissues in both mouse[16] and humans[17] but are distinguished from

doi: 10.1111/j.1749-6632.2011.06284.x
Ann. N.Y. Acad. Sci. 1247 (2012) 1–15 © 2012 New York Academy of Sciences.

**Table 1.** Phenotypes of embryonic and adult LTi in human and mouse

| | Mouse | | Human | |
|---|---|---|---|---|
| | Embryonic LTi | Postnatal LTi | Embryonic LTi | Postnatal LTi |
| Th17 gene | | | | |
| IL-22 | + | + | + | + |
| IL-17A | + | + | + | Low |
| IL-23R | + | + | + | + |
| Transcription factor | | | | |
| RORγt | + | + | + | + |
| ID2 | + | + | + | + |
| AHR | + | + | + | + |
| Surface marker | | | | |
| CD3 | − | − | − | − |
| CD4 | +/− | +/− | − | − (low) |
| CD117 | + | + | + | + |
| IL-7Rα (CD127) | + | + | + | + |
| IL-2Rα (CD25) | + | + | + | + |
| TNFSF | | | | |
| OX40L (TNFSF4) | − | +++ | − | +++ |
| CD30L (TNFSF8) | − | + | − | − |
| TRANCE (TNFSF11) | + | + | + | + |
| TNF, LTα, LTβ | ++ | ++ | ++ | ++ |
| DR3 (TNFRSF25) | + | + | + | + |
| Chemokine receptor | | | | |
| CXCR5 | + | + | + | + |
| CCR7 | + | + | + | + |
| CCR6 | + | + | + | + |

the neonatal population by their expression of high levels of OX40-ligand (OX40L; TNFSF4)[16,17] and in mouse, CD30L (TNFSF8; see Table 1).[16] Our studies have found that CD4+ T cell memory function is highly dependent on signaling through both OX40 and CD30,[18] suggesting additional roles for LTi in the mediation of adaptive CD4+ T cell–dependent immune responses.

The set of characteristics described earlier links LTi with a number of apparently disparate functions. We think that this apparent complexity arises because LTi have a long history, and their function has been modified by the acquisition of new genes over time. Comparison of the immune system of teleosts (bony fish), which diverged from humans some 500 million years ago (Mya), shows that the T and B cell immune system is at least this old. Indeed recent evidence shows that B- and T-like lymphocytes[19] and a primitive thymus[20] were present in the protochordate ancestors of vertebrates. Were

lymphocyte-like LTi also participants in this ancestral immune system?

## Possible origin of LTi cells and evolution of LTi function

Although we have no way of knowing what the 500-million-year-old ancestor's immune system really looked like, genetic phylogeny is prismatic on the sequence of gene evolution. In an ideal world, one would have detailed genomic maps of not only all vertebrate classes including cartilaginous fish, but also the vertebrate ancestors, lamprey and amphioxus. However, as yet, genomes of these animals have not been recorded in the Ensembl database,[a] so we have focused on identifying LTi genes in teleosts (bony fish), which

---

[a]http://useast.ensembl.org/index.html

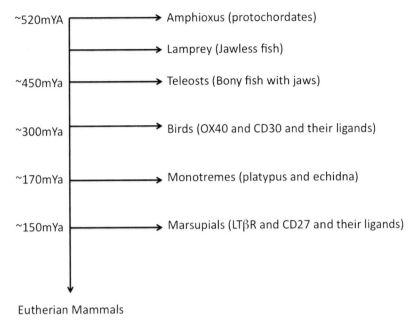

**Figure 1.** Phylogenetic tree depicting the approximate time of divergence of the ancestors of jawed vertebrates, teleosts, birds, monotremes, and marsupial mammals from eutherian placental mammals. Ma, millions of years ago. OX40 and CD30 and their ligands are in bird genomes but not bony fish; LTβR and CD27 are present only in placental mammals.

share a common ancestor with mammals some 450 Ma (Fig. 1). By comparing the genes and genomic organization (synteny) of teleosts with those of higher vertebrates, we discover not only genes common to both but newly evolved genes (Table 1).[21] Commonality of genes and synteny implies that they were present in the common jawed vertebrate ancestor. And indeed, key transcription factors required for LTi development (Ikaros,[22] Tox,[23] RORγt,[24] and Id2[25]) have zebrafish orthologues, and associated genes show synteny between the human and zebrafish genomes.

Other genes essential to the LTi phenotype, however, are present in higher vertebrates but not teleosts, which places their evolution after the establishment of the ancestral vertebrate immune system. Thus, not all of the TNFSF expressed by LTi (TRANCE, LTα₁β₂, and OX40L and CD30L) are ancient, although TRANCE is.[21] OX40L and CD30L and their respective receptors are found only in birds and mammals who share a common ancestor some 300 Ma, but not teleosts.[21] LTβR ligands and their receptor, which programme lymph node development,[10] are exclusive to therian (placental) mammals (including marsupials)[26] but do not occur in monotremes (egg laying mammals of which platy-

pus and echidna are the only extant examples).[27,28] However, if one postulates that LTi had a function in the common vertebrate ancestor in promoting epithelial integrity of the gut through the expression of IL-22, a plausible ancestral function for LTi emerges. In addition to key transcription factors required for LTi development, teleosts have orthologues of the transcription factor AHR,[29] which is required for the expression of IL-22.[30] IL-22 is expressed at high levels in LTi[12] and is also found in zebrafish genomes clustered with interferon gamma (IFN-γ) and IL-26, as it is in higher mammals. Therefore the genes essential for the generation of IL-22–expressing LTi could have been present in the ancestral immune system. An understanding of where these cells might have been and what they might have been doing is provided by their role in the development of cryptopatches.[6]

Cryptopatches are clusters of LTi with DCs located mainly in intestine, as the name suggests, in close proximity to intestinal crypts: the sites of genesis of the epithelial cells that provide the single layer barrier from the bacteria rich gut lumen. Their formation is dependent on TNFRSF1a signals,[31] and in particular on the chemokine, CCL20, which is secreted by intestinal epithelium, and serves as an

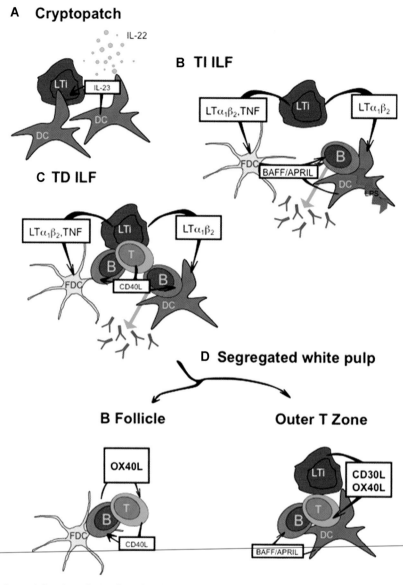

**Figure 2.** Location and function of LTi cells within the adult. LTi cells support both innate and adaptive immune responses. (A) Within the intestine, LTi cells reside within cryptopatches, producing IL-22, critical for maintenance of the gut epithelium. In response to bacterial signals, some cryptopatches form (B and C) ILFs, mediated by $LT\alpha_1\beta_2$ and TNF signals from LTi cells. (B) Within ILFs, LTi cells can further orchestrate T cell-independent production of IgA. (D) Within secondary lymphoid tissue, LTi cells reside at the outer T zone supporting antigen-independent survival of CD4$^+$ T cells through provision of OX40L and CD30L signals. Within follicles, OX40L signals from B cells and DCs support affinity maturation.

attractant for cells, including LTi, bearing its ligand, CCR6. Again, gene orthologues of all of these interacting factors, CCL20, CCR6, and TNFRSF1a, are present in zebrafish. As already mentioned, LTi are rich sources of IL-22,[12] a key function of which is the maintenance of epithelial integrity.[12,14,15,32–34] In many ways, LTi in cryptopatches behave like CD4$^+$ Th17 T cells. At least in mice, they express CD4, and like CD4$^+$ T cells, they cluster with DCs (Fig. 2). There are two essential components to DC function: an antigen-processing component that is clearly irrelevant to LTi, as they lack a T cell receptor (TcR), and an innate sensor component whereby pattern recognition receptors (activated by bacteria in the gut) stimulate the expression of cytokines such as IL-23, which in turn, through interaction with its receptor on LTi, can elicit the secretion of Th17 cytokines.[12]

LTi, therefore, have half of the CD4[+] Th17 T cell equation: they receive signals (by IL-23; zebrafish have orthologues of IL-23R) from DCs, which are specialized to recognize bacterial gene products, and then secrete the cytokines (IL-22, IL-17) that help other cells (in this case, IL-22R–expressing epithelia), in response to this information. This feature, forming multicellular interactions and effecting cooperation between different cell types, remains constant throughout LTi evolution, and parallels the way that CD4[+] T helper cells interact with antigen-presenting cells, and then provide help to other cells through the expression of cytokines.

Could this define the ancestral function of RORγt-dependent LTi in the prejawed vertebrate world before RAG-dependent TcRs? RORγt is also expressed in double positive thymocytes, which are substantially reduced in RORγ[KO] mice. So, is RORγt expressed in teleost thymocytes? This is not currently known, but recent identification of mAbs to fish CD4 and CD8 has allowed the observation that fish resemble RORγ[KO] mice[3,4] in having relatively few double positive (CD8[+]CD4[+]) thymocytes. In contrast, the developing zebrafish shows strong expression of RORγ in the gut, which brings us back to the mammalian cryptopatch, CCR6[+] LTi, and CCL20-expressing epithelia.[24] Therefore, although not proven, it is nonetheless possible that the RORγ-dependent development of IL-22–secreting LTi anticipated RORγ function in T cell development and effector function. Expression profiling of RORγ in zebrafish thymocytes would resolve this issue.

In any case, it is clear that with regard to this aspect of their function, there is an emerging family of innate lymphoid cells (ILCs) whose members secrete cytokines that are normally associated with CD4[+] T cells,[35] for example, the Th2 cytokine, IL-13, and the Th1 cytokine, IFN-γ (genes also present in teleost genomes). These ILCs clearly have effector function. It is tempting to speculate, therefore, that members of the family of ILCs, which like LTi depend on the Id2 gene product for their development,[35] were ancestral innate effector cells with a common lymphocyte progenitor, into which a RAG-dependent TcR was inserted, resulting in adaptive recognition

as we now understand it in conventional T cells. In this respect, it is interesting to note that subsets of CD4[+] T cells selected in the mouse thymus have been identified as being already committed to a Th1/Th2-expressing program[36] or a Th17/IL-22–expressing program.[37] The latter are identified by their upregulation of expression of CCR6, which guides them, as it does LTi, to epithelial sites, where their expression of IL-23R allows them to amplify the secretion of IL-22 for the protection of epithelial integrity. Perhaps these CD4[+] Th17-committed cells selected on thymic epithelium are descendants of the putative LTi that acquired a TcR, now programmed to recognize epithelial antigens associated with class II in the gut, just as many thymus selected invariant gamma delta T cells do for antigens associated with nonconventional MHC molecules.

## Cryptopatch maturation into B cell-rich ILFs

ILFs are the mature progeny of cryptopatches. They develop after birth in response to bacterial colonization in the gut; they recruit predominantly B cells through their expression of CXCR5,[9] but also some T cells by CCR6[38] expression, to form follicular nonencapsulated structures that lack high endothelial venules (HEV), the specialized postcapillary blood vessels seen in lymph nodes.[9] ILFs depend on both TNFRSF1a and LTβR signals; lymph nodes in contrast depend almost exclusively on LTβR.[9] The TNFRSF1a and LTβR genes are closely linked genetically (∼50 kB apart, see Table 2) in the modern therian mammals where both genes occur, but in both poikilothermic animals and endothermic birds, which have orthologues of TNFRSF1a but lack the LTβR gene,[39] there is also evidence for clustering of lymphocytes in the gut. It seems probable that TNFRSF1a signals are sufficient in these nonmammalian animals, lacking the LTβR gene, to foster lymphocyte clustering.

A key step in our understanding of the function of ILFs (summarized in Fig. 2) was a relatively recent paper published by the group of Fagarasan.[40] They had previously observed that mice deficient in the activation-induced cytidine deaminase (AID) gene, which is expressed in B cells and is responsible for their class switch recombination and somatic hypermutation,[41] had abnormal gut flora,[42] and that normal gut bacterial homeostasis was maintained through class switching to IgA. In the more recent

**Table 2.** Chromosomal organization of TNF clusters

| Chromosome 1 | | Chromosome 12 | |
|---|---|---|---|
| TNF cluster 1 | Position (MB) | TNF cluster 2 | Position (MB) |
| GITR | 1.13 | TNFR1[a] | 12:6.3 |
| OX40 | 1.14 | *LTβR* | 12:6.36 |
| HVEM | 2.5 | *CD27* | 12:6.4 |
| DR3[a] | 6.4 | *CD4* | 12:6.7 |
| 4-1BB | 7.9 | C1rs[b] | 12:7.1 |
| MASP2[b] | 11 | AID | 12:8.6 |
| CD30 | 12 | | |
| TNFR2 | 12.1 | | |
| podoplanin | 13.9 | | |

Human TNF receptors on chromosome 1 and 12. Underlined genes show TNF receptors whose ligands are only present in higher vertebrates (birds and mammals); genes marked italics are only present in therian mammals; all others are TNF receptors present in all vertebrates. Genes marked with [b] show the 2 serine proteases that catalytically cleave complement component, C4; those marked with [a] are TNF receptor close paralogues. This is evidence of ancient genome-wide duplication. Data from www.ensembl.org.

paper,[40] they showed that LTi-dependent ILFs were the sites where this AID-dependent but T cell- and CD40-independent IgA class switching occurred.

Here is the earliest demonstration of a helper or orchestrating function for LTi: they foster the generation of IgA-specific plasma cells, which localize to the gut epithelium and secrete IgA antibodies into the lumen. Although at first sight this action does not seem related to IL-22 production, both functions are directed at the maintenance of epithelial integrity. Particularly relevant to the intrinsic nature of LTi is that in fostering plasma cells, they do not appear to provide help to B cells directly, as they do not express CD40-ligand, the molecular link to T cell-dependent class switching in mice[43] and humans.[44]

### Primitive monotremes have ILFs, whereas placental mammals have lymph nodes

ILFs are clearly the ancestors of lymph nodes, as monotremes, whose genome lacks the LTβR gene, have ILFs, not only associated with the gut, but in locations where placental animals have lymph nodes.[27,28] In monotremes, ILFs are located inside lymphatics, and appear to be vascularized. In placental lymph nodes, lymphocytes expressing L-selectin (gene name SELL) enter lymph nodes through HEV. SELL is absent in avian genomes,

which nevertheless have the closely related paralogues, P-(SELP) and E-selectin (SELE), that, due to a mammalian gene duplication, are clustered with SELL on human chromosome 1 in genetic linkage with the TNF cluster containing OX40L. The L-selectin gene is present in monotremes, suggesting that entry into lymphatic related ILFs could occur as in conventional lymph nodes by L-selectin. It is not clear from the original publications whether monotremes have HEVs; it appears unlikely, as the development and persistence of HEV is LTβR-dependent,[45] but it could be readily determined. In any case, the evidence from monotremes indicates that ILFs in lymphatics embedded in fatty tissue were the direct ancestors of the therian lymph nodes that evolved subsequently in the context of the therian-specific LTβR.

### Orthologues of therian IgG and IgE in monotreme immunoglobulin heavy chain locus

The fostering by LTi of AID-dependent class switching to IgA in the gut could quite plausibly be related to the function of centrally located ILFs in monotremes. In addition to having orthologues of IgA, monotremes have an immunoglobulin locus that harbors IgG and IgE orthologues, present only in mammals, and the immunoglobulin heavy

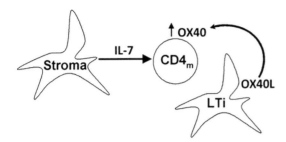

**Figure 3.** Model for how memory CD4⁺ T cells are sustained by IL-7 and OX40-signals from LTi. As memory CD4⁺ T cells (CD4ₘ) recirculate through lymph nodes, they receive IL-7 signals from stromal cells and upregulate expression of OX40. They then receive OX40 signals from OX40L-expressing LTi. This simple scheme ensures the independent regulation of CD4⁺ memory and naive pools.

chain locus is structurally organized in a similar manner to that in mouse and human.[46] The conventional perception of IgG and particularly IgE identifies them as high affinity antibody isotypes dependent on CD40L-expressing CD4⁺ T cells, and on postgerminal center (GC) selection and affinity maturation. However, there is no evidence that monotreme antibody responses undergo affinity maturation, as primary and secondary antibody responses are quantitatively and qualitatively similar.[47] Furthermore, there is no evidence of the spatial and temporal compartmentalization of the primary IgM-dominated responses from the class switched IgG/IgE-dominated secondary immune responses seen in eutherian mammals. We think, therefore, that a plausible scenario in monotremes is that the sites of CD4⁺ T cell- and CD40 ligand-dependent IgG and IgE class switching were centrally located LTi-dependent ILFs. In any case, this suggests that AID-dependent class switching to monomeric immunoglobulins anticipated the significant AID-dependent affinity maturation and memory that are the hallmark of antibody responses in placental mammals. These old studies combined with our current knowledge of the requirement for LTi in the formation of ILFs, portray LTi as likely participants in the evolution of adaptive antibody responses, involving CD40L on CD4⁺ T cells.

## How did monotreme ILFs arise?

The migration of antigen-presenting cells to lymph nodes is dependent on the expression of the T zone localizing chemokine receptor, CCR7, and LTi

express CCR7.[48] Fish genomes have synteneic orthologues for CCR7 but not for the mammalian ligands, CCL19 and CCL21, despite the identification of the synteneic region in zebrafish containing the closely related gene, *IL11RA*. The type 2 mucin, podoplanin,[49] is expressed on lymphatic endothelium and T zone stroma,[50,51] is thought to retain CCL21 for presentation,[52] and is also only present in homoeothermic birds and mammals. Epithelial cancers use this CCR7 pathway to metastasize to lymph nodes.[53] One possible origin of the monotremes' centrally located ILFs is the gut cryptopatch, which is associated with the lacteal rich lymphatic network that absorbs fat. Perhaps in the ancestor of all mammals that had evolved both podoplanin and CCL21, the migration of CCR7-bearing LTi by local lymphatics to sites of CCL21 presentation led to the formation of centrally located ILFs in the gut mesentery, where, during ontogeny, the first proper lymph nodes, the mesenteric lymph nodes, appear?[54] If this is the case, LTi should be found in lymph—and preliminary data suggest that they are (Simon Milling and Stephanie Houston, personal communication).

## Phylogenetic links between lymph node development and CD4⁺ T cell memory

In the embryo LTi are responsible for the formation of secondary lymphoid tissue[3,4] through their expression of five members of the TNFSF: lymphotoxin α (LTα), lymphotoxin β (LTβ), tumor necrosis factor α (TNF-α), LIGHT, and TRANCE. Because the developmental process of secondary lymphoid tissue has been reviewed extensively elsewhere,[54,55] in this review we focus instead on the evolutionary significance of its outcome.

Not quite achieved by the monotremes, the possession of multifollicular encapsulated lymph nodes with segregated B and T cell areas is a feature of both marsupial[26,56] and eutherian immune systems. Neither of the two extant monotreme groups has the capacity to evoke memory CD4⁺ T cell-dependent antibody responses,[47] also characteristic of all eutherians and marsupials,[56] which places the appearance of lymph nodes and the development of classical high affinity CD4⁺ T cell-dependent memory antibody responses in the same time frame: after the divergence of monotremes from other mammals some 166 Ma, and before marsupials and eutherians split approximately 148 Ma.[57] The key gene missing in monotremes is the LTβR gene, which is obviously crucial for LTi-dependent lymph node development, but which is also essential for generating high affinity CD4+ T cell-dependent memory antibody responses.[10] This is because of the provision it makes for CD4+ T cell help for B cells, but the LTβR gene *per se* is not required for the generation of CD4+ T cell memory.[58] Thus, we can identify two key functions for the LTβR gene: not only does it catalyze the fusion of ILFs inside lymphatics into multifollicular lymph nodes where individual B follicles are separated by intranodal lymphatics, it also affects the segregation of B and T cell areas, the essential provision for the affinity maturation of the B cell response in GCs. This is because the affinity maturation of an ongoing antibody response requires iterative GC B cell selection by antigen-specific follicular T helper cells, and depends on the exclusion of T cells of other specificities, which might recognize peptides presented by GC B cells of irrelevant specificity.

## Does genetic proximity favor evolutionary cooperation between cells for multicellular functions?

The genes for CD4 (required for CD4+ T cell selection that then select B cells in GCs), AID (required for the generation of B cell somatic mutants in GCs) and TNFRSF1A (that induces expression of homeostatic chemokines that allow CD4+ T cells and B cells to aggregate), are closely associated genetically in all jawed vertebrates (Table 2). Lower vertebrates, however, never acquired the additional neighborhood presence of LTβR that we see in placental mammalian genomes, and they lack both the lymph nodes and the capacity to make class switched and high affinity antibodies, which requires the segregation of lymphocytes within structured lymphoid tissues. We think that the fact that the LTβR gene is in the close neighborhood of the older gene grouping is no coincidence; linkage by proximity ensures that genes that are functionally related can coevolve. For example, changes in one gene favorable for the evolution of a new function can be stably inherited with the linked genes. These, in turn, can accumulate other favorable mutations, effectively forming favorable haplotypes, which after inbreeding could be fixed in evolving populations consequent on selection. In this regard, although the LTβR gene product is expressed on stromal cells, it is through its induc-

tion of homeostatic chemokines that it provides the environment for the efficient selection by CD4+ T cells of B cells bearing AID-dependent mutated immunoglobulin receptors.

As mentioned earlier, LTβR-deficient mice have CD4+ T cell memory and they have LTi that express both OX40L and CD30L, which we have linked to CD4+ T cell memory formation and maintenance. The OX40L gene is close to the L-selectin gene, whose gene product is required for entry of lymphocytes into lymph nodes by HEVs. The other selectins, P- and E-selectin, are involved in trafficking of CD4+ effector cells to sites of inflammation and infection. Currently, we think of lymph nodes as sites of priming, but they are effector sites in the sense that affinity maturation of the B cell response driven by follicular T helper cells occurs in B follicles inside lymph nodes. Perhaps the proximity of OX40L to the selectin gene cluster favored the evolution of its function in both CD4+ T cell effector and memory function, particularly with respect to the generation of high affinity memory antibodies.

## LTi OX40L and CD30L expression supports CD4+ T cell memory but not effector functions

It is clear from our discussion so far that the evolution of LTβR-signals in therian mammals between 170 and 148 Ma was the key to the evocation of high affinity antibodies, but the genes that we have linked to CD4+ effector and memory function, OX40 and CD30 and their ligands, evolved in the common ancestor of birds and mammals at least 150 million years before, as birds have both the receptors and ligands (Table 2). Many studies have examined the phenotype of mice individually deficient in OX40 and CD30,[59] but because of the coexpression of their ligands on LTi and the sharing of their signaling pathways, indicating possible redundancy, we chose to generate mice deficient in both signals (dKO) by interbreeding CD30-deficient and OX40-deficient mice. We have already shown that OX40-deficient mice had impaired affinity maturation and reduced memory antibody responses.[16] The combined phenotype of OX40 and CD30 deficiency, however, was dramatic:

(a) Not only was affinity maturation of the antibody response grossly impaired, but there was abrogation of memory antibody responses to CD4$^+$ T cell-dependent protein antigens.[18]

(b) By crossing dKO with CD4$^+$ TcR transgenic (TcRtg) mice, we were also able to show that primary antigen-driven proliferation of dKO or singly deficient OX40- or CD30-deficient TcRtg CD4$^+$ T cells was normal, but that their survival was defective both *in vivo* and *in vitro*.

(c) This deficit was not restricted to CD4$^+$ T cell help for B cells, as dKO mice were also deficient in their capacity to clear *Salmonella*, a Th1-dependent CD4$^+$ response.[60]

(d) Studies by the Jenkins group had shown that naive CD4$^+$ T cells reside exclusively in primary lymphoid organs like spleen and lymph node, but a significant fraction of memory CD4$^+$ T cells resides in sites outside conventional lymphoid structures, including the lamina propria (LP) of the gut. In dKO mice, LP CD4$^+$ T cells were grossly depleted in contrast to other LP T cell populations.[61] This was not due to defective proliferation of CD4$^+$ T cells in the mesenteric lymph node, or to defects in their migration to the LP. Although the majority of the CD4$^+$ T cell deficit was attributable to the absence of OX40, significant additional synergy was seen in the additional absence of CD30.

## CD4$^+$ T cell-mediated autoimmunity in FoxP3-KO mice requires OX40 and CD30 but not LTi

To test the requirement for OX40 and CD30 in CD4$^+$ T cell effector function we crossed dKO mice with FoxP3-KO mice. The transcription factor, FoxP3, controls the development of regulatory T cells (T$_{reg}$ cells), which temper T cell effector responses.[62] In mice and humans,[63,64] deficiency of FoxP3 causes fatal CD4$^+$ T cell-driven autoimmune disease mediated by both Th1 and Th2 immunopathology, which develops shortly after birth but not *in utero*. The disease is CD4$^+$ T cell-dependent as it is abrogated by the depletion of CD4$^+$ but not CD8$^+$ T cells, or by rendering FoxP3-KO mice MHC class II- but not class I-deficient.[65]

Once again, a dramatic effect can be produced by the application of a double deficiency of OX40 and CD30 signals: in contrast to FoxP3-KO mice with intact OX40 and CD30 signals, which die aged between three and five weeks, dKO/FoxP3-KO mice fail to develop clinically significant disease and have a normal lifespan.[66] This outcome contrasts favorably with treatment by abrogation of CD28 signals,[67] which delays significantly but does not prevent the development of FoxP3-KO disease. Most of the effect is attributable to OX40 signals, but OX40-deficient mice with intact CD30 signaling still develop fatal disease around six months, so again there is clear synergy between OX40 and CD30 in driving the disease. Furthermore, female dKO/FoxP3-KO mice breed normally across major histocompatibility complex differences, indicating that the absence of OX40 and CD30 obviates the need for the T$_{reg}$ cells contribution to fetomaternal tolerance during normal potentially alloreactive pregnancies.[68] The abrogation of disease by lack of OX40 and CD30 is in part due to impairment of survival rather than of primary proliferation by activated CD4$^+$ T cells. However, the most striking deficit is in the expression of cytokines, both IL-4 and IFN-$\gamma$, in CD4$^+$ but not in CD8$^+$ T cells. This further emphasizes the CD4$^+$ T cell-specific function of these molecules.

Freedom from disease in dKO/FoxP3-KO mice is not simply due to developmental defects in CD4$^+$ T cells consequent on lack of OX40 and CD30, because injection of blocking antibodies to the ligands also prevented disease. Significantly, the effector CD4$^+$ T cell cytokine expression in antibody-blockaded mice was very similar to that observed in dKO/FoxP3-KO mice. In summary, this experiment indicates the essential role of OX40 and to a lesser extent CD30 signals in driving CD4$^+$ T cell effector function, and furthermore indicates that blockade of these signaling pathways in humans could significantly ameliorate human CD4$^+$ T cell-driven autoimmune disease.

The expression of OX40L and CD30L is not restricted to LTi, as activated B cells, DCs, and other nonhemopoietic cells can express them, but the expression on LTi is high and does appear to be independent of antigenic stimulation. To test whether FoxP3-KO disease was LTi-dependent, we crossed FoxP3-KO mice with ROR$\gamma$t-KO mice (lacking LTi, but with essentially normal B and DCs) to generate FoxP3-KO/ROR$\gamma$t-KO mice. Although the onset of FoxP3-KO disease was delayed slightly (our unpublished observations), these mice still developed fatal lymphoproliferative disease, indicating that expression by cells other than LTi of OX40L and CD30L was sufficient to support autoimmune effectors (our unpublished observations).

## Are LTi required for the maintenance of CD4+ T cell memory?

Our work on FoxP3-dependent autoimmunity (above) indicated that CD4+ T cell effector function was dependent on OX40 and CD30, but that the abundance of their ligands on LTi was not by itself driving effector responses. Another context for the relevance of the high constitutive expression of OX40L and CD30L on LTi is the LTi- and LTβR-dependent development of lymph nodes and its co-evolution with the capacity to evoke CD4+ T cell-dependent memory antibody responses.[69] So are LTi required for CD4+ T cell memory? Supportive evidence for this hypothesis is our finding that RORγt-KO mice that are without LTi behave like CD30/OX40 dKO mice: they fail to evoke memory antibody responses, although their primary antibody responses are normal.[70] In contrast to dKO mice, however, affinity maturation in RORγt-KO mice was no different from WT controls, indicating that OX40L[71] and/or CD30L signals from B cells were sufficient for this aspect of the B cell response.

We have also gone on to test directly whether the absence of LTi impairs the generation of CD4+ T cell memory using CD4 tetramers developed by the Jenkins laboratory,[72] and this again supports the contention that LTi are strong contenders for the provision of these signals to memory CD4+ T cells (our unpublished data).

## Location of LTi at sites where CD4+ lymphocytes recirculate

The capacity of memory lymphocytes to recirculate between blood and lymph was established 50 years ago.[73,74] The location of LTi in secondary lymphoid tissues is consistent with the provision of OX40 and CD30 signals to recirculating CD4+ memory T cells. In both spleen and lymph node, LTi are tightly associated with mucosal vascular addressin cell adhesion molecule 1 (MAdCAM-1) expressing cells. In the spleen, this consistent membrane contact between LTi and MAdCAM-1 expressing stromal cells is manifested in the same parts of the

lymphocyte-rich white pulp areas that have been identified by imaging studies to be points of entry for splenic lymphocytes: first the marginal sinus, then the bridging channels.[75] The location of LTi is therefore opportune for interactions with incoming memory CD4+ T cells. In the lymph node, LTi are located in the subcapsular sinus and interfollicular areas where intranodal lymphatics drain lymph to the medulla and efferent lymphatics, again associated with MAdCAM-1 expressing cells, and again positioned to intercept incoming lymphocytes.

## LTi IL-7– and OX40-dependent survival signals support CD4+ T cell memory

Although our data link LTi with CD4+ T cell memory, there is also clear evidence for a role for IL-7 (reviewed in Ref. 76). This is not a contradiction; we have observed that OX40, expressed at low levels on memory but not naive CD4+ T cells, is upregulated by IL-7 only on memory CD4+ T cells.[18] The response of memory CD4+ T cell OX40 expression to IL-7 signals provides a simple antigen-independent contribution to their survival. This model is laid out in Figure 3: memory CD4+ T cells recirculating through secondary lymphoid tissues receive IL-7 signals from IL-7–expressing stromal cell populations in lymph node and spleen,[51,77] which consequently upregulates OX40 and enables the T cells to engage OX40L-expressing LTi, thus providing the survival signals[78] they need to persist. A key advantage of this model is that it suggests an antigen-independent mechanism for the support of memory CD4+ T cells specifically; although both naive and memory populations depend on IL-7,[76] the OX40–OX40L axis provided by LTi constitutes a selective survival niche for CD4+ T cell memory.

## Were lymph nodes and high-affinity class switched antibodies in therian mammals pivotal to evolution of placentation?

Placentation, particularly the eutherian variety, has clearly conferred significant survival advantages to mammals compared with oviparous animals. An appreciable component of the success of nourishing the developing mammalian embryo with a highly vascularized eutherian placenta is the sterilizing immunity in the blood, conferred by the capacity to make high affinity class switched antibody responses. In this regard, lymph nodes provide an additional layer of protection by filtering the lymph of potential pathogens before their entry into the blood stream, a protection amplified by memory responses that are characterized by their sensitivity to trace amounts of the antigen that originally evoked them, their quality (high affinity and class switched), and finally their rapidity of onset. Redistributing both B cell and CD4[+] T cell memory cells to LTi-dependent lymph nodes ensures that sterilizing immunity against previously encountered pathogens protects not only the maternal host but also the next generation—the developing embryo.

Zinkernagel[79] has clearly articulated the view that the most important function of memory antibody responses is to protect the newborn by passive transfer of maternal IgG high affinity neutralizing antibodies. Childhood mortality rates for infectious diseases in the prevaccination era support this view.[80] The majority of infections exhibit an exponential decline in mortality with age, with relative protection seen in the first year of life when maternal antibodies are present in the infant. However, there is also a very significant excess mortality from *de novo* infections in pregnant women, particularly from cytopathic viruses, perhaps best exemplified by the Spanish influenza epidemic of 1918, which killed somewhere between 50 and 100 million people worldwide; although the overall mortality was between 2% and 20%, the mortality in pregnant women was much higher (23–71%).[81] Such excess mortality is not exclusive to influenza; it was also true for smallpox, where on average one third of pregnant women died.[82] In the absence of immune memory all infections are *de novo*, and survival of a primary infection outside of pregnancy does not equate with survival in pregnancy when the maternal immune system is compromised. This indicates that a very potent Darwinian selective pressure for the acquisition of maternal memory antibody was for protection during pregnancy, because for the embryo to survive, the mother must survive.

The maternal susceptibility to *de novo* infection during pregnancy supports the idea that pregnancy is associated with significant immunosuppression, or at least immunomodulation.[83] Immunosuppression/modulation during pregnancy is likely to be a response to the strong evolutionary requirement for tolerance toward the developing allogeneic fetus, and is further supported by the well-documented spontaneous remission of at least some autoimmune diseases in pregnancy, followed by postpartum relapse.[84]

## Embryonic LTi lack expression of OX40L and CD30L

Although OX40L is expressed at high levels on adult LTi, its expression is lacking on embryonic LTi in both mice[85] and humans (Cupedo, personal communication), but it can be upregulated by removal from the fetal environment.[85,86] One obvious possibility is that suppression of expression of these ligands could be a strategy to protect the fetus from potential alloreactive maternal lymphocytes that enter the fetal circulation, as OX40 and CD30 drive CD4[+] T cell effector-driven damage.[66]

## Role of LTi in generation of T cell tolerance in the thymus

The evolution of high affinity memory antibody responses placed an additional burden on the purging of self-reactivity from the emerging T cell repertoire. In respect of this, we have also reported that LTi are implicated in the generation of thymic tolerance. In the thymus, LTi are located adjacent to thymic medullary epithelium (mTEC),[87] which is believed to assist the negative selection of TcRs recognizing tissue restricted antigens through its expression of the autoimmune regulator (AIRE) gene that controls the intrathymic expression of peripheral self-proteins.[88] AIRE deficient humans develop autoantibodies to self-antigens and cytokines.[89] LTi are able to induce AIRE through their expression of RANKL, as RAG-KO mice with LTi retained expression of AIRE, whereas RORγt-KO mice deficient in LTi did not (our unpublished observations). Furthermore, AIRE was induced in mTEC before T cell genesis in the embryonic thymus. Given that as the neonatal period has long been known to represent a key developmental stage in the induction of T cell tolerance, the contribution from LTi cells to thymic medullary development in the fetal/neonatal period is likely to be critical. Indeed, the importance of AIRE-mediated neonatal tolerance has recently been demonstrated by studies in which the deletion of AIRE[+] mTEC is temporally controlled. These findings indicate that intrathymic tolerance to AIRE-dependent peripheral self-antigens is crucial in fetal/neonatal life, and that the deletion of AIRE[+] mTEC in the steady-state adult thymus does not result in tolerance breakdown unless it is accompanied by T lymphopenia.[90] Collectively, these findings suggest that the induction of long lasting T cell tolerance is dependent on the generation of AIRE-expressing microenvironments in the embryonic thymus, which are fostered in part by LTi cells before the emergence of mature αβ T cells.

## Summary

Based on the fact that the key transcription factors are present in all jawed vertebrates, we have suggested in this perspective that IL-22–secreting LTi could have been participants at least in the common ancestor of bony fish and mammals (Fig. 2). We have also provided the phylogenetic evidence that their function in forming ILFs antedated the LTβR-dependent formation of lymph nodes, and have linked LTi in ILFs with AID-dependent immunoglobulin class switching, first in gut-associated lymphoid tissues to IgA, and later, in the common mammalian ancestor, in centrally located ILFs, to IgG and IgE. We have concentrated, however, on the major transition to the modern mammalian immune system that occurred in the common placental ancestor after the split from the monotreme lineage some 170 Ma, a transition that heralded a fundamental change in reproductive strategy key to the long-term survival of mammals. We have also suggested that LTi are excellent candidates for the maintenance of CD4 memory cells, and that by having distinct cells to regulate CD4$^+$ T cell memory, this allows independent regulation of CD4$^+$ T cell effectors. This is pertinent to pregnancy in particular, where CD4$^+$ T cell memory is maintained, whereas CD4$^+$ T cell effector function is regulated to prevent rejection of the developing fetus, with protection of both fetus and mother by maternal immunoglobulin, and rebound of the maternal immune system postpartum.

LTi are, therefore, linked with both innate and adaptive arms of the immune system. Our interest in these cells, however, has focused on their high levels of expression of OX40L in the adult mammal. Because we think that LTi expression of OX40L is not modulated in the same way as on other cells, we propose that evolution has selected for CD4$^+$ T cell memory to be preserved, and for regulation to occur at the level of effector CD4$^+$ T cells. This has

important implications for therapeutic strategies that treat diseases mediated by pathogenic CD4$^+$ T cells. CD28-blockade, currently showing promise in clinical trials for autoimmune disease,[91] may block effector function, but is unlikely to cure autoimmune diseases mediated by CD4$^+$ T cells, because it fails to target the molecular mechanism, OX40L and CD30L, which maintains CD4$^+$ T cell memory. On the other hand, blockade of OX40L, and to a lesser extent CD30L, has the potential to disable not only CD4$^+$ T cell effector function but also memory function. That makes these molecules attractive targets for the treatment and potentially for the cure of human autoimmune diseases.

## Acknowledgments

P.L. and G.A. are supported by program grants from the Medical Research Council and the Wellcome Trust. D.W. is supported by a career development fellowship from the Wellcome Trust.

## Conflicts of interest

The authors declare no conflicts of interest.

## References

1. Mebius, R.E., P. Rennert & I.L. Weissman. 1997. Developing lymph nodes collect CD4+CD3- LTbeta+ cells that can differentiate to APC, NK cells, and follicular cells but not T or B cells. *Immunity* **7:** 493–504.
2. Kelly, K.A. & R. Scollay. 1992. Seeding of neonatal lymph nodes by T cells and identification of a novel population of CD3-CD4+ cells. *Eur. J. Immunol.* **22:** 329–334.
3. Sun, Z. *et al.* 2000. Requirement for RORgamma in thymocyte survival and lymphoid organ development. *Science* **288:** 2369–2373.
4. Kurebayashi, S. *et al.* 2000. Retinoid-related orphan receptor gamma (RORgamma) is essential for lymphoid organogenesis and controls apoptosis during thymopoiesis. *Proc. Natl. Acad. Sci. USA* **97:** 10132–10137.
5. Eberl, G. & D.R. Littman. 2003. The role of the nuclear hormone receptor RORgammat in the development of lymph nodes and Peyer's patches. *Immunol. Rev.* **195:** 81–90.
6. Eberl, G. & D.R. Littman. 2004. Thymic origin of intestinal alphabeta T Cells revealed by fate mapping of RORgammat+ cells. *Science* **305:** 248–251.
7. Kanamori, Y. *et al.* 1996. Identification of novel lymphoid tissues in murine intestinal mucosa where clusters of c-kit+ IL-7R+ Thy1+ lympho-hemopoietic progenitors develop. *J. Exp. Med.* **184:** 1449–1459.
8. Saito, H. *et al.* 1998. Generation of intestinal T cells from progenitors residing in gut cryptopatches. *Science* **280:** 275–278.

9. Eberl, G. 2005. Opinion: inducible lymphoid tissues in the adult gut: recapitulation of a fetal developmental pathway? *Nat. Rev. Immunol.* **5:** 413–420.

10. Futterer, A. *et al.* 1998. The lymphotoxin beta receptor controls organogenesis and affinity maturation in peripheral lymphoid tissues. *Immunity* **9:** 59–70.

11. Kong, Y.Y. *et al.* 1999. OPGL is a key regulator of osteoclastogenesis, lymphocyte development and lymph-node organogenesis. *Nature* **397:** 315–323.

12. Takatori, H. *et al.* 2009. Lymphoid tissue inducer-like cells are an innate source of IL-17 and IL-22. *J. Exp. Med.* **206:** 35–41.

13. Wolk, K. *et al.* 2004. IL-22 increases the innate immunity of tissues. *Immunity* **21:** 241–254.

14. Aujla, S.J. *et al.* 2008. IL-22 mediates mucosal host defense against Gram-negative bacterial pneumonia. *Nat. Med.* **14:** 275–281.

15. Satoh-Takayama, N. *et al.* 2008. Microbial flora drives interleukin 22 production in intestinal NKp46+ cells that provide innate mucosal immune defense. *Immunity* **29:** 958–970.

16. Kim, M.Y. *et al.* 2003. CD4(+)CD3(-) accessory cells costimulate primed CD4 T cells through OX40 and CD30 at sites where T cells collaborate with B cells. *Immunity* **18:** 643–654.

17. Kim, S. *et al.* 2011. CD117(+) CD3(-) CD56(-) OX40L(high) cells express IL-22 and display an LTi phenotype in human secondary lymphoid tissues. *Eur. J. Immunol.* **41:** 1563–1572.

18. Gaspal, F.M. *et al.* 2005. Mice deficient in OX40 and CD30 signals lack memory antibody responses because of deficient CD4 T cell memory. *J. Immunol.* **174:** 3891–3896.

19. Guo, P. *et al.* 2009. Dual nature of the adaptive immune system in lampreys. *Nature* **459:** 796–801.

20. Bajoghli, B. *et al.* 2011. A thymus candidate in lampreys. *Nature* **470:** 90–94.

21. Glenney, G.W. & G.D. Wiens. 2007. Early diversification of the TNF superfamily in teleosts: genomic characterization and expression analysis. *J. Immunol.* **178:** 7955–7973.

22. Georgopoulos, K. *et al.* 1994. The Ikaros gene is required for the development of all lymphoid lineages. *Cell* **79:** 143–156.

23. Aliahmad, P., B. de la Torre & J. Kaye. 2010. Shared dependence on the DNA-binding factor TOX for the development of lymphoid tissue-inducer cell and NK cell lineages. *Nat. Immunol.* **11:** 945–952.

24. Flores, M.V. *et al.* 2007. The zebrafish retinoid-related orphan receptor (ror) gene family. *Gene Expr. Patterns* **7:** 535–543.

25. Yokota, Y. *et al.* 1999. Development of peripheral lymphoid organs and natural killer cells depends on the helix-loop-helix inhibitor Id2. *Nature* **397:** 702–706.

26. Canfield, P.J. & S. Hemsley. 2000. The roles of histology and immunohistology in the investigation of marsupial disease and normal lymphoid tissue. *Dev. Comp. Immunol.* **24:** 455–471.

27. Connolly, J.H. *et al.* 1999. Histological and immunohistological investigation of lymphoid tissue in the platypus (*Ornithorhynchus anatinus*). *J. Anat.* **195**(Pt 2): 161–171.

28. Diener, E. & E.H. Ealey. 1965. Immune system in a monotreme: studies on the Australian echidna (*Tachyglossus aculeatus*). *Nature* **208:** 950–953.

29. Hahn, M.E. *et al.* 1997. Molecular evolution of two vertebrate aryl hydrocarbon (dioxin) receptors (AHR1 and AHR2) and the PAS family. *Proc. Natl. Acad. Sci. USA* **94:** 13743–13748.

30. Veldhoen, M. *et al.* 2008. The aryl hydrocarbon receptor links TH17-cell-mediated autoimmunity to environmental toxins. *Nature* **453:** 106–109.

31. Lorenz, R.G. *et al.* 2003. Isolated lymphoid follicle formation is inducible and dependent upon lymphotoxin-sufficient B lymphocytes, lymphotoxin beta receptor, and TNF receptor I function. *J. Immunol.* **170:** 5475–5482.

32. Zheng, Y. *et al.* 2008. Interleukin-22 mediates early host defense against attaching and effacing bacterial pathogens. *Nat. Med.* **14:** 282–289.

33. Cella, M. *et al.* 2009. A human natural killer cell subset provides an innate source of IL-22 for mucosal immunity. *Nature* **457:** 722–725.

34. Sanos, S.L. *et al.* 2009. RORgammat and commensal microflora are required for the differentiation of mucosal interleukin 22-producing NKp46+ cells. *Nat. Immunol.* **10:** 83–91.

35. Spits, H. & J.P. Di Santo. 2011. The expanding family of innate lymphoid cells: regulators and effectors of immunity and tissue remodeling. *Nat. Immunol.* **12:** 21–27.

36. Li, W. *et al.* 2007. Thymic selection pathway regulates the effector function of CD4 T cells. *J. Exp. Med.* **204:** 2145–2157.

37. Marks, B.R. *et al.* 2009. Thymic self-reactivity selects natural interleukin 17-producing T cells that can regulate peripheral inflammation. *Nat. Immunol.* **10:** 1125–1132.

38. McDonald, K.G. *et al.* 2007. CC chemokine receptor 6 expression by B lymphocytes is essential for the development of isolated lymphoid follicles. *Am. J. Pathol.* **170:** 1229–1240.

39. Zapata, A. & C.T. Ameimiya. 2000. Phylogeny of lower vertebrates and their immunological structures. In *Origin and Evolution of the Vertebrate Immune System.* L. du Pasquier & G.W. Litman, Eds.: 67–110. Springer. Berlin.

40. Tsuji, M. *et al.* 2008. Requirement for lymphoid tissue-inducer cells in isolated follicle formation and T cell-independent immunoglobulin A generation in the gut. *Immunity* **29:** 261–271.

41. Muramatsu, M. *et al.* 2000. Class switch recombination and hypermutation require activation-induced cytidine deaminase (AID), a potential RNA editing enzyme [see comments]. *Cell* **102:** 553–563.

42. Fagarasan, S. *et al.* 2002. Critical roles of activation-induced cytidine deaminase in the homeostasis of gut flora. *Science* **298:** 1424–1427.

43. Grewal, I.S. & R.A. Flavell. 1996. The role of CD40 ligand in costimulation and T-cell activation. *Immunol. Rev.* **153:** 85–106.

44. DiSanto, J.P. *et al.* 1993. CD40 ligand mutations in x-linked immunodeficiency with hyper-IgM. *Nature* **361:** 541–543.

45. Browning, J.L. *et al.* 2005. Lymphotoxin-beta receptor signaling is required for the homeostatic control of HEV differentiation and function. *Immunity* **23:** 539–550.

46. Zhao, Y. *et al.* 2009. Ornithorhynchus anatinus (platypus) links the evolution of immunoglobulin genes in eutherian

mammals and nonmammalian tetrapods. *J. Immunol.* **183:** 3285–3293.

47. Wronski, E.V., G.M. Woods & B.L. Munday. 2003. Antibody response to sheep red blood cells in platypus and echidna. *Comp. Biochem. Physiol. A Mol. Integr. Physiol.* **136:** 957–963.

48. Kim, M.Y. *et al.* 2008. Heterogeneity of lymphoid tissue inducer cell populations present in embryonic and adult mouse lymphoid tissues. *Immunology* **124:** 166–174.

49. Farr, A.G. *et al.* 1992. Characterization and cloning of a novel glycoprotein expressed by stromal cells in T-dependent areas of peripheral lymphoid tissues. *J. Exp. Med.* **176:** 1477–1482.

50. Forster, R., A.C. Davalos-Misslitz & A. Rot. 2008. CCR7 and its ligands: balancing immunity and tolerance. *Nat Rev Immunol.* **8:** 362–371.

51. Link, A. *et al.* 2007. Fibroblastic reticular cells in lymph nodes regulate the homeostasis of naive T cells. *Nat. Immunol.* **8:** 1255–1265.

52. Kerjaschki, D. *et al.* 2004. Lymphatic neoangiogenesis in human kidney transplants is associated with immunologically active lymphocytic infiltrates. *J. Am. Soc. Nephrol.* **15:** 603–612.

53. Muller, A. *et al.* 2001. Involvement of chemokine receptors in breast cancer metastasis. *Nature* **410:** 50–56.

54. Mebius, R.E. 2003. Organogenesis of lymphoid tissues. *Nat. Rev. Immunol.* **3:** 292–303.

55. van de Pavert, S.A. & R.E. Mebius. 2010. New insights into the development of lymphoid tissues. *Nat. Rev. Immunol.* **10:** 664–674.

56. Shearer, M.H. *et al.* 1995. Humoral immune response in a marsupial *Monodelphis domestica*: anti-isotypic and anti-idiotypic responses detected by species-specific monoclonal anti-immunoglobulin reagents. *Dev. Comp. Immunol.* **19:** 237–246.

57. Warren, W.C. *et al.* 2008. Genome analysis of the platypus reveals unique signatures of evolution. *Nature* **453:** 175–183.

58. Fu, Y.X. *et al.* 2000. Lymphotoxin-alpha-dependent spleen microenvironment supports the generation of memory B cells and is required for their subsequent antigen-induced activation. *J. Immunol.* **164:** 2508–2514.

59. Croft, M. 2009. The role of TNF superfamily members in T-cell function and diseases. *Nat. Rev. Immunol.* **9:** 271–285.

60. Gaspal, F. *et al.* 2008. Critical synergy of CD30 and OX40 signals in CD4 T cell homeostasis and Th1 immunity to salmonella. *J. Immunol.* **180:** 2824–2829.

61. Withers, D.R. *et al.* 2009. The survival of memory CD4+ T cells within the gut lamina propria requires OX40 and CD30 signals. *J. Immunol.* **183:** 5079–5084.

62. Fontenot, J.D., M.A. Gavin & A.Y. Rudensky. 2003. Foxp3 programs the development and function of CD4+CD25 +regulatory T cells. *Nat. Immunol.* **4:** 330–336.

63. Bennett, C.L. *et al.* 2001. The immune dysregulation, polyendocrinopathy, enteropathy, X-linked syndrome (IPEX) is caused by mutations of FOXP3. *Nat. Genet.* **27:** 20–21.

64. Wildin, R.S. *et al.* 2001. X-linked neonatal diabetes mellitus, enteropathy and endocrinopathy syndrome is the human equivalent of mouse scurfy. *Nat. Genet.* **27:** 18–20.

65. Blair, P.J. *et al.* 1994. CD4+CD8- T cells are the effector cells in disease pathogenesis in the scurfy (sf) mouse. *J Immunol.* **153:** 3764–3774.

66. Gaspal, F.M. *et al.* 2011. Abrogation of CD30 and OX40 signals prevents autoimmune disease in FoxP3 deficient mice. *J. Exp. Med.* **208:** 1579–1584.

67. Singh, N. *et al.* 2007. Role of CD28 in fatal autoimmune disorder in scurfy mice. *Blood.* **110:** 1199–1206.

68. Aluvihare, V.R., M. Kallikourdis & A.G. Betz. 2004. Regulatory T cells mediate maternal tolerance to the fetus. *Nat. Immunol.* **5:** 266–271.

69. Lane, P.J., F.M. Gaspal & M.Y. Kim. 2005. Two sides of a cellular coin: CD4(+)CD3- cells regulate memory responses and lymph-node organization. *Nat Rev Immunol.* **5:** 655–660.

70. Withers, D.R. *et al.* 2011. Role of OX40 and CD30 in murine CD4 effector and memory function. *Immunol. Rev.* **244:** 134–138.

71. Kim, M.Y. *et al.* 2005. OX40 signals during priming on dendritic cells inhibit CD4 T cell proliferation: IL-4 switches off OX40 signals enabling rapid proliferation of Th2 effectors. *J. Immunol.* **174:** 1433–1437.

72. Pepper, M. *et al.* 2010. Different routes of bacterial infection induce long-lived TH1 memory cells and short-lived TH17 cells. *Nat. Immunol.* **11:** 83–89.

73. Gowans, J.L. 1959. The recirculation of lymphocytes from blood to lymph in the rat. *J. Physiol.* **146:** 54–69.

74. Gowans, J.L. & J.W. Uhr. 1966. The carriage of immunological memory by small lymphocytes in the rat. *J. Exp. Med.* **124:** 1017–1030.

75. Bajenoff, M., N. Glaichenhaus & R.N. Germain. 2008. Fibroblastic reticular cells guide T lymphocyte entry into and migration within the splenic T cell zone. *J. Immunol.* **181:** 3947–3954.

76. Surh, C.D. & J. Sprent. 2008. Homeostasis of naive and memory T cells. *Immunity* **29:** 848–862.

77. Repass, J.F. *et al.* 2009. IL7-hCD25 and IL7-Cre BAC transgenic mouse lines: new tools for analysis of IL-7 expressing cells. *Genesis* **47:** 281–287.

78. Rogers, P.R. *et al.* 2001. OX40 promotes Bcl-xL and Bcl-2 expression and is essential for long- term survival of CD4 T cells. *Immunity* **15:** 445–455.

79. Zinkernagel, R.M. & H. Hengartner. 2006. Protective 'immunity' by pre-existent neutralizing antibody titers and preactivated T cells but not by so-called 'immunological memory'. *Immunol. Rev.* **211:** 310–319.

80. Martin, W.J. 1945. Mortality in childhood during 1920–38. *Br. Med. J.* **1:** 363–365.

81. Barry, J.M. 2004. *The Great Influenza*. Penguin Viking, New York.

82. Nishiura, H. 2006. Smallpox during pregnancy and maternal outcomes. *Emerg. Infect. Dis.* **12:** 1119–1121.

83. Wegmann, T.G. *et al.* 1993. Bidirectional cytokine interactions in the maternal-fetal relationship: is successful pregnancy a TH2 phenomenon? *Immunol. Today* **14:** 353–356.

84. Ostensen, M. & P.M. Villiger. 2002. Immunology of pregnancy-pregnancy as a remission inducing agent in rheumatoid arthritis. *Transpl. Immunol.* **9:** 155–160.

85. Kim, M.-Y. *et al.* 2005. OX40-ligand and CD30-ligand are expressed on adult but not neonatal CD4+CD3- inducer cells: evidence that IL7 signals regulate CD30-ligand but not OX40-ligand expression. *J. Immunol.* **174:** 6686–6691.

86. Kim, M.Y. *et al.* 2006. Neonatal and adult CD4+CD3- cells share similar gene expression profile, and neonatal cells up-regulate OX40 ligand in response to TL1A (TNFSF15). *J. Immunol.* **177:** 3074–3081.

87. Rossi, S.W. *et al.* 2007. RANK signals from CD4(+)3(-) inducer cells regulate development of AIRE-expressing epithelial cells in the thymic medulla. *J. Exp. Med.* **204:** 1267–1272.

88. Metzger, T.C. & M.S. Anderson. 2011. Control of central and peripheral tolerance by AIRE. *Immunol. Rev.* **241:** 89–103.

89. Aaltonen, J. & P. Bjorses. 1999. Cloning of the APECED gene provides new insight into human autoimmunity. *Ann. Med.* **31:** 111–116.

90. Guerau-de-Arellano, M. *et al.* 2009. Neonatal tolerance revisited: a perinatal window for AIRE control of autoimmunity. *J. Exp. Med.* **206:** 1245–1252.

91. Poirier, N., G. Blancho & B. Vanhove. 2010. Alternatives to calcineurin inhibition in renal transplantation: belatacept, the first co-stimulation blocker. *Immunotherapy* **2:** 625–636.

Ann. N.Y. Acad. Sci. ISSN 0077-8923

ANNALS OF THE NEW YORK ACADEMY OF SCIENCES
Issue: *The Year in Immunology*

# Regulation of mature T cell responses by the Wnt signaling pathway

Hai-Hui Xue[1,2] and Dong-Mei Zhao[1,3]

[1]Department of Microbiology, Carver College of Medicine, University of Iowa, Iowa City, Iowa. [2]Interdisciplinary Immunology Graduate Program, Carver College of Medicine, University of Iowa, Iowa City, Iowa. [3]Department of Internal Medicine, Carver College of Medicine, University of Iowa, Iowa City, Iowa

Address for correspondence: Hai-Hui Xue, 51 Newton Rd. BSB 3-710, Iowa City, IA 52246. hai-hui-xue@uiowa.edu

The canonical Wnt signaling pathway is evolutionarily conserved and plays key roles during development of many organ systems. This pathway utilizes TCF/LEF transcription factors, $\beta$-catenin coactivator, and TLE/GRG corepressors to achieve balanced regulation of its downstream gene expression. It is well established that several Wnt ligands and their effector proteins are crucial for normal T cell development. Recent studies have also revealed critical requirements for TCF-1 in generation and persistence of functional memory CD8$^+$ T cells, and in promoting Th2-differentiation and suppressing Th17-differentiation of activated CD4$^+$ T cells. Activation of $\beta$-catenin facilitated CD8$^+$ memory T cell formation, with enhanced protective capacity and extended survival of CD4$^+$CD25$^+$ regulatory T cells. Upregulation of Wnt ligands was observed in *Drosophila* in response to Toll signaling as well as in mammalian dendritic cells and macrophages upon microbial stimulation. These new findings suggest that modulating the activity of Wnt pathway may be a powerful approach to enhance protective immunity and treat autoimmune diseases.

Keywords: Wnt signaling pathway; TCF-1; LEF-1; $\beta$-catenin; memory CD8$^+$ T cells; CD4$^+$ T cell differentiation

## Introduction

The Wnt signaling pathway is evolutionarily conserved and is involved in a large variety of developmental processes including specification of cell fate and maintenance of stem cell pluripotency.[1,2] There are 19 known Wnt family members and 10 Frizzled receptors in mammals, but the specific interaction/affinity between individual Wnt ligands and Frizzled receptors has remained largely unmapped.[3] In addition to the Frizzled receptors, some Wnt ligands require coreceptors, such as low-density lipoprotein receptor-related protein 5 (LRP5) and LRP6, and some others act on receptor tyrosine kinases including Ryk and Ror2.[4,5] Interaction between Wnt and its various receptors can activate several signaling cascades including $\beta$-catenin, c-Jun N-terminal kinase (JNK), and Ca$^{2+}$-nuclear factor associated with T cells (NFAT).[4,5] Specific to T lymphocytes, both JNK and Ca$^{2+}$-NFAT pathways are induced upon stimulation of T cell receptors

(TCRs), however, it has not been determined if they can be elicited by certain Wnt proteins. In this review, we therefore focus on the better-characterized $\beta$-catenin cascade, also known as the canonical Wnt pathway.

$\beta$-catenin functions as a coactivator that cooperates with DNA sequence-specific transcription factors, T cell factor (TCF)/lymphoid enhancer binding factor (LEF) proteins.[6] $\beta$-catenin can also interact with CBP/p300 histone acetyl transferases and several other molecules to enhance its gene regulatory function.[7] One key feature of $\beta$-catenin is that its protein level is subject to posttranslational regulation by a multimolecular destruction complex.[5] The destruction complex contains two scaffolding proteins, adenomatous polyposis coli and axis inhibition protein (Axin), and two serine/threonine protein kinases, casein kinase 1 (CK1) and glycogen synthase kinase 3$\beta$ (GSK3$\beta$). The kinases phosphorylate $\beta$-catenin on four N-terminal Ser33, Ser37, Thr41, and Ser45 residues and thus mark it for

doi: 10.1111/j.1749-6632.2011.06302.x

 Ann. N.Y. Acad. Sci. 1247 (2012) 16–33 © 2012 New York Academy of Sciences.

ubiquitination and proteosome-mediated degradation. In the presence of active Wnt signaling, the destruction complex is disrupted and the kinases inactivated, leading to β-catenin dephosphorylation and stabilization. The accumulated β-catenin in its de- or underphosphorylated form is then translocated into the nucleus, where it interacts with TCF/LEF factors to regulate gene expression (Fig. 1).[5,8]

In T lymphocytes, the predominantly expressed TCF/LEF factors are TCF-1 and LEF-1 (encoded by *Tcf7* and *Lef1*, respectively). Both proteins are expressed in multiple isoforms due to differential promoter usage and alternative splicing.[9] All TCF-1 and LEF-1 isoforms contain a conserved high-mobility group (HMG) DNA binding domain, which recognizes a consensus TCF/LEF binding motif, 5'-TCAAAG, also known as Wnt responsive element (WRE). The HMG domain and adjacent central region of TCF/LEF interact with the pleiotropic repressor, transducin-like enhancer/Groucho-related gene (TLE/GRG) proteins,[10] and the TCF/LEF–TLE/GRG complex suppresses expression of Wnt target genes. The long isoforms of TCF-1 (such as p45) and LEF-1 that are transcribed from respective distal promoters all contain an N-terminal β-catenin-interaction domain. On the other hand, the short isoforms of TCF-1 (such as p33) and LEF-1 that are transcribed from the proximal promoters lack the ability to bind β-catenin and are considered to have dominant negative effects against the long isoforms. When the canonical Wnt cascade is described, it is usually stated that in the absence of Wnt signaling, TCF/LEF factors suppress gene transcription via constant association with the TLE/GRG corepressors, and upon Wnt stimulation, the stabilized β-catenin displaces TLE/GRG from TCF/LEF and activates Wnt target genes. At least in T lineage cells, β-catenin can be readily detected in freshly isolated cells,[11–13] suggesting that T cells have a substantial pool of β-catenin under homeostatic conditions. In addition, different isoforms of TCF-1 and LEF-1 proteins are abundant in both thymocytes and mature T cells.[9,11,14,15] Rather than a complete "on" or "off" state, the expression of Wnt target genes in T cells is likely determined by a binding equilibrium between β-catenin–associated TCF-1/LEF-1 long isoforms and TLE/GRG-associated short isoforms with WREs (Fig. 1). In line with this notion, Wnt reporters, either driven by multimerized WREs as a transgene or knock-in in the *Axin2* locus, were detectable in developing thymocytes and splenic CD4[+] T cells *ex vivo*.[12,13] Thus, the expression of Wnt target genes in T cells can be regulated through a shift of equilibrium in response to Wnt-induced β-catenin stabilization. It is noteworthy that the equilibrium can be influenced by pre-TCR/TCR- or cytokine-derived signals that alter the expression levels of different TCF-1 and LEF-1 isoforms, with pre-TCR/TCR shown to stabilize β-catenin in T lineage cells as well (discussed later).

The involvement of Wnt, TCF, and β-catenin pathway in immune regulation is evolutionary conserved. *Drosophila* larvae mount immune responses to parasites by increased number of circulating hemocytes and generation of lamellocytes, a special class of hemocytes that participate in parasite encapsulation.[16] Forced expression of a dominant-negative isoform of TCF/Pangolin or Shaggy, a negative regulator of β-catenin/Armadillo, potentiated hemocyte and lamellocyte responses.[17] In contrast to the extensive knowledge gained on Wnt pathway-mediated regulation of T cell development, the roles for Wnt signal transducers in regulation of mammalian immune responses have not been known until relatively recently. In this review, we will briefly discuss the involvement of Wnt signaling pathway in T cell development and some outstanding issues. We will then summarize the novel advances in understanding the roles of canonical Wnt pathway in shaping CD4[+] and CD8[+] T cell-mediated immune responses and bridging the innate and adaptive immune systems.

## Wnt signal transducers and T cell development

A critical requirement for the Wnt pathway in normal T cell development has been well established and the readers are referred to recent reviews by Staal,[5] Misra Sen,[18,19] and colleagues. Concerning the Wnt ligands, Wnt4 and Wnt5a, both acting through β-catenin–independent pathways, appeared to have opposing effect on T cell development, with Wnt4 enhancing thymopoiesis and Wnt5a promoting thymocyte apoptosis.[20,21] A more recent study demonstrated that the most widely used canonical Wnt3a is required for normal size of thymic rudiment in embryos and normal thymic cellularity in fetal thymic organ culture (FTOC).[22]

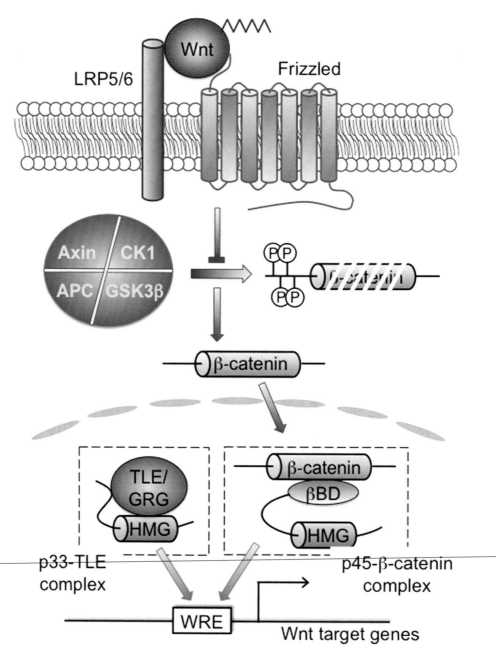

**Figure 1.** The canonical Wnt signaling pathway in T lineage cells. β-catenin is posttranscriptionally regulated via phosphorylation by the CK1 and GSK3β kinases in the destruction complex and proteosome-mediated degradation. Wnt stimulation of its receptor complex consisting of seven transmembrane Frizzled receptor and coreceptors LRP5/6 leads to inactivation of the destruction complex and ensuing β-catenin stabilization. The accumulated β-catenin is then translocated into the nucleus, where it displaces TLE/GRG corepressors and binds to TCF-1/LEF-1 long isoforms through their N-terminal β-catenin binding domain (βBD). The TCF-1/LEF-1 short isoforms cannot bind β-catenin but can interact with the TLE/GRG corepressors. These two types of complexes can both bind to Wnt response elements (WREs) via the HMG domains in TCF-1 and LEF-1, and their binding equilibrium determines the expression levels of Wnt target genes. For the purpose of clarity, depicted in the figure are p45 TCF-1 long isoform (containing both βBD and HMG DNA binding domain) complexed with β-catenin and p33 TCF-1 short isoform (containing HMG domain only) complexed with TLE/GRG. Similar complexes should occur for other TCF-1 and LEF-1 isoforms depending on the presence of βBD. It should be noted that depending on Wnt signal strength and the relative abundance of nuclear β-catenin and TLE/GRG, p45-TLE/GRG complex may also exist and contribute to regulation of Wnt target genes.

As for Wnt signal transducers in the nucleus, TCF-1 deficiency resulted in incomplete arrest of T cell development at early stages including double negative 1 (DN1), DN3, and immature single positive (ISP).[13,23] Whereas targeting LEF-1 alone did not severely impact T cell development, mice that are deficient for LEF-1 and hypomorphic for TCF-1 had a complete block at ISP with impaired TCRα rearrangements,[24] suggesting functional redundancy between TCF-1 and LEF-1. It is noteworthy that $Wnt3a^{-/-}$ fetal liver cells initially gave rise to thymocytes at all developmental stages in FTOC, however, the thymocyte development exhibited a progressive block at the ISP stage after prolonged culture.[22] This similarity in T cell developmental defects resulting from TCF-1 and Wnt3a deficiencies suggests that Wnt3a might be one of the dominant Wnt ligands that act through TCF-1/LEF-1 in developing thymocytes. A most recent progress came from the observations that during early stages of T cell specification and commitment, TCF-1 was upregulated by Notch signaling, and forced expression of TCF-1 was sufficient to direct bone marrow (BM) progenitors to T cell lineage even in the absence of Notch signals.[25]

In most tissues/cell types (such as epithelia), ablation of TCF/LEF factors or β-catenin produced consistent phenotypes.[26,27] However, the relationship between the TCF/LEF factors and β-catenin cofactor is somehow dissociated in developing T cells. Lck-Cre–mediated inactivation of β-catenin reduced T cellularity and partly blocked T cell development at the DN3 stage;[28] albeit the impact was less severe than germline deletion of all TCF-1 isoforms. On the other hand, when β-catenin was inactivated by induced Mx1-Cre activity in BM cells, the BM chimeric mice reconstituted with β-catenin-deficient cells exhibited no detectable T cell developmental defects.[29] In addition, activation of a T cell program in BM progenitors by ectopic expression of TCF-1 was not affected by induced inactivation of β-catenin.[25] A compensatory role by a β-catenin homologue, γ-catenin (also known as plakoglobin), was postulated; however, combined deletion of β-catenin (via Mx1-Cre) and γ-catenin (germline-targeted) did not apparently affect T cell development.[12,30] Several explanations have been proposed, including that timing of β-catenin inactivation at the hematopoietic stem cell (HSC) stage or in the DN3 thymocyte could make a difference,[18,19]

and that there could be an additional β-catenin–like Wnt signal transducer protein.[31] The latter view was inferred from the observations that forced expression of the p45 but not p33 TCF-1 isoform in $Tcf7^{-/-}$ mice partly overcame the developmental blocks,[14] and Wnt reporter activity was substantially compromised by TCF-1 deficiency but relatively unaffected by loss of both β- and γ-catenin.[12] It should be noted that the two different strains of β-catenin–targeted mice used in these studies were generated by floxing exons 2–6 or exons 3–6 in the $Ctnnb1$ gene (encoding β-catenin),[26,32] and the remaining transcript in both strains can be translated from an in-frame ATG in exon 7 and thus generates a 52 kDa protein, a phenomenon that appeared to be specific to hematopoietic cells.[12] It remains to be determined if this truncated form of β-catenin is functional $in vivo$, and further studies including generating a true β-catenin–null mutant in hematopoietic cells are needed to further clarify this important issue.

Although the TCF/LEF transcription factors have not been studied in detail in HSCs, contradictory observations have been reported regarding the effects of Wnt ligand stimulation or β-catenin gene manipulation on HSC proliferation and repopulation capacity. Critical assessments of the literature on this subject have been published elsewhere.[5,33] Relevant to this review, Mx1-Cre–mediated inactivation of β-catenin in adults HSCs did not impact overall hematopoiesis.[12,30] However, deletion of β-catenin from fetal stage by Vav-Cre compromised HSC repopulation capacity under competitive regenerative conditions,[34] highlighting the necessity of investigating and interpreting a gene's function in the context of embryo/organ developmental stages. Therefore, the existing data showing lack of strong effects upon β-catenin deletion should not be held as evidence to deny a regulatory role of the Wnt pathway in regulating thymocyte maturation. Ectopic expression of stabilized β-catenin in thymocytes, either by transgenes or deletion of exon 3 in the $Ctnnb1$ gene, did exhibit dominant effects including bypassing pre-TCR signaling at the DN3 stage, promoting positive selection at the $CD4^+CD8^+$ double positive (DP) stage, and extending thymocyte survival.[35–37] Thus, β-catenin may not be necessary but is sufficient to mediate regulation of T cell development at different stages.

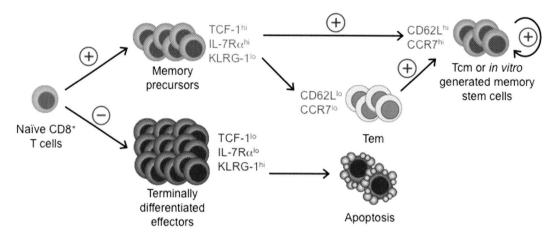

**Figure 2.** Regulation of CD8[+] T cell responses by the Wnt signaling pathway. Upon activation, naive CD8[+] T cells undergo clonal expansion and generate both terminally differentiated effectors and memory precursors. The differentiated effectors succumb to apoptosis during the contraction phase, and the memory precursors give rise to $T_{em}$ and/or $T_{cm}$, with $T_{cm}$ being capable of self-renewal and prolonged protection. "+" marks indicate positive regulation by TCF-1 alone or in combination with β-catenin, including generation of memory precursors, $T_{cm}$ maturation, and memory T cell persistence. The "–" mark indicates negative regulation. It is of note that $T_{cm}$ cells could be derived directly from the memory precursors or through differentiation from $T_{em}$ based on current literature.[41] Regardless of the origin, existing evidence supports a positively regulatory role of TCF-1 for $T_{cm}$ maturation.[60,61]

## Wnt signal transducers and CD8[+] T cells

The cytotoxic CD8[+] T cells are vital in defense against viruses and intracellular bacteria.[38–40] Activation of antigen-specific naive CD8[+] T cells requires TCR stimulation, costimulation, and proinflammatory cytokines from antigen-presenting cells and other innate immune cells. The activated T cells then undergo massive clonal expansion, giving rise to >10,000-fold more antigen-specific effector CD8[+] T cells that are equipped with cytokines such as interferon-γ (IFN-γ) and cytolytic molecules, including granzymes and perforin. In the contraction phase, 90–95% of the effector T cells succumb to apoptosis, and only a small portion transition into memory CD8[+] T cells, capable of providing enhanced protection against the same pathogen. The memory CD8[+] T cells undergo maturation from effector memory ($T_{em}$) to central memory ($T_{cm}$), with Tcm being more efficient in homeostatic self-renewal and secondary proliferation (Fig. 2).[41] How to maximize the beneficial effect of the immunological memory has been a subject of intensive investigation, given its direct relevance to the design and application of vaccines.[42] It is generally accepted that memory precursors can be derived from fully activated effector T cells,[43] one unanswered question is how early the fate of a memory precursor is determined. Is it during the first division of the activated T cell due to asymmetrical partition of key proteins between the two daughter cells, or is it gradually acquired during the expansion phase, factoring in the strength and duration of TCR, costimulation, and cytokines?[44] Whereas a definitive answer awaits further investigation, accumulating evidence indicates that the memory precursors are enriched in a subset of effector CD8[+] T cells expressing higher levels of interleukin-7 receptor α chain (IL-7Rα) and low levels of killer cell lectin-like receptor G1 (KLRG1).[45,46] Follow-up studies to overexpress IL-7Rα or inactivate KLRG1 show little effect in improving CD8[+] memory formation,[47–49] suggesting that these cell-surface molecules did not provide instructive signals for effector to memory transition. Nonetheless, the IL-7Rα$^{hi}$KLRG-1$^{lo}$ cells may have a distinct intrinsic capability to integrate signals from environmental cues and navigate to a memory fate. Here, we summarize recent evidence supporting the involvement of Wnt signaling pathway in promoting generation of memory CD8[+] T cells.

### Sufficiency of Wnt pathway in promoting memory CD8[+] T cell formation

TCF-1 and LEF-1 transcription factors are highly expressed in naive CD8[+] T cells. When examined at the bulk population level, they are both substantially downregulated in antigen-specific effector CD8[+] T cells.[50] TCF-1 and LEF-1 expression was subsequently upregulated as the effector population transitioned into memory CD8[+] T cells but remained lower compared with that in their naive status.[50] This is consistent with the observation that antigen-experienced human memory CD8[+] T cells (isolated based on CCR7 and CD45RA markers) expressed lower TCF-1 and LEF-1 than naive T cells.[51] Interestingly, in an acute viral infection setting, the IL-7Rα[hi]KLRG-1[lo] memory precursors expressed 10-fold more TCF-1 than the terminally differentiated IL-7Rα[lo]KLRG-1[hi] effector CD8[+] T cells,[46,52] suggesting a positive correlation of TCF-1 expression with a memory fate. By crossing previously established transgenic strains expressing a p45 isoform of TCF-1 (p45-Tg) and stabilized β-catenin (βCat-Tg),[14,36] we obtained double transgenic mice in which T cells had constitutively active Wnt signaling, infected them with attenuated *Listeria monocytogenes*-expressing chicken ovalbumin (LM-Ova) and then tracked Ova-specific CD8[+] T cells.[50] Expression of both transgenes limited clonal expansion of Ova-specific effector T cells, but expanded the memory CD8[+] T cell pool, which may partly result from reduced cell death during the contraction phase.[50] The increased quantity of memory CD8[+] T cells gave rise to larger numbers of secondary effector T cells when the immune mice were rechallenged with a virulent version of LM-Ova, conferring enhanced protection. Infection of p45 and βCat double transgenic mice with lymphocytic choriomeningitis virus (LCMV) and vaccinia virus expressing Ova confirmed that activation of Wnt signaling favors memory CD8[+] T cell formation independently of pathogen types or epitopes.[50]

Restifo and colleagues used GSK3β inhibitors or Wnt3a to activate the Wnt signaling pathway in murine CD8[+] T cells primed *in vitro*. This treatment arrested effector T cell differentiation but promoted acquisition of memory-like CD8[+] T cells with stem cell-like features (termed "CD8[+] memory stem cells") including the expression of Sca-1, which is usually associated with hematopoietic stem/progenitor cells.[53] These CD8[+] memory stem cells demonstrated increased homeostatic proliferation when transferred into a lymphopenic environment, enhanced IFN-γ production and proliferation upon reencounter with the same antigen. The authors also generated CD8[+] memory stem cells from Pmel-1 TCR transgenic CD8[+] T cells specific for a B16 melanoma antigen gp100; and upon adoptive transfer in combination with gp100 vaccine and IL-2, the Pmel-1 CD8[+] memory stem cells completely protected the hosts bearing B16 tumors.[53] This set of studies, however, has been questioned by others. Gajewski and colleagues confirmed that CD8[+] T cells primed in the presence of a GSK3β inhibitor acquired a CD62L[high]CD44[low] phenotype, but they did not find a similar effect with T cells primed in the presence of Wnt3a or T cells expressing adenovirus-delivered stabilized β-catenin.[54] They also showed that B16 tumor cells with forced expression of Wnt3a did not elicit stronger T cell responses upon transfer into syngeneic hosts.[54] Prlic and Bevan also reported failure to reproduce the memory stem cell phenotype after priming CD8[+] T cells in the presence of low concentrations of GSK3β inhibitor, and they further showed that the "memory stem cell" phenotype was instead associated with partially activated or nondividing cells when a high concentration of GSK3β inhibitor was used.[55] The exact nature of discrepancy in the *in vitro* studies is currently unclear and requires further investigation. Nevertheless, our findings through *in vivo* infection of transgenic models suggest that the TCF-1–β-catenin axis could be one of the intrinsic molecular switches that facilitate the transition of effectors to memory T cells (Fig. 2).[50,53]

A consensus finding in currently available data is that constitutive activation of the Wnt signaling pathway reduced effector CD8[+] T cell expansion.[50,53] Another recent study by Gajewski and colleagues confirmed this finding and further demonstrated that forced expression of stabilized β-catenin in naive T cells interfered with proximal TCR signaling including phosphorylation of the adaptor protein LAT and activation of phospholipase C-γ1.[56] It thus appears that downregulation of TCF-1 and hence attenuation of Wnt signaling are necessary for optimal expansion of terminally differentiated effector T cells (Fig. 2). However, the inhibition of effector expansion by Wnt signaling did not have a negative impact on function or secondary expansion of memory CD8[+] T cells.[50,53] For translational application, such data are promising. In vaccination, adjuvants are critical components used to stimulate the innate immune system and aid generation of robust adaptive immunological memory.[57,58] Because

Wnt proteins can be produced by DCs and other innate immune cells (discussed later), Wnt could potentially be used during vaccination to generate durable CD8[+] memory without eliciting substantial inflammation. In considering the origin and identity of memory precursors, it is tempting to speculate that the memory precursors are a subset of effector CD8[+] T cells that have less pronounced or limited downregulation of TCF-1 during initial clonal expansion phase; that sustain responsiveness to Wnt ligands which may restrain them from vigorous proliferation; that manifest cell surface markers that coincide with the IL-7Rα[hi]KLRG-1[lo] phenotype; and that persist during the contraction phase to become memory CD8[+] T cells. As discussed above, TCR-, costimulation-, and cytokine-derived signals are all involved in influencing output of memory CD8[+] T cells, and these signals may act through critical transcription factors such as T-bet, Eomes, and Blimp-1.[46,52,59] Lower expression of T-bet and Blimp-1 was associated with the IL-7Rα[hi]KLRG-1[lo] subset and, of particular interest, Blimp-1–deficient effector CD8[+] T cells predominantly exhibited this memory precursor phenotype with 10-fold increase in the *Tcf7* transcripts over the control cells.[52] Although no single pathway has been identified to be the sole determinant, it is plausible to conclude that the interplay of the Wnt–TCF-1–β-catenin axis with other key transcription factors collectively programs CD8[+] memory fate.

## Necessity of Wnt pathway in maturation and persistence of memory CD8[+] T cells

Early studies suggested that TCF-1 is dispensable for T cell proliferation and certain antiviral responses.[23] To further explore the physiological role of TCF-1 in regulating CD8[+] T cell responses, Held and colleagues and our group used LCMV and LM-Ova infection models, respectively, to track the behavior of *Tcf7[−/−]* CD8[+] T cells.[60,61] The consensus conclusions of these two studies include (1) lack of TCF-1 did not affect initial T cell activation but moderately reduced expansion of antigen-specific effector CD8[+] T cells; (2) *Tcf7[−/−]* effector T cells were not compromised in production of IFN-γ, tumor necrosis factor α (TNF-α), or granzyme-B; Held and colleagues also showed that the *Tcf7[−/−]* effectors were capable of controlling LCMV titers in infected mice and killing peptide-pulsed target cells *in vitro*; (3) the *Tcf7[−/−]* effector T cells contained

greatly diminished portion of the IL-7Rα[hi]KLRG-1[lo] memory precursor cells with concomitant increase in terminally differentiated effector T cells; (4) the *Tcf7[−/−]* memory CD8[+] T cells were not compromised in cytotoxicity as measured by *in vivo* killing assays but exhibited a sustained T$_{em}$ phenotype, being CD62L[lo]CCR7[lo] and with reduced IL-2 production; and (5) the ability of *Tcf7[−/−]* memory CD8[+] T cells to generate secondary effectors after bacterial or viral rechallenge was greatly diminished. Due to incomplete developmental blocks, *Tcf7[−/−]* mice exhibited moderate lymphopenia, with splenic T cells reduced to about one-third to one-half of littermate controls.[23] As a result of homeostatic proliferation, an increased portion of *Tcf7[−/−]* mature T cells showed a CD44[hi]CD62L[lo] phenotype but a substantial faction remained as CD44[lo]CD62L[hi] naive T cells.[61] We confirmed that the naive *Tcf7[−/−]* CD8[+] T cells did not produce IFN-γ upon brief exposure to TCR stimulation *in vitro* and transferred the sorted naive *Tcf7[−/−]* OT-I CD8[+] T cells into naive hosts followed by LM-Ova infection. *Tcf7[−/−]* memory CD8[+] T cells derived from these naive precursors exhibited similar defects, as unsorted input population, including diminished T$_{cm}$ maturation, excluding the possibility of a secondary effect.[61] These observations indicate a nonredundant role of TCF-1 in promoting maturation of memory CD8[+] T cells to a more durable T$_{cm}$ phenotype and sustaining their capacity for secondary expansion (Fig. 2).

Although not dramatically decreased at early memory stage (30–40 days postinfection), *Tcf7[−/−]* memory CD8[+] T cells exhibited time-dependent attrition, resulting in >10-fold decrease in cell numbers at 100+ days postinfection.[61] Mechanistically, we demonstrated that TCF-1 directly regulates Eomes expression via a Wnt-dependent mechanism, and that TCF-1–mediated induction of Eomes is critical for sustained IL-2 receptor β chain (IL-2Rβ) expression and, hence, IL-15 responsiveness.[61] Consistent with our finding, Prlic and Bevan showed that Wnt-mediated Eomes induction is dependent on β-catenin.[55] We also showed that forced expression of Eomes in *Tcf7[−/−]* memory CD8[+] T cells partly restored IL-2Rβ expression and protected them from time-dependent loss. However, maturation of *Tcf7[−/−]* memory CD8[+] T cells to T$_{cm}$ was not improved by ectopic Eomes expression, suggesting that additional TCF-1–dependent genes/pathways are required to sufficiently rectify memory T cell defects caused by TCF-1 ablation. Indeed, Myc expression was impaired in $Tcf7^{-/-}$ memory CD8[+] T cells, and Myc was previously reported to act downstream of IL-15 and to contribute to CD8[+] memory maintenance.[62] Interestingly, Myc expression was not induced by Wnt stimulation in naive or memory CD8[+] T cells, suggesting that TCF-1 may have Wnt-independent effects in this context. It has been shown that Smad transcription factors downstream of the transforming growth factor (TGF)-β pathway directly interact with LEF-1 in *Xenopus*, and this interaction can act independently or synergistically with the Wnt pathway to activate TCF/LEF target genes.[63,64] Further molecular dissection is needed to elucidate TCF-1 downstream mediators at the memory stage that promote $T_{cm}$ maturation and sustain intact secondary expansion.

Given the apparent dissociation between TCF-1 and β-catenin in T cell development discussed above, it is not surprising that deletion of β-catenin did not phenocopy the defects observed in TCF-1 deficiency during mature CD8[+] T cell responses. Gajewski and colleagues showed that *in vitro* priming of β-catenin–deficient CD8[+] T cells in the presence of a GSK3β inhibitor did not affect acquisition of some of the memory stem cell markers.[54] More recently, Prlic and Bevan reported that CD8[+] T cell responses were essentially indistinguishable in β-catenin–targeted and control mice, using various viral and bacterial infection models and different infection routes.[55] It should be noted that these β-catenin–mutant T cells may express the 52 kDa truncated form of β-catenin protein, and thus a definitive conclusion requires evaluation of a true β-catenin–null mutant. On the other hand, using gene complementation approaches Held and colleagues showed that forced expression of p45, but not p33, TCF-1 isoform at least partly rescued TCF-1 deletion-derived defects, including diminished frequency of IL-7Rα[hi]KLRG-1[lo] memory precursors at the effector phase, arrested maturation to $T_{cm}$ phenotype at the memory phase, and inefficient generation of secondary effectors in response to rechallenge.[60] These results indicate that the ability of TCF-1 to interact with β-catenin or a β-catenin–like protein is essential for generation of functional memory CD8[+] T cells. In addition, the authors also showed that double deficiency of both β- and γ-catenin did compromise the secondary expansion of memory CD8[+] T cells.[60] Detailed phenotypic analyses of effector and memory T cells lacking both β- and γ-catenin would be critical to determine if γ-catenin is *the* other factor compensating for loss of β-catenin in mature CD8[+] T cells, or if there are additional TCF-1-interacting molecules whose expression and/or activity can be modulated by Wnt stimulation or GSK3β inhibition. Complete resolution of this issue awaits further investigation of T cell biology and hematopoiesis.

## Wnt signal transducers and CD4[+] T cells

Upon activation by cognate antigens, CD4[+] T cells differentiate to distinct T helper (Th) populations, and each Th subset secretes a different set of cytokines, providing help to antibody-producing B lymphocytes and CD8[+] cytotoxic T cells as well as activation of innate immune cells. The binary Th1/Th2 paradigm has been well established and characterized. Th1 cells produce IFN-γ and are critical in confining intracellular microorganisms, whereas Th2 cells produce IL-4, IL-5, and IL-13 are required for controlling helminths and other extracellular pathogens.[65] New additions to the Th lineage include Th17 cells, which secrete IL-17a, IL-17f, and IL-22,[66] regulatory T cells ($T_{reg}$ cells),[67] IL-9–producing Th9 cells, and IL-21–producing T follicular helper cells.[68,69] Summarized below are recent advances linking Wnt signaling pathway with Th lineage differentiation.

### Wnt pathway and Th2

Initiation of Th2 differentiation depends on upregulation of the Gata3 transcription factor, which is critical for initial production of IL-4. IL-4 will in turn augment Gata3 expression via a STAT6-dependent manner and thus enforce a Th2 fate.[70–72] Gata3 is transcribed from two promoters, with a distal promoter driving transcription from noncoding exon1a (*Gata3*–1a) and a proximal promoter from another noncoding exon1b (*Gata3*–1b). Notch signaling has been shown to activate Gata3 transcription from *Gata3*–1a.[73,74] Two recent reports demonstrated the critical requirements of the Wnt-β–catenin pathway for Th2 differentiation.[75,76] Misra Sen and colleagues showed that when CD4[+] T cells are activated in a neutral (nonpolarizing) condition, the *Gata3*–1b transcripts were upregulated more rapidly and more abundantly than *Gata3*–1a transcripts.[75] Both the upregulation of *Gata3*–1b and subsequent induction of IL-4 were diminished by TCF-1 deficiency, overexpression of β-catenin-interacting protein (ICAT), which binds β-catenin and impairs its interaction with TCF-1, and forced expression of a mutant TCF-1, which is equivalent to short isoforms lacking the N-terminal β-catenin interaction domain. Conversely, the induction of *Gata3*–1b and *Il4* was promoted by forced expression of a stabilized β-catenin, and the effect by β-catenin was independent of IL-4–Stat6 and Notch signaling pathways. The authors further showed direct occupancy of both TCF-1 and β-catenin on a WRE upstream of *Gata3*-1b. These observations demonstrated that TCF-1 and its interaction with β-catenin are critically required by CD4[+] T cells to adopt a Th2 fate. This conclusion was further substantiated in a mouse model of allergic asthma, where *Tcf7*[−/−] animals exhibited diminished inflammation in the perivascular and more pronouncedly in the peribronchial areas in the lung.[75]

In line with these findings, Galande and colleagues showed that under Th2 polarizing conditions for human CD4[+] T cells isolated from umbilical cord blood, inclusion of Wnt inhibitor Dickkopf (Dkk1) in the culture or siRNA-mediated knockdown of β-catenin diminished Gata3 expression as well as production of Th2 cytokines, including IL-4 and IL-13.[76] Significantly, knockdown of SATB1 (special AT-rich binding protein 1) in Th2-differentiating CD4[+] T cells showed a similar effect as knockdown of β-catenin, including diminished Gata3 transcription and IL-4/13 production. SATB1 is a well-characterized global genome organizer that anchors chromatin at specialized DNA sequences, thus contributing to organization of chromatin into three-dimensional folded architecture.[77] SATB1 is predominantly expressed in developing thymocytes, diminished in resting mature T cells, and can be increased in expression in activated T cells. It has been shown that upregulation of SATB1 in activated CD4[+] T cells is required for compacting the Th2 cytokine locus encompassing *Il4*, *Il5*, and *Il13* genes into dense loops, a chromatin configuration that allows active transcription of the Th2 cytokines.[78] In the studies by Galande and colleagues, the C-terminus of β-catenin was found to physically interact with SATB1, and stabilization of β-catenin in primary human thymocytes induced a fraction of SATB1 target genes, accompanied by enhanced SATB1 binding to these gene loci.[76] In

Th2-polarized CD4[+] T cells, enriched binding of both β-catenin and SATB1 was found at a potential SATB1 binding region located at 600–900 bp upstream of the human *GATA3* transcription initiation site. Based on our sequence alignment and conservation analysis, this β-catenin/SATB1 cooccupied region in the human *GATA3* gene contains a WRE, which corresponds to the one upstream of mouse *Gata3*–1b, identified by Misra Sen and colleagues.[75] Although it appears that stabilized β-catenin is partitioned between SATB1 and TCF factors, it is possible that these factors may act in a cooperative fashion to initiate Gata3 induction in activated CD4[+] T cells and promote their differentiation to Th2 lineage (Fig. 3).

Similar to TCF-1 in CD8[+] T cells, TCF-1 expression is modulated by cytokine and TCR signaling in CD4[+] T cells. Expression of IL-4 receptor α chain (IL-4Rα) on naive CD4[+] T cells makes them responsive to IL-4 stimulation prior to TCR activation. The early exposure to IL-4 appears to prepare naive CD4[+] T cells for Th2 differentiation because IL-4 stimulation of human naive CD4[+] T cells specifically downregulates the shorter isoforms of TCF-1, which may otherwise negatively affect Gata3 induction.[15] This effect is likely direct as Stat6 was shown to bind *in vivo* to several putative binding sites in the *TCF7* locus in an IL-4–dependent manner.[15] On the other hand, TCR stimulation alone moderately downregulated TCF-1 on transcript level in both human and mouse CD4[+] T cells.[15,75] However, under Th2-polarizing conditions (i.e., the combination of TCR and IL-4 stimulation), TCF-1 was further diminished at both transcript and protein levels.[15,79] Given the caveat that these observations were made *in vitro* with CD4[+] T cells exposed to prolonged TCR stimulation and high concentrations of cytokines, one plausible explanation of these observations is that during the initiation stage of Th2 responses, innate immune cell-derived IL-4 may prime the antigen-specific CD4[+] T cells to downregulate inhibitory isoforms of TCF-1, and upon cognate antigen encounter, these CD4[+] T cells may utilize the full-length TCF-1 as well as upregulated SATB1 to induce Gata3, which helps to commit to a Th2 fate. In this context, further downregulation of all TCF-1 isoforms in fully differentiated Th2 cells (by TCR and IL-4) may serve as a way to tune down Gata3–IL-4 feed-forward responses.

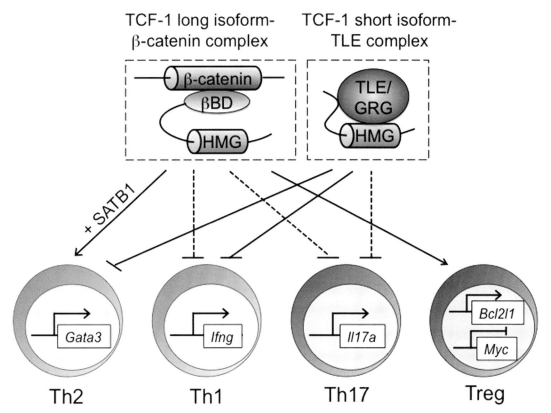

**Figure 3.** A hypothetical model of regulation of CD4$^+$ T cell differentiation by the Wnt signaling pathway. Possible regulatory roles of TCF-1 in different CD4$^+$ lineages are depicted based on current literature. Arrows denote positive regulation and lines ending with bars denote negative regulation. Solid lines indicate regulatory roles supported by reported experimental data, and dashed lines are possible regulation. Genes that are modulated by TCF-1 in expression are shown for each CD4$^+$ lineage. Note that only *Gata3* and *Il17a* have been shown to be potential direct targets for TCF-1. *Ifng* and *Bcl2l1* encode IFN-γ and Bcl-X$_L$, respectively.

It has been clear that TCF-1 and LEF-1 have partly overlapping roles in thymocyte maturation; however, existing experimental data suggest that LEF-1 may have a distinct, or even TCF-1–opposing, role in CD4$^+$ T cell differentiation. By a proteomics screening, LEF-1 was found to directly interact with Gata3 via its HMG box domain.[80] Like TCF-1, LEF-1 is downregulated in Th2-polarized cells. Forced expression of LEF-1 in Th2 cells resulted in diminished production of IL-4, IL-5, and IL-13.[80] In contrast, expression of a mutant form of LEF-1 that lacks the HMG domain and C-terminus alleviated the repression. These data were interpreted as LEF-1–Gata3 interaction negatively controls Th2 responses; however, one cannot exclude other possibilities such as deletion of the HMG domain in LEF-1 may abrogate its interaction with GRG/TLE corepressors or overexpression of LEF-1 may compete for β-catenin with

TCF-1 as well as SATB1. Another report described a potential LEF-1 binding site in the *Il4* gene upstream regulatory region and also showed reduction of IL-4 expression upon siRNA-mediated knockdown of LEF-1 in Jurkat cells.[79] Since germline targeting of LEF-1 resulted in perinatal lethality, a conditionally targeted *Lef1* allele is needed to further elucidate the role of LEF-1 in CD4$^+$ differentiation.

### Wnt pathway, Th1, and Th17

Although the TCF-1/β-catenin complex positively regulates Th2 initiation and further differentiation, TCF-1 represses alternative Th1 and Th17 fates in activated CD4$^+$ T cells, and these effects appear to be independent of β-catenin (Fig. 3).[75,81] Under nonpolarizing conditions, TCF-1–deficient CD4$^+$ T cells gave rise to more IFN-γ–producing cells than WT CD4$^+$ T cells, and forced expression of a short isoform of TCF-1 was sufficient to reduce IFN-γ–producing cells.[75] Consistent with a negative regulatory role of TCF-1 in Th1 polarization, a recent study reported that in Th1-differentiating CD4$^+$ T cells, T-bet and Bcl6 cooperatively repress the expression of TCF-1.[82] Interestingly, single nucleotide polymorphisms in the *TCF7* allele were found to be associated with type I diabetes, an autoimmune disease with apparent involvement of Th1 cytokines. Among these, the C883A polymorphism in *TCF7* exon 2, resulting in single amino acid substitution of proline with threonine, was significantly associated with type I diabetes patients who do not carry the high risk HLA genotype DR3/DR4.[83] It would be interesting to determine if the Pro–Thr substitution in TCF-1 favors differentiation of CD4$^+$ T cells to Th1 lineage. It is of note that although both TCF-1 and LEF-1 were substantially downregulated in fully differentiated Th2 cells, the expression of LEF-1, but not TCF-1, was sustained in Th1 cells.[79] One possible role for continued presence of LEF-1 in Th1-differentiating CD4$^+$ T cells might be to repress IL-4,[79] a notion that deserves more investigation.

Under Th17-polarizing conditions, a larger fraction of *Tcf7$^{-/-}$* CD4$^+$ T cells expressed IL-17a, with concomitant increase in *Il17f* and *Il22* transcripts. In the experimental autoimmune encephalomyelitis (EAE) mouse model, which has been shown to be causally associated with pathological Th17 responses, *Tcf7$^{-/-}$* mice exhibited exacerbated clinical scores with increased IL-17a–producing CD4$^+$ cells detected in both lymph nodes and spleens compared with WT controls.[81] Exhaustive searches for TCF-1 targets required for Th17 differentiation excluded an impact of TCF-1 on known cytokines, cytokine receptors, and transcriptional regulators, such as RORγt, but suggested that TCF-1 may directly suppress *Il17a* gene transcription via direct binding to intronic TCF-1 consensus motifs (or WREs).[81] The authors also showed that forced expression of stabilized β-catenin or ICAT (which interrupts TCF and β-catenin interaction) had little impact on Th17 differentiation, in contrast to active involvement of β-catenin in generating Th2 cells (Fig. 3). These findings raised an interesting possibility that different TCF-1 isoforms may have distinct roles in directing CD4$^+$ helper cells to proper lineages. Since the *Tcf7$^{-/-}$* mice lack all TCF-1 isoforms, detailed mapping of TCF-1 isoform-specific functions may

provide more mechanistic insights into this important biological process.

## Wnt pathway and T$_{reg}$ cells

T$_{reg}$ cells are vital in maintaining self-tolerance and curtailing excessive immune responses. The impact of TCF-1 or β-catenin deficiency on naturally occurring T$_{reg}$ cells (nT$_{reg}$) or induced T$_{reg}$ cells has not been specifically addressed. Lafaille and colleagues introduced a different version of stabilized β-catenin (all 3 Ser and 1 Thr phosphorylation sites in the N-terminus of β-catenin were replaced with Ala[84]) into CD4$^+$CD25$^+$ nT$_{reg}$ cells via retroviral transduction after brief TCR priming *in vitro*.[85] The expression of active β-catenin extended T$_{reg}$ cell survival without evoking proliferation and cytokine production, and this effect was mediated by upregulation of Bcl-X$_L$ and suppression of Myc (Fig. 3). Furthermore, the β-catenin–transduced nT$_{reg}$ cells exhibited enhanced protection against disease when adoptively transferred into a mouse model of autoimmune colitis. In line with these findings, treatment of nT$_{reg}$ cells *in vitro* with a GSK3β inhibitor led to β-catenin stabilization and prolonged expression of Foxp3 and Bcl-X$_L$.[86] In an allotransplant mouse model in which pancreatic islets were transplanted into recipients with induced diabetes, systematic administration of a GSK3β inhibitor moderately extended the survival of islet grafts.[86] These findings suggest that the β-catenin pathway can be modulated to enhance T$_{reg}$ cell activity, which may have important implications in treatment of autoimmune diseases and transplant rejection.

The effect of stabilized β-catenin on non-T$_{reg}$ CD4$^+$ cells is, however, controversial. In a study by Lafaille and colleagues, transduction of the active β-catenin into CD4$^+$CD25$^-$ T cells was shown to result in anergy, with decreased proliferation and reduced capacity to induce severe pathology in autoimmune colitis mouse model.[85] This effect might be specific to the experimental conditions used in this study, because an initial TCR priming of the CD4$^+$ T cells *in vitro* was necessary to make them permissive to retrovirus-mediated delivery of the active β-catenin. In contrast, Misra Sen and colleagues reported that CD4$^+$ T cells from β-catenin transgenic mice showed increased *Gata3*–1b transcripts and IL-4 production,[75] and these cells did not seem to be impeded in proliferation after prolonged culture (6 days) under nonpolarizing conditions. Using our *in vivo* infection studies, we infected β-catenin transgenic mice and littermate controls with attenuated *Listeria monocytogenes*, which predominantly elicited Th1 CD4[+] responses. By monitoring Listeriolysin O (LLO)-specific CD4[+] T cells, we found similar expansion of effector CD4[+] T cells at day 7 postinfection in both βCat-Tg and control mice, as measured by LLO peptide-stimulated IFN-γ production.[50] After 40+ days of infection, similar numbers of antigen-specific memory CD4[+] T cells were detected in both βCat-Tg and control mice, and these memory T cells exhibited similar secondary expansion and IFN-γ production capacity upon rechallenge with virulent *Listeria monocytogenes*.[50] Thus, β-catenin activation may not be associated with anergy of non-T$_{reg}$ CD4[+] T cells under physiological conditions. Nonetheless, this does not negate the potential translational use of suppressing the responsiveness of pathogenic CD4[+] T cells by manipulating β-catenin activity *in vitro*.

## Sources of Wnt ligands and cross-talk with other signaling pathways in T cells

Given the sufficiency and/or necessity of TCF-1 and β-catenin in modulating mature T cell responses (discussed above), a critical question is how this pathway is activated and utilized in mammalian immune systems. Wnt ligands are naturally the most potent stimulating factors to activate β-catenin. WntD, one member of the *Drosophila* Wnt family, was found to be under control of Toll signaling, and increased levels of WntD negatively modulated the NF-κB/Dorsal pathway and a subset of antimicrobial peptide expression.[87] In mammals, likely sources of Wnt ligands may include cells with direct contact with T cells during inflammatory responses, such as antigen presenting cells, via paracrine, or T cells themselves, via autocrine mechanisms. In a high-throughput gene expression profiling of human CD14[+] monocyte-derived macrophages and DCs, Wnt5a exhibited consistent upregulation in response to stimulation by *Mycobacterium tuberculosis*, helminths, and three other phylogenetically distinct protozoa.[88] An independent study showed that during monocyte differentiation, DCs exhibited sustained Wnt5a upregulation prior to any microbial stimulation.[89] The increased Wnt5a expression was also confirmed in stimulated human primary macrophages in re-

sponse to *mycobacteria*, as well as conserved bacteria structures such as lipopolysaccharide (LPS), and this induction was found to be dependent on Toll-like receptor signaling and the NF-κB pathway.[90] Both stimulated macrophages and TCR-ligated T cells upregulated the expression of Fzd5, a known receptor for Wnt5a.[91] Importantly, antibody-mediated blocking of Wnt5a–Fzd5 interaction reduced IL-12 production by macrophages and IFN-γ production by T cells.[90] In addition, resident macrophages were also found to express Wnt transcripts, such as Wnt7b and Wnt10b in ocular macrophages,[92] and Wnt3a, 5b, 7a, 8b, and 11 in intestinal lamina propria macrophages as well as DCs.[93] In addition to antigen-presenting cells, endothelial cells were found to express multiple Wnt transcripts including Wnt1, Wnt2b, Wnt4, Wnt5a, and Wnt8b.[94] Among these, Wnt1 was shown to induce expression of matrix metalloproteinases in activated T cells in a β-catenin–dependent fashion and hence enhance transmigration of T cells to inflammatory sites.[94] Whereas expression of CXCL12 in BM stromal cells is negatively regulated by Wnt3a but not Wnt5a,[95] T cells can produce Wnt5a in response to the CXCL12 chemokine, and the autocrine Wnt5a in turn augmented CXCL12-directed T cell migration without involving β-catenin.[96] Thus, Wnt proteins derived from multiple sources during systematic or local immune responses impact T cell migration and influence T cell fate determination and cytokine production.

Although not reviewed in detail here, it is important to note that several recent studies indicate critical involvement of Wnt/β-catenin pathway in differentiation and functionality of antigen presenting cells. It has been demonstrated that β-catenin is required for differentiation of conventional DCs and that β-catenin activation in DCs contributes to balancing proinflammatory and tolerogenic T cell responses.[93,97,98] In addition, β-catenin is implicated in macrophage survival and secretion of IFN-β by macrophages via interaction with cytosolic nucleic acid-sensing proteins.[99,100] In experimental settings using mycobacterium infection or LPS stimulation, Wnt5a augmented, whereas Wnt3a suppressed, production of proinflammatory cytokines by either human monocyte-derived or murine BM-derived macrophages.[101,102] Wnt proteins thus emerge as evolutionarily conserved key players bridging the innate and adaptive immunity and may have far-reaching roles in modulating the activity of cellular immune responses.[103–105]

Increasing evidence has suggested crosstalk between Wnt pathway and TCR-elicited signaling cascades. β-catenin in T cells can also be stabilized by TCR stimulation. This was shown in DN thymocytes undergoing β-selection,[106] as well as in CD4+CD8+ DP thymocytes undergoing positive selection.[107] In mature CD4+ T cells, TCR stimulation increased β-catenin protein by approximately twofold,[28,81] and this may account for the initial induction of Gata3–1b transcripts in Th2-destined cells before TCF-1 and LEF-1 are downregulated.[75] TCR-induced stabilization of β-catenin was also observed in human T cells;[108] however, the accumulated β-catenin by TCR was phosphorylated on its N-terminal Ser/Thr residues and failed to induce the known Wnt target genes such as *Axin2* and *Dkk1*.[108] This is in contrast to lithium-mediated accumulation of β-catenin, which is free of N-terminal Ser/Thr phosphorylation and capable of inducing *Axin2*. Whereas it remains to be determined if similar events are occurring in murine thymocytes and mature T cells, these observations raised a possibility that TCR and Wnt may utilize β-catenin in distinct ways to regulate their specific target genes. It has been suggested that TCR signaling pathway may converge with Wnt on GSK3β, because TCR coupled with costimulation activates phosphoinositide 3-kinase (PI3-K) and Akt,[109] and Akt can phosphorylate Ser9 in GSK3β, leading to GSK3β inactivation and β-catenin accumulation.[110] Akt was also reported to directly phosphorylate β-catenin on its C-terminal Ser552 residue in intestinal stem cells, resulting in β-catenin stabilization and nuclear localization.[111] Several other pathways were reported to lead to β-catenin stabilization and/or nuclear localization, including p38 mitogen-activated protein kinase-mediated phosphorylation of Thr390(human)/Ser389(mouse) in GSK3β,[112] Rac1 small GTPase-induced activation of JNK, which phosphorylates β-catenin on Ser191 and Ser605,[113] protein kinase C-mediated direct phosphorylation of N-terminal serine residues in β-catenin,[114] and a potential link between Pyk2 and tyrosine phosphorylation of β-catenin.[115] There is only limited knowledge as to whether these signaling events are occurring in T lineage cells,[116] and the few studies using pharmacological inhibitors of different pathways generated conflicting conclusions, partly because the cells tested were at different developmental stages.[106–108] More investigation is needed to determine TCR downstream events that lead to modulation of β-catenin quantity and activity, and importantly, how modulation of β-catenin by TCR impacts functional output of activated T cells. It is of interest to note that TGF-β–elicited signals have critical regulatory roles in thymocyte development and Th lineage differentiation[117] and that extensive crosstalk between TGF-β and Wnt signaling cascades has been described.[118] Smad transcription factors—the key TGF-β signal mediators—have been reported to interact with Axin and/or GSK3β in the cytoplasm and form a complex with β-catenin and TCF/LEF transcription factors in the nucleus (reviewed in Ref. 118). Validation of such crosstalk in T lineage cells may yield interesting insights into how these pathways cooperatively influence T cell-mediated immunity.

Another converging point of Wnt, TCR, and cytokine crosstalk is the TCF-1 and LEF-1 transcription factors. Both transcription factors were downregulated rapidly in both human and murine CD8+ T cells upon TCR stimulation *in vitro*,[51,61,108] and downregulation was also observed in antigen-specific CD8+ T cells generated *in vivo* in infected mice.[50] Interestingly, when CD8+ T cells were primed in the presence of a GSK3β inhibitor *in vitro*, TCF-1 and LEF-1 expression was elevated.[53] The sustained (or even elevated) TCF-1/LEF-1 expression, along with stabilized β-catenin, may thus cooperatively redirect activated T cells from effector to stem cell-like memory CD8+ T cells. In addition to TCR, IL-15 reduced, whereas TGF-β increased, *Tcf7* and *Lef1* transcripts in naive CD8+ T cells isolated from human cord blood without TCR priming.[51] On the other hand, antigen-primed effector CD8+ T cells exhibited downregulation of TCF-1/LEF-1 expression in response to IL-2 and IL-15, but upregulated both transcripts when exposed to IL-21.[119] TCF-1 and LEF-1 expression was also downregulated in CD4+ T cells by TCR, but the downregulation appeared to follow slower kinetics and was influenced by IL-4.[15,75,79] It is thus conceivable that the cytokine milieu, depending on infection types, may impinge on TCF-1 and LEF-1 expression, influence Wnt responsiveness, and function of effector T cells.

## Concluding remarks

Our knowledge on the novel roles of Wnt pathway in regulating immune responses has greatly advanced during the past few years. The regulatory roles of Wnt pathways range from activation of antigen-presenting DCs, memory $CD8^+$ T cell formation and persistence, to $CD4^+$ T helper lineage differentiation. Together with vaccine, the inclusion of Wnt ligands or GSK3β inhibitors to activate the Wnt signaling cascade may help elicit more potent and/or durable memory T cells against pathogens.[120,121] In T cell-based immunotherapies to treat cancer, generation of memory stem cell-like cells through modulation of Wnt signaling holds potential for improved efficacy in eliminating cancer cells.[121,122] Enhancing $T_{reg}$ survival and functionality via the β-catenin pathway has critical implications in inducing allotransplant tolerance or treating autoimmune conditions.[123] Of note is that lithium, a known GSK3-β inhibitor, is already clinically approved, and more selective GSK3-β inhibitors are in clinical trials.[124] Remarkably, administration of lithium substantially ameliorated EAE,[125] and this is at least partly consistent with a role of TCF-1 in inhibiting overexuberant Th17 responses.[81] Although current data demonstrated a dissociation of β-catenin with TCF-1 for their requirements in T lineage cells, gain-of-function approaches using GSK3β inhibitors or forced expression of stabilized β-catenin by a transgene or retroviral transduction did show a clear impact on memory $CD8^+$ T cell formation, Th2 differentiation, and $T_{reg}$ functionality.[50,75,85] Thus, β-catenin stabilization may not be necessary but is sufficient to influence T cell activity and fate choice, and the lack of necessity for β-catenin should not compromise the promise of modulating the Wnt signaling pathway to foster immunity against pathogens or tumors and to divert from harmful autoimmunity.

This review has focused on key molecules utilized by the canonical Wnt pathway, which are best studied in T lineage cells; however, what remains unexplored territory are the noncanonical Wnt pathways leading to activation of JNK and $Ca^{2+}$ signaling cascades, which are downstream of TCR ligation and have clear relevance in T cell biology. A key unanswered question is which Wnt ligand or what combination of Wnt ligands has the most critical impact on regulating T cell activation, differentiation, and memory formation. The field will benefit from the generation of quality antibodies to reliably detect Wnt proteins and Fzd receptors in immune cells. We have learned a great deal through analysis of animal models lacking key Wnt signal transducers, however, the insufficiency in these existing models has become evident. For example, a true β-catenin–null mutant in hematopoietic cells could help resolve the too-often-observed controversies regarding a role of Wnt–β-catenin pathway in T cell development, mature T cell responses, and HSC functionality. Whereas both TCF-1 and LEF-1 are the most abundantly expressed Wnt effector transcription factors in T cells, most current studies utilize TCF-1 knockout mice. The roles of LEF-1 in mature T cells are not sufficiently addressed due to lack of a proper animal model. In addition, both factors may have isoform-specific and/or β-catenin–independent function, given that forced expression of a TCF-1 short isoform in T cells primed *in vitro* suppresses expression of IFN-γ.[75] The existing germline-targeted TCF-1 knockout mice lack all TCF-1 isoforms, and thus new animal models are needed. Furthermore, next generation sequencing coupled with chromatin immunoprecipitation has been applied to transcription factors to map their genome-wide binding locations, and this has been done for TCF-4 and β-catenin in colorectal cancer cells.[126,127] Mapping TCF-1, LEF-1, and β-catenin in $CD8^+$ T cells at different stages of immune response or in $CD4^+$ T cells differentiated to distinct lineages should generate molecular insights into their critical roles in regulating cellular immune responses. More in-depth knowledge on Wnt ligands and Wnt signal transducers in T cells will undoubtedly provide important information for directing different T subsets to beneficial translational applications.

## Acknowledgments

We thank Drs. John Harty (University of Iowa), Jyoti Misra Sen (NIA), and Jinfang Zhu (NIAID) for critical reading of this manuscript and the Xue lab members for useful discussion. This work is supported by NIH Grants (HL095540 and AI080966) and funds from the American Cancer Society (RSG-11-161-01-MPC).

## Conflicts of interest

The authors declare no conflicts of interest.

# References

1. Logan, C.Y. & R. Nusse. 2004. The Wnt signaling pathway in development and disease. *Annu. Rev. Cell Dev. Biol.* **20:** 781–810.

2. Clevers, H. 2006. Wnt/beta-catenin signaling in development and disease. *Cell* **127:** 469–480.

3. Khan, N.I. & L.J. Bendall. 2006. Role of WNT signaling in normal and malignant hematopoiesis. *Histol. Histopathol.* **21:** 761–774.

4. van Amerongen, R., A. Mikels & R. Nusse. 2008. Alternative wnt signaling is initiated by distinct receptors. *Sci. Signal.* **1:** re9.

5. Staal, F.J., T.C. Luis & M.M. Tiemessen. 2008. WNT signalling in the immune system: WNT is spreading its wings. *Nat. Rev. Immunol.* **8:** 581–593.

6. Arce, L., N.N. Yokoyama & M.L. Waterman. 2006. Diversity of LEF/TCF action in development and disease. *Oncogene* **25:** 7492–7504.

7. Mosimann, C, G. Hausmann & K. Basler. 2009. Beta-catenin hits chromatin: regulation of Wnt target gene activation. *Nat. Rev. Mol. Cell Biol.* **10:** 276–286.

8. Staal, F.J., M. Noort Mv, G.J. Strous & H.C. Clevers. 2002. Wnt signals are transmitted through N-terminally dephosphorylated beta-catenin. *EMBO Rep.* **3:** 63–68.

9. Van de Wetering, M., J. Castrop, V. Korinek & H. Clevers. 1996. Extensive alternative splicing and dual promoter usage generate Tcf-1 protein isoforms with differential transcription control properties. *Mol. Cell Biol.* **16:** 745–752.

10. Daniels, D.L. & W.I. Weis. 2005. Beta-catenin directly displaces Groucho/TLE repressors from Tcf/Lef in Wnt-mediated transcription activation. *Nat. Struct. Mol. Biol.* **12:** 364–371.

11. Weerkamp, F., M.R. Baert, B.A. Naber, *et al.* 2006. Wnt signaling in the thymus is regulated by differential expression of intracellular signaling molecules. *Proc. Natl. Acad. Sci. USA* **103:** 3322–3326.

12. Jeannet, G., M. Scheller, L. Scarpellino, *et al.* 2008. Long-term, multilineage hematopoiesis occurs in the combined absence of beta-catenin and gamma-catenin. *Blood* **111:** 142–149.

13. Goux, D., J.D. Coudert, D. Maurice, *et al.* 2005. Cooperating pre-T-cell receptor and TCF-1-dependent signals ensure thymocyte survival. *Blood* **106:** 1726–1733.

14. Ioannidis, V., F. Beermann, H. Clevers & W. Held. 2001. The beta-catenin–TCF-1 pathway ensures CD4(+)CD8(+) thymocyte survival. *Nat. Immunol.* **2:** 691–697.

15. Maier, E., D. Hebenstreit, G. Posselt, *et al.* 2001. Inhibition of suppressive T cell factor 1 (TCF-1) isoforms in naive CD4+ T cells is mediated by IL-4/STAT6 signaling. *J. Biol. Chem.* **286:** 919–928.

16. Hoffmann, J.A. & J.M. Reichhart. 2002. Drosophila innate immunity: an evolutionary perspective. *Nat. Immunol.* **3:** 121–126.

17. Zettervall, C.J., I. Anderl, M.J. Williams, *et al.* 2004. A directed screen for genes involved in Drosophila blood cell activation. *Proc. Natl. Acad. Sci. USA* **101:** 14,192–14,197.

18. Yu, Q., A. Sharma & J.M. Sen. 2010. TCF1 and beta-catenin regulate T cell development and function. *Immunol. Res.* **47:** 45–55.

19. Staal, F.J. & J.M. Sen. 2008. The canonical Wnt signaling pathway plays an important role in lymphopoiesis and hematopoiesis. *Eur. J. Immunol.* **38:** 1788–1794.

20. Louis, I., K.M. Heinonen, J. Chagraoui, *et al.* 2008. The signaling protein Wnt4 enhances thymopoiesis and expands multipotent hematopoietic progenitors through beta-catenin-independent signaling. *Immunity* **29:** 57–67.

21. Liang, H., A.H. Coles, Z. Zhu, *et al.* 2007. Noncanonical Wnt signaling promotes apoptosis in thymocyte development. *J. Exp. Med.* **204:** 3077–3084.

22. Luis, T.C., F. Weerkamp, B.A. Naber, *et al.* 2009. Wnt3a deficiency irreversibly impairs hematopoietic stem cell self-renewal and leads to defects in progenitor cell differentiation. *Blood* **113:** 546–554.

23. Schilham, M.W., A. Wilson, P. Moerer, *et al.* 1998. Critical involvement of Tcf-1 in expansion of thymocytes. *J. Immunol.* **161:** 3984–3991.

24. Okamura, R.M., M. Sigvardsson, J. Galceran, *et al.* 1998. Redundant regulation of T cell differentiation and TCRalpha gene expression by the transcription factors LEF-1 and TCF-1. *Immunity* **8:** 11–20.

25. Weber, B.N., A.W. Chi, A. Chavez, *et al.* 2011. A critical role for TCF-1 in T-lineage specification and differentiation. *Nature* **476:** 63–68.

26. Huelsken, J., R. Vogel, B. Erdmann, *et al.* 2001. beta-Catenin controls hair follicle morphogenesis and stem cell differentiation in the skin. *Cell* **105:** 533–545.

27. Kratochwil, K., M. Dull, I. Farinas, *et al.* 1996. Lef1 expression is activated by BMP-4 and regulates inductive tissue interactions in tooth and hair development. *Genes Dev.* **10:** 1382–1394.

28. Xu, Y., D. Banerjee, J. Huelsken, *et al.* 2003. Deletion of beta-catenin impairs T cell development. *Nat. Immunol.* **4:** 1177–1182.

29. Cobas, M., A. Wilson, B. Ernst, *et al.* 2004. Beta-catenin is dispensable for hematopoiesis and lymphopoiesis. *J. Exp. Med.* **199:** 221–229.

30. Koch, U., A. Wilson, M. Cobas, *et al.* 2008. Simultaneous loss of beta- and gamma-catenin does not perturb hematopoiesis or lymphopoiesis. *Blood* **111:** 160–164.

31. Huelsken, J. & W. Held. 2009. Canonical Wnt signalling plays essential roles. *Eur. J. Immunol.* **39:** 3582–3583; author reply 3583–3584.

32. Brault, V., R. Moore, S. Kutsch, *et al.* 2001. Inactivation of the beta-catenin gene by Wnt1-Cre-mediated deletion results in dramatic brain malformation and failure of craniofacial development. *Development* **128:** 1253–1264.

33. Malhotra, S. & P.W. Kincade. 2009. Wnt-related molecules and signaling pathway equilibrium in hematopoiesis. *Cell Stem Cell.* **4:** 27–36.

34. Zhao, C., J. Blum, A. Chen, *et al.* 2007. Loss of beta-catenin impairs the renewal of normal and CML stem cells in vivo. *Cancer Cell.* **12:** 528–541.

35. Gounari, F., I. Aifantis, K. Khazaie, *et al.* 2001. Somatic activation of beta-catenin bypasses pre-TCR signaling and TCR selection in thymocyte development. *Nat. Immunol.* **2:** 863–869.

36. Xie, H., Z. Huang, M.S. Sadim & Z. Sun. 2005. Stabilized beta-catenin extends thymocyte survival by up-regulating Bcl-xL. *J. Immunol.* **175:** 7981–7988.

37. Yu, Q. & J.M. Sen. 2007. Beta-catenin regulates positive selection of thymocytes but not lineage commitment. *J. Immunol.* **178:** 5028–5034.

38. Kaech, S.M. & E.J. Wherry. 2007. Heterogeneity and cell-fate decisions in effector and memory CD8+ T cell differentiation during viral infection. *Immunity* **27:** 393–405.

39. Harty, J.T. & V.P. Badovinac. 2008. Shaping and reshaping CD8+ T-cell memory. *Nat. Rev. Immunol.* **8:** 107–119.

40. Williams, M.A. & M.J. Bevan. 2007. Effector and memory CTL differentiation. *Annu. Rev. Immunol.* **25:** 171–192.

41. Lefrancois, L. & A.L. Marzo. 2006. The descent of memory T-cell subsets. *Nat. Rev. Immunol.* **6:** 618–623.

42. Pulendran, B. & R. Ahmed. 2006. Translating innate immunity into immunological memory: implications for vaccine development. *Cell* **124:** 849–863.

43. Bannard, O., M. Kraman & D.T. Fearon. 2009. Secondary replicative function of CD8+ T cells that had developed an effector phenotype. *Science* **323:** 505–509.

44. Ahmed, R., M.J. Bevan, S.L. Reiner & D.T. Fearon. 2009. The precursors of memory: models and controversies. *Nat. Rev. Immunol.* **9:** 662–668.

45. Sarkar, S., V. Kalia, W.N. Haining, *et al.* 2008. Functional and genomic profiling of effector CD8 T cell subsets with distinct memory fates. *J. Exp. Med.* **205:** 625–640.

46. Joshi, N.S., W. Cui, A. Chandele, *et al.* 2007. Inflammation directs memory precursor and short-lived effector CD8(+) T cell fates via the graded expression of T-bet transcription factor. *Immunity* **27:** 281–295.

47. Haring, J.S., X. Jing, J. Bollenbacher-Reilley, *et al.* 2008. Constitutive expression of IL-7 receptor alpha does not support increased expansion or prevent contraction of antigen-specific CD4 or CD8 T cells following Listeria monocytogenes infection. *J. Immunol.* **180:** 2855–2862.

48. Hand, T.W., M. Morre & S.M. Kaech. 2007. Expression of IL-7 receptor alpha is necessary but not sufficient for the formation of memory CD8 T cells during viral infection. *Proc. Natl. Acad. Sci. USA* **104:** 11730–11735.

49. Grundemann, C., S. Schwartzkopff, M. Koschella, *et al.* 2010. The NK receptor KLRG1 is dispensable for virus-induced NK and CD8+ T-cell differentiation and function in vivo. *Eur. J. Immunol.* **40:** 1303–1314.

50. Zhao, D.M., S. Yu, X. Zhou, *et al.* 2010. Constitutive activation of Wnt signaling favors generation of memory CD8 T cells. *J. Immunol.* **184:** 1191–1199.

51. Willinger, T., T. Freeman, M. Herbert, *et al.* 2006. Human naive CD8 T cells down-regulate expression of the WNT pathway transcription factors lymphoid enhancer binding factor 1 and transcription factor 7 (T cell factor-1) following antigen encounter in vitro and in vivo. *J. Immunol.* **176:** 1439–1446.

52. Rutishauser, R.L., G.A. Martins, S. Kalachikov, *et al.* 2009. Transcriptional repressor Blimp-1 promotes CD8(+) T cell terminal differentiation and represses the acquisition of central memory T cell properties. *Immunity* **31:** 296–308.

53. Gattinoni, L., X.S. Zhong, D.C. Palmer, *et al.* 2009. Wnt signaling arrests effector T cell differentiation and generates CD8+ memory stem cells. *Nat. Med.* **15:** 808–813.

54. Driessens, G., Y. Zheng & T.F. Gajewski. 2010. Beta-catenin does not regulate memory T cell phenotype. *Nat. Med.* **16:** 513–514; author reply 514–515.

55. Prlic, M. & M.J. Bevan. 2011. Cutting Edge: {beta}-Catenin is dispensable for T cell effector differentiation, memory formation, and recall responses. *J. Immunol.* **187:** 1542–1546.

56. Driessens, G., Y. Zheng, F. Locke, *et al.* 2011. Beta-catenin inhibits T cell activation by selective interference with linker for activation of T cells-phospholipase C-gamma1 phosphorylation. *J. Immunol.* **186:** 784–790.

57. Pashine, A., N.M. Valiante & J.B. Ulmer. 2005. Targeting the innate immune response with improved vaccine adjuvants. *Nat. Med.* **11:** S63–S68.

58. Klebanoff, C.A., N. Acquavella, Z. Yu & N.P. Restifo. 2011. Therapeutic cancer vaccines: are we there yet? *Immunol. Rev.* **239:** 27–44.

59. Banerjee, A., S.M. Gordon, A.M. Intlekofer, *et al.* 2010. Cutting edge: the transcription factor eomesodermin enables CD8+ T cells to compete for the memory cell niche. *J. Immunol.* **185:** 4988–4992.

60. Jeannet, G., C. Boudousquie, N. Gardiol, *et al.* 2010. Essential role of the Wnt pathway effector Tcf-1 for the establishment of functional CD8 T cell memory. *Proc. Natl. Acad. Sci. USA* **107:** 9777–9782.

61. Zhou, X., S. Yu, D.M. Zhao, *et al.* 2010. Differentiation and persistence of memory CD8(+) T cells depend on T cell factor 1. *Immunity* **33:** 229–240.

62. Bianchi, T., S. Gasser, A. Trumpp & H.R. MacDonald. 2006. c-Myc acts downstream of IL-15 in the regulation of memory CD8 T-cell homeostasis. *Blood* **107:** 3992–3999.

63. Nishita, M., M.K. Hashimoto, S. Ogata, *et al.* 2000. Interaction between Wnt and TGF-beta signalling pathways during formation of Spemann's organizer. *Nature* **403:** 781–785.

64. Labbe, E., A. Letamendia & L. Attisano. 2000. Association of Smads with lymphoid enhancer binding factor 1/T cell-specific factor mediates cooperative signaling by the transforming growth factor-beta and wnt pathways. *Proc. Natl. Acad. Sci. USA* **97:** 8358–8363.

65. Zhu, J., H. Yamane & W.E. Paul. 2010. Differentiation of effector CD4 T cell populations (*). *Annu. Rev. Immunol.* **28:** 445–489.

66. Dong C. 2008. TH17 cells in development: an updated view of their molecular identity and genetic programming. *Nat. Rev. Immunol.* **8:** 337–348.

67. Josefowicz, S.Z. & A. Rudensky. 2009. Control of regulatory T cell lineage commitment and maintenance. *Immunity* **30:** 616–625.

68. Veldhoen, M., C. Uyttenhove, J. van Snick, *et al.* 2008. Transforming growth factor-beta 'reprograms' the differentiation of T helper 2 cells and promotes an interleukin 9-producing subset. *Nat. Immunol.* **9:** 1341–1346.

69. King, C., S.G. Tangye & C.R. Mackay. 2008. T follicular helper (TFH) cells in normal and dysregulated immune responses. *Annu. Rev. Immunol.* **26:** 741–766.

70. Zheng, W. & R.A. Flavell. 1997. The transcription factor GATA-3 is necessary and sufficient for Th2 cytokine gene expression in CD4 T cells. *Cell* **89:** 587–596.

71. Zhu, J., B. Min, J. Hu-Li, *et al.* 2004. Conditional deletion of Gata3 shows its essential function in T(H)1-T(H)2 responses. *Nat. Immunol.* **5:** 1157–1165.

72. Yamane, H., J. Zhu & W.E. Paul. 2005. Independent roles for IL-2 and GATA-3 in stimulating naive CD4+ T cells to generate a Th2-inducing cytokine environment. *J. Exp. Med.* **202:** 793–804.

73. Amsen, D., A. Antov, D. Jankovic, *et al.* 2007. Direct regulation of Gata3 expression determines the T helper differentiation potential of Notch. *Immunity* **27:** 89–99.

74. Fang, T.C., Y. Yashiro-Ohtani, C. Del Bianco, *et al.* 2007. Notch directly regulates Gata3 expression during T helper 2 cell differentiation. *Immunity* **27:** 100–110.

75. Yu, Q., A. Sharma, S.Y. Oh, *et al.* 2009. T cell factor 1 initiates the T helper type 2 fate by inducing the transcription factor GATA-3 and repressing interferon-gamma. *Nat. Immunol.* **10:** 992–999.

76. Notani, D., K.P. Gottimukkala, R.S. Jayani, *et al.* 2008. Global regulator SATB1 recruits beta-catenin and regulates T(H)2 differentiation in Wnt-dependent manner. *PLoS Biol.* **8:** e1000296.

77. Galande, S., P.K. Purbey, D. Notani & P.P. Kumar. 2007. The third dimension of gene regulation: organization of dynamic chromatin loopscape by SATB1. *Curr. Opin. Genet. Dev.* **17:** 408–414.

78. Cai, S., C.C. Lee & T. Kohwi-Shigematsu. 2006. SATB1 packages densely looped, transcriptionally active chromatin for coordinated expression of cytokine genes. *Nat. Genet.* **38:** 1278–1288.

79. Hebenstreit, D., M. Giaisi, M.K. Treiber, *et al.* 2008. LEF-1 negatively controls interleukin-4 expression through a proximal promoter regulatory element. *J. Biol. Chem.* **283:** 22,490–22,497.

80. Hossain, M.B., H. Hosokawa, A. Hasegawa, *et al.* 2008. Lymphoid enhancer factor interacts with GATA-3 and controls its function in T helper type 2 cells. *Immunology* **125:** 377–386.

81. Yu, Q., A. Sharma, A. Ghosh & J.M. Sen. 2011. T cell factor-1 negatively regulates expression of IL-17 family of cytokines and protects mice from experimental autoimmune encephalomyelitis. *J. Immunol.* **186:** 3946–3952.

82. Oestreich, K.J., A.C. Huang & A.S. Weinmann. 2011. The lineage-defining factors T-bet and Bcl-6 collaborate to regulate Th1 gene expression patterns. *J. Exp. Med.* **208:** 1001–1013.

83. Erlich, H.A., A.M. Valdes, C. Julier, *et al.* 2009. Evidence for association of the TCF7 locus with type I diabetes. *Genes Immun.* **10**(Suppl 1): S54–S59.

84. Barth, A.I., D.B. Stewart & W.J. Nelson. 1999. T cell factor-activated transcription is not sufficient to induce anchorage-independent growth of epithelial cells expressing mutant beta-catenin. *Proc. Natl. Acad. Sci. USA* **96:** 4947–4952.

85. Ding, Y., S. Shen, A.C. Lino, *et al.* 2008. Beta-catenin stabilization extends regulatory T cell survival and induces anergy in nonregulatory T cells. *Nat. Med.* **14:** 162–169.

86. Graham, J.A., M. Fray, S. de Haseth, *et al.* 2010. Suppressive regulatory T cell activity is potentiated by glycogen synthase kinase 3{beta} inhibition. *J. Biol. Chem.* **285:** 32852–32859.

87. Gordon, M.D., M.S. Dionne, D.S. Schneider & R. Nusse. 2005. WntD is a feedback inhibitor of Dorsal/NF-kappaB in Drosophila development and immunity. *Nature* **437:** 746–749.

88. Chaussabel, D., R.T. Semnani, M.A. McDowell, *et al.* 2003. Unique gene expression profiles of human macrophages and dendritic cells to phylogenetically distinct parasites. *Blood* **102:** 672–681.

89. Lehtonen, A., H. Ahlfors, V. Veckman, *et al.* 2007. Gene expression profiling during differentiation of human monocytes to macrophages or dendritic cells. *J. Leukoc. Biol.* **82:** 710–720.

90. Blumenthal, A., S. Ehlers, J. Lauber, *et al.* 2006. The Wingless homolog WNT5A and its receptor Frizzled-5 regulate inflammatory responses of human mononuclear cells induced by microbial stimulation. *Blood* **108:** 965–973.

91. He, X., J.P. Saint-Jeannet, Y. Wang, *et al.* 1997. A member of the Frizzled protein family mediating axis induction by Wnt-5A. *Science* **275:** 1652–1654.

92. Lobov, I.B., S. Rao, T.J. Carroll, *et al.* 2005. WNT7b mediates macrophage-induced programmed cell death in patterning of the vasculature. *Nature* **437:** 417–421.

93. Manicassamy, S., B. Reizis, R. Ravindran, *et al.* 2010. Activation of beta-catenin in dendritic cells regulates immunity versus tolerance in the intestine. *Science* **329:** 849–853.

94. Wu, B., S.P. Crampton & C.C. Hughes. 2007. Wnt signaling induces matrix metalloproteinase expression and regulates T cell transmigration. *Immunity* **26:** 227–239.

95. Tamura, M., M.M. Sato & M. Nashimoto. 2011. Regulation of CXCL12 expression by canonical Wnt signaling in bone marrow stromal cells. *Int. J. Biochem. Cell Biol.* **43:** 760–767.

96. Ghosh, M.C., G.D. Collins, B. Vandanmagsar, *et al.* 2009. Activation of Wnt5A signaling is required for CXC chemokine ligand 12-mediated T-cell migration. *Blood* **114:** 1366–1373.

97. Jiang, A., O. Bloom, S. Ono, *et al.* 2007. Disruption of E-cadherin-mediated adhesion induces a functionally distinct pathway of dendritic cell maturation. *Immunity* **27:** 610–624.

98. Zhou, J., P. Cheng, J.I. Youn, *et al.* 2009. Notch and wingless signaling cooperate in regulation of dendritic cell differentiation. *Immunity* **30:** 845–859.

99. Otero, K., I.R. Turnbull, P.L. Poliani, *et al.* 2009. Macrophage colony-stimulating factor induces the proliferation and survival of macrophages via a pathway involving DAP12 and beta-catenin. *Nat. Immunol.* **10:** 734–743.

100. Yang, P., H. An, X. Liu, *et al.* 2010. The cytosolic nucleic acid sensor LRRFIP1 mediates the production of type I interferon via a beta-catenin-dependent pathway. *Nat. Immunol.* **11:** 487–494.

101. Neumann, J., K. Schaale, K. Farhat, *et al.* 2010. Frizzled1 is a marker of inflammatory macrophages, and its ligand Wnt3a is involved in reprogramming Mycobacterium tuberculosis-infected macrophages. *FASEB J.* **24:** 4599–4612.

102. Pereira, C., D.J. Schaer, E.B. Bachli, *et al.* 2008. Wnt5A/CaMKII signaling contributes to the inflammatory response of macrophages and is a target for the antiinflammatory action of activated protein C and interleukin-10. *Arterioscler. Thromb. Vasc. Biol.* **28**: 504–510.

103. Schaale, K., J. Neumann, D. Schneider, *et al.* 2011. Wnt signaling in macrophages: augmenting and inhibiting mycobacteria-induced inflammatory responses. *Eur. J. Cell Biol.* **90**: 553–559.

104. Sen, M. & G. Ghosh. 2008. Transcriptional outcome of Wnt-Frizzled signal transduction in inflammation: evolving concepts. *J. Immunol.* **181**: 4441–4445.

105. Pereira, C.P., E.B. Bachli G. Schoedon. 2009. The wnt pathway: a macrophage effector molecule that triggers inflammation. *Curr. Atheroscler. Rep.* **11**: 236–242.

106. Xu, M., A. Sharma, D.L. Wiest & J.M. Sen. 2009. Pre-TCR-induced beta-catenin facilitates traversal through beta-selection. *J. Immunol.* **182**: 751–758.

107. Kovalovsky, D., Y. Yu, M. Dose, *et al.* 2009. Beta-catenin/Tcf determines the outcome of thymic selection in response to alphabetaTCR signaling. *J. Immunol.* **183**: 3873–3884.

108. Lovatt, M. & M.J. Bijlmakers. 2010. Stabilisation of beta-catenin downstream of T cell receptor signalling. *PLoS One.* **5**.

109. Diehn, M., A.A. Alizadeh, O.J. Rando, *et al.* 2002. Genomic expression programs and the integration of the CD28 costimulatory signal in T cell activation. *Proc. Natl. Acad. Sci. USA* **99**: 11796–11801.

110. Cross, D.A., D.R. Alessi, P. Cohen, *et al.* 1995. Inhibition of glycogen synthase kinase-3 by insulin mediated by protein kinase B. *Nature* **378**: 785–789.

111. He, X.C., T. Yin, J.C. Grindley, *et al.* 2007. PTEN-deficient intestinal stem cells initiate intestinal polyposis. *Nat. Genet.* **39**: 189–198.

112. Thornton, T.M., G. Pedraza-Alva, B. Deng, *et al.* 2008. Phosphorylation by p38 MAPK as an alternative pathway for GSK3beta inactivation. *Science* **320**: 667–670.

113. Wu, X., X. Tu, K.S. Joeng, *et al.* 2008. Rac1 activation controls nuclear localization of beta-catenin during canonical Wnt signaling. *Cell* **133**: 340–353.

114. Gwak, J., M. Cho, S.J. Gong, *et al.* 2006. Protein-kinase-C-mediated beta-catenin phosphorylation negatively reg- ulates the Wnt/beta-catenin pathway. *J. Cell Sci.* **119**: 4702–4709.

115. van Buul, J.D., E.C. Anthony, M. Fernandez-Borja, *et al.* 2005. Proline-rich tyrosine kinase 2 (Pyk2) mediates vascular endothelial-cadherin-based cell-cell adhesion by regulating beta-catenin tyrosine phosphorylation. *J. Biol. Chem.* **280**: 21129–21136.

116. Voskas, D., L.S. Ling & J.R. Woodgett. 2010. Does GSK-3 provide a shortcut for PI3K activation of Wnt signalling? *F1000 Biol Rep.* **2**: 82.

117. Li, M.O. & R.A. Flavell. 2008. TGF-beta: a master of all T cell trades. *Cell* **134**: 392–404.

118. Guo, X. & X.F. Wang. 2009. Signaling cross-talk between TGF-beta/BMP and other pathways. *Cell Res.* **19**: 71–88.

119. Hinrichs, C.S., R. Spolski, C.M. Paulos, *et al.* 2008. IL-2 and IL-21 confer opposing differentiation programs to CD8+ T cells for adoptive immunotherapy. *Blood* **111**: 5326–5333.

120. Paley, M.A. & E.J. Wherry. 2010. TCF-1 flips the switch on Eomes. *Immunity* **33**: 145–147.

121. Koehn, B.H. & S.P. Schoenberger. 2009. Tumor immunotherapy: making an immortal army. *Nat. Med.* **15**: 731–732.

122. Gattinoni, L., Y. Ji, N.P. Restifo. 2010. Wnt/beta-catenin signaling in T-cell immunity and cancer immunotherapy. *Clin. Cancer Res.* **16**: 4695–4701.

123. Bluestone, J.A. & M. Hebrok. 2008. Safer, longer-lasting regulatory T cells with beta-catenin. *Nat. Med.* **14**: 118–119.

124. Martinez A. 2008. Preclinical efficacy on GSK-3 inhibitors: towards a future generation of powerful drugs. *Med. Res. Rev.* **28**: 773–796.

125. De Sarno, P, R.C. Axtell, C. Raman, *et al.* 2008. Lithium prevents and ameliorates experimental autoimmune encephalomyelitis. *J. Immunol.* **181**: 338–345.

126. Bottomly, D., S.L. Kyler, S.K. McWeeney & G.S. Yochum. 2010. Identification of {beta}-catenin binding regions in colon cancer cells using ChIP-Seq. *Nucl. Acids Res.* **38**: 5735–5745.

127. Hatzis, P., L.G. van der Flier, M.A. van Driel, *et al.* 2008. Genome-wide pattern of TCF7L2/TCF4 chromatin occupancy in colorectal cancer cells. *Mol. Cell Biol.* **28**: 2732–2744.

Ann. N.Y. Acad. Sci. ISSN 0077-8923

# Development and function of interleukin 17–producing γδ T cells

Thomas Korn and Franziska Petermann

Klinikum rechts der Isar, Department of Neurology, Technical University Munich, Ismaninger, Munich, Germany

Address for correspondence: Thomas Korn, M.D., Klinikum rechts der Isar, Department of Neurology, Technical University Munich, Ismaninger Str. 22, 81675 Munich, Germany. korn@lrz.tum.de

Interleukin (IL) 17 is a phylogenetically ancient cytokine that has been adopted by the adaptive immune system, and the investigation of adaptive T helper (Th) 17 cells has substantially contributed to our understanding of the molecular requirements for the induction, regulation, and function of IL-17. However, IL-17 is in fact produced by a large variety of innate immune cells and exerts its most significant biological functions at the interface of the organism with its environment, such as, for example, at epithelial surfaces, where γδ T cells are a prominent source of IL-17. In this review, we will give an overview on the concepts of commitment of γδ T cells to effector phenotypes, focusing on IL-17–producing γδ T cells (γδT17 cells). The role of γδT17 cells in animal models of autoimmunity will be discussed as well as the prerequisites for the development of human γδT17 cells and their potential importance for human disease conditions.

Key words: γδ T cells; T cell lineage; interleukin17; experimental autoimmune encephalomyelitis

## Introduction

γδ T cells are lymphocytes whose T cell receptor is composed of a γ chain and a δ chain instead of α and β chains as in conventional T cells. γδ T cells rapidly respond to TCR signals but also to pattern recognition receptor signals by secretion of cytokines or cytotoxic activity. Their fast response dynamics and capacity to sense danger signals define their function as players of the innate immune system. However, γδ T cells also exhibit some degree of immunological memory formation, a classic feature of adaptive immune responses. Thus, γδ T cells are often considered to bridge innate and adaptive immune responses. Since there are at least four different classification systems for the designation of γ and δ chains, the literature is at times difficult to understand. Here, we refer to the nomenclature that has been coined by Heilig and Tonegawa.[1] We will discuss the biology of γδ T cells with a focus on the recently described IL-17–producing γδ T cells (γδT17 cells)[2,3] and highlight the conditions of their development and their potential role in inflamma-

tory responses in murine models of autoimmunity. In addition, we will review the literature on human γδT17 cells.

## γδ T cell development in the thymus

In the thymus, γδ T cells develop from CD4⁻CD8⁻, i.e., double negative (DN) thymocytes. The development of γδ thymocytes branches off at the transition of thymocytes from the DN3 to the DN4 stage.[4] Before that, in the DN2 and DN3 stages, the genes encoding for the TCR-β, TCR-γ, and TCR-δ chains are rearranged. Recombination of the *Tcrb* locus leads to the expression of a TCR-β chain, which associates with the invariant pre-TCR–α to form a pre-TCR. However, successful recombination of both the *Tcrd* and *Tcrg* locus will promote the assembly of a γδ TcR in DN thymocytes. Restricted pairing of distinct TCR-γ chains with TCR-δ chains, that is, partial allelic exclusion of some TCR-γ chains, suggests that the *Tcrd* locus might be open for active transcription prior to the *Tcrg* locus.[5] The temporal sequence of somatic rearrangement of the *Tcrd* and *Tcrg* locus,

doi: 10.1111/j.1749-6632.2011.06355.x

as well as its dependency on IL-7 signaling, have been studied in detail[6] (for review, see Ref. 7). Models of selective and instructive "decision making" in favor of the $\gamma\delta$ versus $\alpha\beta$ lineages have been proposed on the basis of either TCR signal strength or Notch signaling, respectively.[8] In this scenario, high signal strength through the $\gamma\delta$ TCR heterodimer in the absence of Notch signals prevents transition of a DN thymocyte to the $CD4^+CD8^+$ (double-positive, DP) state and induces commitment to the $\gamma\delta$ lineage, whereas low signal strength via the pre-TCR in the presence of strong Notch signaling promotes thymocyte transition from DN to DP and commitment to the $\alpha\beta$ lineage.[9,10] Upon initiation of TCR-$\alpha$ chain rearrangement in the DP stage, further expression of TCR-$\delta$ chains is prevented because the *Tcrd* locus is incorporated into the *Tcra* locus and is thus physically excised during *Tcra* rearrangement. However, in about 1% of DP thymocytes, rearrangement of the *Tcra* locus occurs monoallelically.[11] Therefore, it is possible that a small subset of thymocytes—in addition to their functional $\alpha\beta$ TCR—continue to express a TCR-$\delta$ chain (see also Ref. 12).

While $\alpha\beta$ TCR$^+$ DP cells continue to become single-positive (SP) CD4 or CD8 thymocytes and pass through MHC-restricted negative selection, it is a matter of debate whether commitment to the $\gamma\delta$ lineage also involves clonal deletion events based on TCR signal strength.[7,13,14] Ligand recognition by the $\gamma\delta$ TCR is not restricted by polymorph MHC molecules because neither $\beta2$ microglobulin-deficient nor MHC class II–deficient mice show defects in the generation or function of $\gamma\delta$ T cells.[15,16] Moreover, as positive selection in the embronic thymus can convert into "negative selection" of adult $\gamma\delta$ T cell precursor cells with the same $\gamma\delta$ TCR, it has been suggested that TCR-independent, ontogenetically regulated signals contribute to the thymic selection process of $\gamma\delta$ T cells.[17] $\gamma\delta$ thymocytes remain DN (CD4$^-$CD8$^-$) and exit the thymus as mature $\gamma\delta$ T cells. Even those $\gamma\delta$ T cells that have recently left the thymus express markers that are associated with antigen-experienced T cells. Thus, "naive" $\gamma\delta$ T cells may not exist. Yet, similar to T helper (Th) cell subsets, distinct functional phenotypes of $\gamma\delta$ T cells have recently been identified, and current observations suggest that the commitment of $\gamma\delta$ T cells to particular effector subsets occurs already in the thymus (Fig. 1).

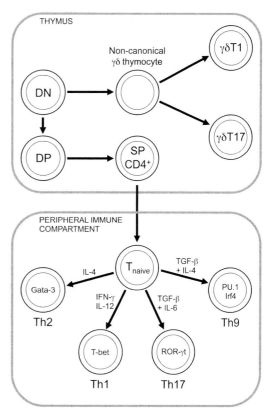

**Figure 1.** Commitment of $\gamma\delta$ T cells to cytokine phenotypes. The development of $\gamma\delta$ T cells in the thymus branches off from common thymocyte precursor cells at the DN 3 stage and the commitment of $\gamma\delta$ thymocytes to produce either IFN-$\gamma$ ($\gamma\delta$T1) or IL-17 ($\gamma\delta$T17) occurs in the thymus. In contrast, SP $\alpha\beta$ T cells that have passed negative selection leave the thymus as naive peripheral T cells. Naive T cells can then differentiate into T helper type 1 (Th1), Th2, Th17, or Th9 cells depending on the cytokine environment at the time of their encounter of cognate antigen in secondary lymphoid tissues. The transcription factors Gata3, T-bet, ROR-$\gamma$t or PU.1, and IRF4, are, among others, required for the induction of Th2, Th1, Th17, or Th9 cells, respectively.

## Functional subsets of T helper cells

Conventional $\alpha\beta$ T cells leave the thymus in a naive state and are committed to effector T cells with distinct functional phenotypes upon encounter of antigen in secondary lymphoid organs (Fig. 1). The commitment to a particular effector "lineage" is determined by the cytokine milieu that is present during the priming process of conventional T cells. For example, IFN-$\gamma$ and IL-12 induce naive T cells to develop into the Th1 lineage and the presence of IL-4 results in the commitment of naive T cells to

Th2 cells during antigen specific sensitization, while TGF-β plus IL-6 (or IL-21) are required to commit naive T cells to the Th17 lineage.[18] Th17 cells but not Th1 and Th2 cells express the IL-23 receptor (IL-23R), and the sensing of IL-23 stabilizes the production of IL-17 by Th17 cells and may confer additional pathogenic properties to this Th lineage that define their exquisite role in tissue inflammation and autoimmunity.[19] The functional phenotypes of conventional CD4$^+$ T cells have received major attention. First, on the molecular level, they are distinct, and commitment to one lineage can occur in the genetic absence of transcription factors required for another phenotype; and second, on the functional level, they orchestrate different types of inflammation that are appropriate for distinct types of pathogens in host defense. These modes of inflammation are also accompanied by different degrees of immunopathology and thus lead to distinct types of tissue damage during autoimmune reactions.[20] The biology of the effector Th cell subsets has been extensively analyzed in a series of experimental models for host defense, autoimmunity, chronic inflammation, and tumor immunity (for review, see Refs. 21–23).

## Functional subsets of γδ T cells

Noncanonical (conventional) γδ T cells do not express fixed TCR chains but have a broader TCR repertoire than canonical (niche-restricted) γδ T cells, and they home to secondary lymphoid tissues. We and others have observed that noncanonical γδ T cells participate in immune reactions distant from their original site of residence, and they traffic to sites of inflammation in solid organs in large numbers.[24–26] Thus, the question of self-renewal and homeostasis of γδ T cells in lymph nodes and the spleen needs to be determined. It is likely that there must be some replenishment of the lymph node pool of noncanonical γδ T cells by thymic emigrants throughout the life span of an individual.

Moreover, similar to CD4$^+$ T helper cells, subsets of γδ T cells can be defined based on distinct cytokine profiles. Indeed, IFN-γ–producing (γδT1) and IL-17–producing γδ T (γδT17) cells constitute distinct functional phenotypes of γδ T cells. The expression of NK1.1 and CD27 versus Scart-2 and CCR6 segregate with the commitment of γδ T cells to produce IFN-γ and IL-17, respectively.[3,27,28] More recently, constitutive expression of the IL-23R

has also been identified in a subset of noncanonical γδ T cells.[29] Like Scart-2$^+$ γδ T cells, IL-23R$^+$ γδ T cells exhibit a restricted γδ TCR repertoire that is strongly skewed toward the γ4 chain.[3,24] Thus, Scart-2$^+$CCR6$^+$γ4$^+$ γδ T cells—or γδT17 cells— have an almost complete overlap with IL-23R$^+$ γδ T cells in the peripheral lymph nodes.

γδT17 cells express some of the transcription factors that have been identified as master regulators of the Th17 transcriptional program, such as ROR-γt. ROR-γt, together with Sox13, drives the differentiation of γδ thymocytes toward an IL-17-producing phenotype (Fig. 2). It appears that the γδT17-associated transcriptional program must be actively suppressed by an Egr3, NFAT, NF-κB gene regulatory network in order to commit γδ thymocytes to T-bet expression and production of IFN-γ[30] (Fig. 2). In the adult thymus, this process requires the engagement of the γδ TCR (see below).

IFN-γ production has previously been regarded as the default phenotype of γδ T cells, because even under conditions of IL-4 exposure, splenic γδ T cells (enriched from *Tcrb*$^{-/-}$ mice) continue to express IL-12Rβ2,[31] which determines their tonic responsiveness to IL-12. This concept was developed when a strict dichotomic classification of T helper cells into Th1 and Th2 fostered the idea that γδ T cells might also be classified according to either production of IFN-γ (γδT1) or IL-4 (γδT2).[31–33]

In contrast to αβ T cells, which are primed upon antigen recognition in the peripheral immune compartment, the commitment of γδ T cells to functional subsets takes place in the thymus. In elegant experiments, it was recently suggested that thymic commitment of γδ T cells to an IFN-γ– or an IL-17–producing phenotype was based on whether or not the γδ TCR had been engaged during thymic development.[25] Ligand recognition through the TCR was not required for the thymic selection process *per se* but determined the cytokine phenotype of thymus-derived γδ T cells. γδ T cells that had encountered their cognate antigen in the thymus acquired the capacity to produce IFN-γ, while ligand-naive γδ T cells produced IL-17.[25] Given the observation that γδT17 cells may not require γδ TCR ligand-mediated selection in the thymus, it is currently not very well understood why γδT17 cells use a strongly restricted TCR-γ repertoire (Vγ4).[3,24,34]

Lymphotoxin (LT) signals in the thymus are likely to be permissive for the commitment of γδ T cells to the expression of T-bet and production of IFN-γ because the expression of CD27 segregates with IFN-γ production in γδ T cells, and CD27 induces the LTβ receptor.[28] By interaction with its ligand CD70 (expressed on DCs and thymic epithelial cells as well as on DP thymocytes), CD27 conveys an intrathymic cue that licenses CD27+ γδ T cells for production of IFN-γ (*trans*-conditioning). In contrast, CD27⁻ γδ thymocytes are induced to express ROR-γt and Runx-1, and represent the precursor pool for γδT17 cells.[28,35] However, the role of LT signaling in γδ T cells for thymic commitment to cytokine phenotypes remains controversial. While CD27, which is associated with IFN-γ production in γδ T cells, controls the expression of LTβ receptor, it has recently been reported that LTβ receptor expression on γδ T cells, and its downstream signaling via the NF-κB family member RelB (noncanonical NF-κB pathway), is required for the expression of ROR-γt and ROR-α4, and for the production of IL-17, but not IFN-γ, in γδ T cells.[36]

Another pathway implicated in the thymic development and peripheral maintenance of γδT17 cells is the Notch/Hes1 pathway. CD27⁻IL-17+ γδ thymocytes selectively express Hes1, and IL-17+ γδ thymocytes were virtually absent in fetal thymi of Hes1-deficient mice.[35] In the same study, Shibata *et al.* refute the idea that Stat3 is required for the initial commitment of γδ thymocytes to γδT17 cells because—similar to IL-6–deficient mice[2]—*Tie2-Cre x Stat3^flox/flox* mice that lack expression of Stat3 in endothelial cells and hematopoietic cells failed to show reduced numbers of γδT17 cells in the thymus.[35] Stat3 appears to be required for the extrathymic expansion of γδT17 cells because the fraction of γδT17 cells in the peripheral immune compartment is reduced in mice that lack IL-6 and IL-23R, which signal through Stat3.[24] Finally, γδT17 cell precursors might also have to respond to TGF-β for their lineage commitment in the thymus, since *Tgfb⁻/⁻* mice and *Smad3⁻/⁻* mice harbor strongly reduced numbers of IL-17+ γδ thymocytes.[37] Taken together, the development of functionally distinct noncanonical γδ T cell subsets, as defined by "master transcription factors" and distinct cytokine profiles, is initiated as early as in the embryonic thymus, reaches a steady state around embryonic day 18, and continues postnatally.

Once exported into the peripheral immune compartment, γδT17 cells further expand upon encounter of specific γδ TCR ligands or cytokine signals such as IL-6 and IL-23.[24] IL-2 has also been proposed to be necessary for the maintenance of γδT17 cells in the peripheral immune

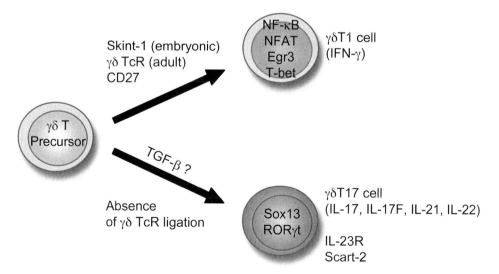

**Figure 2.** Molecular cues that determine the commitment of γδ T cells to distinct transcriptional programs. It is believed that a γδ thymocyte stably expresses CD27 and differentiates into an IFN-γ–producing γδ T1 cell when either its γδ TCR is engaged or when the γδ thymocyte senses the expression of Skint-1 on thymic epithelial cells. In the absence of γδ TCR ligation and probably upon sensing of TGF-β, a γδ thymocyte is committed to a transcriptional program that results in the production of IL-17 driven by ROR-γt (γδT17 cells). It appears that the expression of ROR-γt and Sox13 is actively suppressed by NF-κB, NFAT, and Egr3 that promote the expression of T-bet in γδ T1 cells.

compartment and specific niches because γδT17 cells (but not IFN-γ–producing γδ T cells) express the high affinity IL-2 receptor CD25; in addition, the peripheral γδ T cell compartment of $Il2^{-/-}$ mice, as well as of $Cd25^{-/-}$ mice, is selectively depleted of γδT17 cells.[38] Although IL-2 inhibits the development of Th17 cells,[39] its role in γδT17 cell development might be different because γδT17 cells are already firmly committed to their transcriptional program upon exit of the thymus. IL-21, which—like IL-2—signals through a receptor that uses the common γ chain of cytokine receptors, might also be required for the maintenance and functional modulation of γδT17 cells in the peripheral immune compartment.[40]

In summary, commitment of γδ T cells to functional subsets occurs in the thymus. It will now be important to understand how the interaction of TCR signaling and TCR-independent cues of the thymic environment are integrated on the molecular level to result in the initiation of distinct transcriptional programs and cytokine phenotypes in γδ thymocytes.

## Canonical γδ T cells

Canonical γδ T cells are exported from the thymus during embryonic development (but no longer during adulthood) and populate specific niches of the organism, such as the epidermal layer of the skin (dendritic epidermal T cells, DETC) and the mucosal surfaces of the urogenital tract and intestine (IEL). Most data suggest that for thymic selection of canonical γδ T cells—at least for DETC—TCR-mediated ligand recognition is required.[41] Canonical γδ T cells are characterized by restricted TCR Vγ usage. For example, γδ T cells that home to the epidermis (DETC) express Vγ5; γδ T cells that reside in the reproductive tract and the tongue express Vγ6; and IEL of the intestine are Vγ7 positive.[7]

Because canonical γδ T cells are generated by the embryonic but not the adult thymus, and because within their peripheral niche γδ T cells respond vigorously to environmental stimuli and are not constantly replenished, the hypothesis of extrathymic development of some canonical γδ T cells has been raised. For example, it is possible that in the small intestine extrathymic development of γδ T cells takes place in cryptopatches.[42]

Although DETC likely have experienced a TCR signal during selection in the thymus, this is less clear for intestinal IELs and lamina propria γδ T cells. Based on studies in TCR signaling–deficient mice ($Itk^{-/-}$) or TCR ligand–deficient mice with transgenic γδ TCRs ($b2m^{-/-} \times$ T10 or T22), the hypothesis was raised that sensing of a TCR signal by γδ thymocytes not only leads to their positive selection but also endows them with expression of S1P1, chemokine receptors (CCR10 and CCR4), and E/P selectins that direct the γδ thymocytes to the epidermal compartment of the skin.[43,44] In contrast, intestinal IEL or γδ T cells residing in the lamina propria of the intestine express CCR9.[45,46] Notably, DETC and intestinal IELs are IFN-γ producers, while a large fraction of lamina propria γδ T cells secrete IL-17.[29,47–49]

These findings support the idea that γδ T cells are committed to a distinct cytokine phenotype based on whether or not their γδ TCR has been "triggered" during thymic development. Because DETC are positively selected in the thymus, then, are they committed to production of IFN-γ?

In early studies, murine DETC were indeed shown to fail to survive in an IL-4–enriched environment and to produce IFN-γ but not IL-4 directly *ex vivo* upon mitogenic stimulation;[50,51] IL-2, IL-3, GM-CSF, and TNF-α are expressed by DETC after stimulation.[52] *In vitro*, DETC respond by cytokine production to constituents of Gram-negative but not Gram-positive bacteria.[53] More recently, the commitment of Vγ5+Vδ1+ γδ T cells (DETC) to the production of IFN-γ in the embryonic thymus was found to be induced by Skint-1, a ligand expressed on thymic epithelial cells.[30] In view of these data, it has been surprising that in an *in vivo* model of skin infection with *S. aureus*, TCR Vγ5+ T cells (and thus presumably DETC) produced IL-17 in response to TLR2, IL-1, and IL-23 stimuli. DETC-derived IL-17 was essential for host defense in this model, as IL-17R–deficient and TCR-δ–deficient mice, but not $Tcrb^{-/-}$ mice, developed exaggerated disease.[54] These data suggested that DETC were able to adopt a γδT17 phenotype and were not restricted to IFN-γ responses. However, this is a controversial idea, and it remains to be determined whether the detection of IL-17 production in DETCs is due to plasticity of TCR Vγ5+ γδ T cells that have previously been committed to the production of IFN-γ or whether it results from the presence of a heterogeneous population of γδ T cells in the experimental preparation of the epidermal compartment.[55] In fact, the purity of DETC preparations is always an issue, and contamination of DETCs by dermal γδ T cells that produce IL-17 must be excluded. Interestingly, although IL-22 is clearly produced by conventional γδ T cells in response to IL-23 (see below), IL-22 production was not observed by skin-resident TCR Vγ5[+] DETC, and this might provide a means to resolve the question of plasticity versus heterogeneity of niche-restricted γδ T cell pools.[56]

## γδ T cell responses in the peripheral lymphoid compartment

In the secondary lymphoid organs, γδ T cells comprise about 1–2% of all CD3[+] T cells, and about 10% of the γδ T cells express the IL-23R in wild-type mice. Upon activation, γδ T cells deploy immediate effector functions. In mice, several γδ TCR specificities have been described, including low affinity recognition of MHC class II epitopes (I-E) (clone LBK5[57]), nonclassical MHC class I epitopes (the class IB molecules T10 and T22) (clones G8 and KN6[58,59]), the Herpes simplex virus glycoprotein I (clone TgI4.4), and antigens derived from purified protein derivative from *Mycobacterium tuberculosis*.[60] In contrast to DETCs, conventional γδ T cells in secondary lymphoid organs express CD28, and it is likely that in addition to a TCR stimulus they have to sense a costimulatory signal for optimum activation. However, in contrast to naive αβ T cells, γδ T cells seem to also be able to respond to cytokine signals and either TLR or dectin stimuli in the absence of TCR ligation. In fact, a subset of peripheral γδ T cells expresses TLR1, TLR2, and dectin-1 (but not TLR4) and responds to Pam$_3$CSK$_4$ (TLR1 and 2 ligand) and curdlan (TLR2 and dectin-1 ligand) with production of IL-17.[34] It should be pointed out, however, that Ribot *et al.* suggested that the IL-17 response to TLR ligands of CD27[−] γδ T cells was indirect via TLR-mediated induction of IL-1β and IL-23 and not a direct effect of sensing TLR ligands by γδ T cells.[61] IL-23 and IL-1β—and IL-18 in part via induction of IL-1β—enhance production of IL-17 from purified γδ T cells in the absence of TCR stimuli.[26,62] Although IL-18 has been shown to facilitate and enhance the secretion of IFN-γ in antigen experienced/committed Th1 cells, IL-18 promotes expression of IL-17, rather than IFN-γ, by γδ T cells. One way of interpreting these data

would be that γδ T cells that have been committed to the production of IL-17 in the thymus are more susceptible to cytokine signals that converge on the MyD88 pathway than are IFN-γ–producing γδT1 cells. Notably, MyD88 deficiency severely affects IL-17 responses by γδ T cells, but spares IFN-γ responses.[61] Instead, a productive IFN-γ response by γδ T cells requires triggering of the γδ TCR and CD27 activation, in a malaria infection model.[61] These data suggest that the dichotomous conditions for thymic generation of IL-17[+] and IFN-γ[+] γδ T cells translate into a differential requirement for optimum activation of these distinct γδ T cell subsets in the peripheral immune compartment.

Similar to Th17 cells, γδT17 cells express ROR-γt, IL-23R, and the arylhydrocarbon receptor (Ahr) in secondary lymphoid organs.[34,63,64] Expression of Ahr by γδ T cells has been suggested to be absolutely required for IL-23–driven expression of IL-22 in γδT17 cells, as *Ahr*[−/−] γδT17 cells continue to express IL-17 but fail to produce IL-22.[34] Expression and activation of the Ahr system is also necessary for the expression of IL-22 in γδ T cells, in a model of *Bacillus subtilis*–induced pneumonitis.[65] Because DETCs do not secrete IL-22 in various cutaneous infection models, it has been surprising that DETCs are still found to express Ahr. However, GM-CSF, which is produced by DETCs, and c-kit, which is required for the homeostatic proliferation of DETCs, are targets of Ahr in DETCs.[66] Thus, Ahr may have different functions in secondary lymphoid organ γδ T cells, compared with DETCs. The specific relevance of Ahr with regard to the induction of IL-22 remains to be determined.

## γδ T cells in induced models of autoimmunity

In certain instances, γδ T cell responses are essential and nonredundant, such as in host defense at epithelial surfaces. For example, the early control of infection with *Nocardia* and *Listeria* most likely involves direct effector functions of γδ T cells.[67–69] However, due to their proposed antigen specificity for "altered self" (see below) and, more recently, to the observation that γδ T cells are a major source of IL-17, γδ T cells have been assumed to play a role in autoimmunity as well. Indeed, in early studies, γδ T cells were detected in multiple sclerosis (MS) lesions and appeared clonally expanded based on restricted usage of TCR variable chain segment Vγ9 (see Ref.

70). Furthermore, the fraction of γδ T cells in circulating blood, most of which are Vγ9 positive,[71] is a predictor of disease activity in MS patients, as measured by magnetic resonance imaging.[72]

The role of conventional γδ T cells has been tested in a variety of models of induced autoimmunity. The method of induction of experimental autoimmune encephalomyelitis (EAE), a model for human MS, and of collagen-induced arthritis (CIA), a model for human rheumatoid arthritis, by immunization with an autoantigen emulsified in complete Freund's adjuvant (CFA, which contains *Mycobacterium* extract), leads not only to the priming of autoantigen-specific adaptive T helper cell responses but also activates γδ T cells at the site of antigen injection[73] and in the draining lymph nodes.[24] The majority of studies identified a disease-promoting effect of γδ T cells in EAE [74–76] and CIA.[77,78] However, some studies are difficult to interpret because the conclusions are uniquely based on the application of "depleting" anti-γδ T cell antibodies,[79–81] of which all available clones (for example, GL-3 or UC7-13D5) are directed against the γδ TCR. With the help of Tcrd-H2b-eGFP.KI reporter mice, in which γδ T cells can be tracked due to GFP expression, it has recently been shown that the monoclonal antibodies that were used to deplete γδ T cells are actually functionally depleting, blocking, or even activating, rather than physically depleting *in vivo*.[82]

Upon immunization with myelin oligodendrocyte glycoprotein (MOG) peptide in CFA, γδ T cells expand in the secondary lymphoid tissue and migrate to the central nervous system (CNS) in a β2 integrin–independent manner. The largest accumulation of γδ T cells in the CNS is observed shortly before the peak of clinical signs of disease,[24,73] followed by their rapid contraction. IFN-γ and TNF-α were believed to be γδ T cell–derived cytokines required to promote local immunopathology in the CNS during EAE.[73] However, other mechanisms of action of γδ T cells have been suggested in models of induced autoimmunity, including presentation of antigen to CD4+ T helper cells in an MHC class II-restricted manner,[83] activation of third-party antigen presenting cells in the peripheral immune compartment,[76] and Fas ligand-mediated killing of target cells, including encephalitogenic T cells in the CNS.[84]

γδ T17 cells were first described in a model of lung infection with *M. tuberculosis*.[85] It took three

more years to establish a connection between the presence of γδT17 cells in the CNS and the disease mechanism in MOG$_{35-55}$/CFA-induced EAE.[24,26] At the onset of disease, the majority of γδ T cells that can be found in the CNS parenchyma express the TCR-γ4 chain, are IL-23R-positive, and secrete IL-17,[24] whereas IL-23R+ γδ T cells are outnumbered by IL-23R− γδ T cells in the peripheral immune compartment.

Since we have observed that IL-12 and IL-23 expand IL-23R− and IL-23R+ γδ T cells, respectively, we proposed that in the CNS γδ T cells must "sense" IL-23 during the development of EAE. However, the role of IL-23 for the biology of γδ T cells during an inflammatory response *in vivo* has not yet been entirely clarified. Using a fate tracking system based on IL-17A–Cre-mediated labeling of historic IL-17 producers, Stockinger *et al.* have reported that about half of Th17 cells, and still about 5–10% of historic γδT17 cells, express IFN-γ in the CNS parenchyma.[86] Although the expression of IL-17 and IFN-γ is clearly more distinct in γδ T cells than in Th17 cells, i.e., there are few double producers in the γδ T cell compartment, it is possible that IL-23 has other functions besides stabilizing the secretion of IL-17 in γδ T cells.

Thus far, the role of IL-23 for γδ T cell–mediated effects *in vivo* has only been discussed in terms of inducing Th17-associated cytokines (IL-17, IL-17F, IL-21, and IL-22) in γδ T cells, which might license APCs to activate αβ T cells.[26] Yet, although we did not observe a priming defect of encephalitogenic αβ T cells in *Tcrd*$^{−/−}$ mice, we identified enhanced regulatory T cell (T$_{reg}$ cell) responses in the absence of γδ T cells. IL-23 responsive γδ T cells are particularly suited to suppress the development and function of Foxp3+ T$_{reg}$ cells.[24] IL-23 has no direct effect on T$_{reg}$ cells that do not express the IL-23R. Thus, via activation of γδ T cells, IL-23 can promote adaptive effector T cell responses by inhibiting T$_{reg}$ cell responses in an indirect manner. Although the mechanism of how γδ T cells are armed by IL-23 to suppress the conversion of conventional αβ T cells into Foxp3+ T$_{reg}$ cells remains to be elucidated on the molecular level, it appears that IL-23R+ γδ T cells secrete soluble mediators (other than IL-17, IL-21, or IL-22) that prevent the development of induced T$_{reg}$ cells during an adaptive immune response. Subsequently, the basis for the attenuated EAE phenotype in *Tcrd*$^{−/−}$ mice is an exaggerated

$T_{reg}$ cell response, which is consistent with the finding that the antigen-specific priming of T helper cells isolated from $Tcrd^{-/-}$ mice is not impaired in an αβ effector T cell intrinsic manner.

Overall, the data obtained from experimental models of induced autoimmunity support the idea that γδ T cells—in a niche-restricted way—accelerate and enhance the response of tissue antigen-specific T helper cells. The function of γδ T cells might be particularly relevant at epithelial surfaces and, perhaps, in neuroectodermal tissue. The concept of lymphoid stress surveillance response by γδ T cells has recently been discussed in more detail.[87]

## Human γδ T cells in inflammatory disorders

The laboratories of Adrian Hayday and James Allison discovered that human IELs ($V_\gamma 1V_\delta 1$) respond to MHC class I chain–related (MIC) antigens A and B and heat shock proteins that are expressed by epithelial cells as a stress response.[88] MICA is recognized by the $V_\gamma 1V_\delta 1$ TCR and by NKG2D, an activating receptor that is expressed on human γδ T cells. Because mice do not express MICA, the biological significance of MICA recognition—as potential "altered self recognition"—has not been tested *in vivo*. Unfortunately, the known specificities of human systemic γδ T cells and IELs also differ fundamentally from the γδ TCR specificities that have been described in mice. Systemic human γδ T cells recognize mostly small nonpeptidic molecules; $V_\gamma 2V_\delta 2$ cells are highly reactive against isopentenyl pyrophosphate (IPP). Besides phosphoantigen, alkyl amines activate $V_\gamma 9V_\delta 2$ cells, the best characterized γδ T cell subset in human peripheral blood.[89] Phosphoantigens and alkyl amines also might be natural ligands because they are catabolites of plant compounds and exist as constituents of bacteria such as *Mycobacteria*, *Listeria*, and *Borrelia*, as well as fungi and parasites. Although like in murine γδ T cells, antigen recognition by human γδ T cells is not MHC-restricted: indeed, antigens need to be fixed on surfaces in order to be recognized by γδ T cells. However, the functional relevance of antigens *in vivo* is not very well understood because of lack of knowledge regarding their mode of antigen presentation to γδ T cells. In addition, a meaningful animal model likely cannot be produced because

many human γδ TCR reactivities do not exist in mice.

A promising approach to understanding the role of γδ T cells in human conditions emerged with the concept that γδ T cells—irrespective of their specificity—might play distinct roles defined by their functional phenotype, i.e., as a result of their tissue localization and cytokine profile. For example, it is likely that similar to the situation in mice, human γδ T cells participate in lymphoid stress surveillance responses. The majority of circulating γδ T cells in humans are $V_\gamma 9_\delta 2$ and 80% of them are IFN-γ producers, while less than 1% produce IL-17.[90] Notably, on the population level, IL-17 production can be induced in human $V_\gamma 9_\delta 2$ cells upon IPP activation in the presence of a cocktail of cytokines comprising TGF-β, IL-1β, IL-6, and IL-23, followed by a week of culture in differentiation medium supplemented in IL-2. In this protocol, the presence of IL-6 in the differentiation culture made the most difference in enhancing the fraction of γδT17 cells,[91] a result that has also been found for cord blood γδ T cells.[90] The potency of TGF-β plus IL-6 in inducing IL-17 production from purified murine γδ T cells is certainly much reduced compared with the human situation and with naive αβ T cells, for which TGF-β plus IL-6 are the classic Th17 differentiation factors.[24,92,93] It is unclear whether, akin to murine γδ T cells, commitment of human γδ T cells to distinct cytokine phenotypes takes place in the thymus, with limited plasticity in the peripheral immune compartment, or whether human γδ T cells can adopt *de novo* transcriptional programs or be "reprogrammed" in the periphery. Interestingly, in contrast to healthy individuals, up to 30% of *M. tuberculosis*–reactive $V_\delta 2$ γδ T cells and 40% of *Candida albicans*–reactive $V_\delta 1$ γδ T cells were found to be double positive for both IFN-γ and IL-17 in HIV patients.[94] IFN-γ/IL-17 double-producing cells expressed both ROR-γt and T-bet and were positive for CD161, CCR7, CCR4, and CCR6.[94] In patients with pulmonary tuberculosis, peripheral blood γδ T cells contained 20% IL-17 producers, although in this Chinese study the healthy control cohort also harbored an unusually high number (∼8%) of IL-17+ γδ T cells.[95] In children with bacterial meningitis, up to two-thirds of peripheral blood $V_\gamma 9_\delta 2$ γδ T cells and 80% of cerebrospinal fluid $V_\gamma 9_\delta 2$ γδ T cells were IL-17 producers.[91] In this study, human $V_\gamma 9_\delta 2$ γδT17 cells expressed IL-17, but neither IL-22 nor IFN-γ. Similar to murine γδT17 cells, human γδT17 cells are also positive for CCR6, granzyme B, TRAIL, and FasL. A specific marker, restricted to human cells, that is strongly associated with IL-17 production appears to be CD161, which is expressed by human γδT17 cells and by IL-17–producing NK cells, CD8[+], and CD4[+] αβ T cells.[96–98]

The functional relevance of γδT17 cells in humans has not been proven, although it is likely that by secretion of IL-17 at sites of inflammation (perhaps primarily at epithelial surfaces), γδT17 cells directly shape the inflammatory infiltrate, for example, by attracting neutrophils. It is possible that other γδT17-associated mediators like IL-22, which is secreted by $V_\gamma 2_\delta 2$ γδ T cells, also participate in promoting epithelial barrier functions and tissue repair.[90] However, cellular functions of γδ T cells like professional antigen presentation[99] or cytotoxicity[100] have not yet been formally investigated for human γδT17 cells.

## Concluding remarks

Despite marked differences in the TCR specificities of murine and human γδ T cells, the frequencies of effector phenotypes of γδ T cells, namely IFN-γ–producing and IL-17–producing γδ T cells in the circulating blood and various lymphoid compartments as well as their transcription factor profile appear to be strikingly similar. Thus, interventional strategies to study the function of these γδ T cell subsets in mice are likely to be relevant for the understanding of human disease conditions where prominent fractions of γδT17 cells are detected, such as, for example, juvenile rheumatoid arthritis, bacterial meningitis, Lyme disease, *M. tuberculosis* infection, and HIV infection. Moreover, by comparing the transcriptional machinery and regulation of IL-17 in innate and adaptive immune cells, we might be able to learn why it appeared evolutionarily wise for the phylogenetically modern system of adaptive immunity to usurp the ancient IL-17 as an effector cytokine and, conversely, what mechanisms have to fail in order for adaptive Th17 cells to induce severe autoimmunity and chronic inflammation.

## Acknowledgments

We would like to thank Dr. Immo Prinz for fruitful discussions. TK is supported by the DFG (KO 2964/3-1, 4-1, 5-1) and by the Gemeinnützige Hertie-Stiftung (1.01.1/10/010).

## Conflicts of interest

The authors declare no conflicts of interest.

## References

1. Heilig, J.S. & S. Tonegawa. 1986. Diversity of murine gamma genes and expression in fetal and adult T lymphocytes. *Nature* **322:** 836–840.
2. Lochner, M. *et al.* 2008. In vivo equilibrium of proinflammatory IL-17+ and regulatory IL-10+ Foxp3+ RORgamma t+ T cells. *J. Exp. Med.* **205:** 1381–1393.
3. Kisielow, J., M. Kopf & K. Karjalainen. 2008. SCART scavenger receptors identify a novel subset of adult gammadelta T cells. *J. Immunol.* **181:** 1710–1716.
4. Prinz, I. *et al.* 2006. Visualization of the earliest steps of gammadelta T cell development in the adult thymus. *Nat. Immunol.* **7:** 995–1003.
5. Bouconter, L. *et al.* 2005. Mechanisms controlling termination of V-J recombination at the TCRgamma locus: implications for allelic and isotypic exclusion of TCRgamma chains. *J. Immunol.* **174:** 3912–3919.
6. Dik, W.A. *et al.* 2005. New insights on human T cell development by quantitative T cell receptor gene rearrangement studies and gene expression profiling. *J. Exp Med.* **201:** 1715–1723.
7. Hayday, A.C. & D.J. Pennington. 2007. Key factors in the organized chaos of early T cell development. *Nat. Immunol.* **8:** 137–144.
8. Washburn, T. *et al.* 1997. Notch activity influences the alphabeta versus gammadelta T cell lineage decision. *Cell* **88:** 833–843.
9. Haks, M. C. *et al.* 2005. Attenuation of gammadeltaTCR signaling efficiently diverts thymocytes to the alphabeta lineage. *Immunity* **22:** 595–606.
10. Hayes, S.M., L. Li & P.E. Love. 2005. TCR signal strength influences alphabeta/gammadelta lineage fate. *Immunity* **22:** 583–593.
11. Davodeau, F. *et al.* 2001. The tight interallelic positional coincidence that distinguishes T-cell receptor Jalpha usage does not result from homologous chromosomal pairing during ValphaJalpha rearrangement. *EMBO J.* **20:** 4717–4729.
12. Terrence, K. *et al.* 2000. Premature expression of T cell receptor (TCR)alphabeta suppresses TCRgammadelta gene rearrangement but permits development of gammadelta lineage T cells. *J. Exp. Med.* **192:** 537–548.
13. Schweighoffer, E. & B.J. Fowlkes. 1996. Positive selection is not required for thymic maturation of transgenic gamma delta T cells. *J. Exp. Med.* **183:** 2033–2041.
14. Pennington, D.J., B. Silva-Santos & A.C. Hayday. 2005. Gammadelta T cell development—having the strength to get there. *Curr. Opin. Immunol.* **17:** 108–115.
15. Correa, I. *et al.* 1992. Most gamma delta T cells develop normally in beta 2-microglobulin-deficient mice. *Proc. Natl. Acad. Sci. USA* **89:** 653–657.
16. Bigby, M. *et al.* 1993. Most gamma delta T cells develop normally in the absence of MHC class II molecules. *J. Immunol.* **151:** 4465–4475.

17. Jin, Y. *et al*. 2010. Cutting edge: intrinsic programming of thymic gammadelta T cells for specific peripheral tissue localization. *J. Immunol*. **185:** 7156–7160.

18. Korn, T. *et al*. 2007. Th17 cells: effector T cells with inflammatory properties. *Semin. Immunol*. **19:** 362–371.

19. Kastelein, R.A., C.A. Hunter & D.J. Cua. 2007. Discovery and biology of IL-23 and IL-27: related but functionally distinct regulators of inflammation. *Annu. Rev. Immunol*. **25:** 221–242.

20. Petermann, F. & T. Korn. 2011. Cytokines and effector T cell subsets causing autoimmune CNS disease. *FEBS Lett*. **585:** 3747–3757.

21. Murphy, K.M. & S.L. Reiner. 2002. The lineage decisions of helper T cells. *Nat. Rev. Immunol*. **2:** 933–944.

22. Weaver, C.T. *et al*. 2006. Th17: an effector CD4 T cell lineage with regulatory T cell ties. *Immunity* **24:** 677–688.

23. Korn, T. *et al*. 2009. IL-17 and Th17 Cells. *Annu. Rev. Immunol*. **27:** 485–517.

24. Petermann, F. *et al*. 2010. Gammadelta T cells enhance autoimmunity by restraining regulatory T cell responses via an interleukin-23-dependent mechanism. *Immunity* **33:** 351–363.

25. Jensen, K.D. *et al*. 2008. Thymic selection determines gammadelta T cell effector fate: antigen-naive cells make interleukin-17 and antigen-experienced cells make interferon gamma. *Immunity* **29:** 90–100.

26. Sutton, C.E. *et al*. 2009. Interleukin-1 and IL-23 induce innate IL-17 production from gammadelta T cells, amplifying Th17 responses and autoimmunity. *Immunity* **31:** 331–341.

27. Haas, J.D. *et al*. 2009. CCR6 and NK1.1 distinguish between IL-17A and IFN-gamma-producing gammadelta effector T cells. *Eur. J. Immunol*. **39:** 3488–3497.

28. Ribot, J.C. *et al*. 2009. CD27 is a thymic determinant of the balance between interferon-gamma- and interleukin 17-producing gammadelta T cell subsets. *Nat. Immunol*. **10:** 427–436.

29. Awasthi, A. *et al*. 2009. Cutting edge: IL-23 receptor gfp reporter mice reveal distinct populations of IL-17-producing cells. *J. Immunol*. **182:** 5904–5908.

30. Turchinovich, G. & A.C. Hayday. 2011. Skint-1 identifies a common molecular mechanism for the development of interferon-gamma-secreting versus interleukin-17-secreting gammadelta T cells. *Immunity* **35:** 59–68.

31. Yin, Z. *et al*. 2000. Dominance of IL-12 over IL-4 in gamma delta T cell differentiation leads to default production of IFN-gamma: failure to down-regulate IL-12 receptor beta 2-chain expression. *J. Immunol*. **164:** 3056–3064.

32. Zuany-Amorim, C. *et al*. 1998. Requirement for gammadelta T cells in allergic airway inflammation. *Science* **280:** 1265–1267.

33. Yin, Z. & J. Craft. 2000. Gamma delta T cells in autoimmunity. *Springer Semin. Immunopathol*. **22:** 311–320.

34. Martin, B. *et al*. 2009. Interleukin-17-producing gammadelta T cells selectively expand in response to pathogen products and environmental signals. *Immunity* **31:** 321–330.

35. Shibata, K. *et al*. 2011. Notch-Hes1 pathway is required for the development of IL-17-producing gammadelta T cells. *Blood* **118:** 586–593.

36. Powolny-Budnicka, I. *et al*. 2011. RelA and RelB transcription factors in distinct thymocyte populations control lymphotoxin-dependent interleukin-17 production in gammadelta T cells. *Immunity* **34:** 364–374.

37. Do, J.S. *et al*. 2010. Cutting edge: spontaneous development of IL-17-producing gamma delta T cells in the thymus occurs via a TGF-beta 1-dependent mechanism. *J. Immunol*. **184:** 1675–1679.

38. Shibata, K. *et al*. 2008. Identification of CD25+ gamma delta T cells as fetal thymus-derived naturally occurring IL-17 producers. *J. Immunol*. **181:** 5940–5947.

39. Laurence, A. *et al*. 2007. Interleukin-2 signaling via STAT5 constrains T helper 17 cell generation. *Immunity* **26:** 371–381.

40. Nurieva, R. *et al*. 2007. Essential autocrine regulation by IL-21 in the generation of inflammatory T cells. *Nature* **448:** 480–483.

41. Lewis, J.M. *et al*. 2006. Selection of the cutaneous intraepithelial gammadelta+ T cell repertoire by a thymic stromal determinant. *Nat. Immunol*. **7:** 843–850.

42. Ishikawa, H. *et al*. 2007. Curriculum vitae of intestinal intraepithelial T cells: their developmental and behavioral characteristics. *Immunol. Rev*. **215:** 154–165.

43. Xiong, N., C. Kang & D.H. Raulet. 2004. Positive selection of dendritic epidermal gammadelta T cell precursors in the fetal thymus determines expression of skin-homing receptors. *Immunity* **21:** 121–131.

44. Xia, M. *et al*. 2010. Differential roles of IL-2-inducible T cell kinase-mediated TCR signals in tissue-specific localization and maintenance of skin intraepithelial T cells. *J. Immunol*. **184:** 6807–6814.

45. Wurbel, M.A. *et al*. 2001. Mice lacking the CCR9 CC-chemokine receptor show a mild impairment of early T- and B-cell development and a reduction in T-cell receptor gammadelta(+) gut intraepithelial lymphocytes. *Blood* **98:** 2626–2632.

46. Uehara, S. *et al*. 2002. Characterization of CCR9 expression and CCL25/thymus-expressed chemokine responsiveness during T cell development: CD3(high)CD69+ thymocytes and gammadeltaTCR+ thymocytes preferentially respond to CCL25. *J. Immunol*. **168:** 134–142.

47. Malinarich, F.H. *et al*. 2010. Constant TCR triggering suggests that the TCR expressed on intestinal intraepithelial gammadelta T cells is functional in vivo. *Eur. J. Immunol*. **40:** 3378–3388.

48. Gao, Y. *et al*. 2003. Gamma delta T cells provide an early source of interferon gamma in tumor immunity. *J. Exp. Med*. **198:** 433–442.

49. Asigbetse, K.E., P.A. Eigenmann & C.P. Frossard. 2010. Intestinal lamina propria TcRgammadelta+ lymphocytes selectively express IL-10 and IL-17. *J. Invest. Allergol. Clin. Immunol*. **20:** 391–401.

50. Erb, K.J. *et al*. 1995. Impaired survival of T cell receptor V gamma 3+ cells in interleukin-4 transgenic mice. *Eur. J. Immunol*. **25:** 1442–1445.

51. Matsue, H. *et al*. 1993. Profiles of cytokine mRNA expressed by dendritic epidermal T cells in mice. *J. Invest. Dermatol*. **101:** 537–542.

52. Macleod, A.S. & W.L. Havran. 2011. Functions of skin-resident gammadelta T cells. *Cell. Mol. Life Sci.: CMLS* **68:** 2399–2408.

53. Leclercq, G. & J. Plum. 1995. Stimulation of TCR V gamma 3 cells by gram-negative bacteria. *J. Immunol.* **154:** 5313–5319.

54. Cho, J.S. *et al.* 2010. IL-17 is essential for host defense against cutaneous Staphylococcus aureus infection in mice. *J. Clin. Invest.* **120:** 1762–1773.

55. Gray, E.E., K. Suzuki & J.G. Cyster. 2011. Cutting edge: identification of a motile IL-17-producing gammadelta T cell population in the dermis. *J. Immunol.* **186:** 6091–6095.

56. Mabuchi, T., T. Takekoshi & S.T. Hwang. 2011. Epidermal CCR6 +{gamma}{delta} T cells are major producers of IL-22 and IL-17 in a murine model of Psoriasiform dermatitis. *J. Immunol.* **187:** 5026–5031.

57. Schild, H. *et al.* 1994. The nature of major histocompatibility complex recognition by gamma delta T cells. *Cell* **76:** 29–37.

58. Bonneville, M. *et al.* 1989. Recognition of a self-major histocompatibility complex TL region product by gamma delta T-cell receptors. *Proc. Natl. Acad. Sci. USA* **86:** 5928–5932.

59. Weintraub, B.C., M.R. Jackson & S.M. Hedrick. 1994. Gamma delta T cells can recognize nonclassical MHC in the absence of conventional antigenic peptides. *J. Immunol.* **153:** 3051–3058.

60. O'Brien, R.L. *et al.* 1989. Stimulation of a major subset of lymphocytes expressing T cell receptor gamma delta by an antigen derived from Mycobacterium tuberculosis. *Cell* **57:** 667–674.

61. Ribot, J.C. *et al.* 2010. Cutting edge: adaptive versus innate receptor signals selectively control the pool sizes of murine IFN-gamma- or IL-17-producing gammadelta T cells upon infection. *J. Immunol.* **185:** 6421–6425.

62. Lalor, S.J. *et al.* 2011. Caspase-1-processed cytokines IL-1beta and IL-18 promote IL-17 production by gammadelta and CD4 T cells that mediate autoimmunity. *J. Immunol.* **186:** 5738–5748.

63. Veldhoen, M. *et al.* 2008. The aryl hydrocarbon receptor links TH17-cell-mediated autoimmunity to environmental toxins. *Nature* **453:** 106–109.

64. Quintana, F.J. *et al.* 2008. Control of T(reg) and T(H)17 cell differentiation by the aryl hydrocarbon receptor. *Nature* **453:** 65–71.

65. Simonian, P.L. *et al.* 2010. gammadelta T cells protect against lung fibrosis via IL-22. *J. Exp. Med.* **207:** 2239–2253.

66. Kadow, S. *et al.* 2011. Aryl hydrocarbon receptor is critical for homeostasis of invariant {gamma}{delta} T cells in the murine epidermis. *J. Immunol.* **187:** 3104–3110.

67. King, D.P. *et al.* 1999. Cutting edge: protective response to pulmonary injury requires gamma delta T lymphocytes. *J. Immunol.* **162:** 5033–5036.

68. Skeen, M.J. & H.K. Ziegler. 1993. Induction of murine peritoneal gamma/delta T cells and their role in resistance to bacterial infection. *J. Exp. Med.* **178:** 971–984.

69. Riol-Blanco, L. *et al.* 2010. IL-23 receptor regulates unconventional IL-17-producing T cells that control bacterial infections. *J. Immunol.* **184:** 1710–1720.

70. Wucherpfennig, K.W. *et al.* 1992. Gamma delta T-cell receptor repertoire in acute multiple sclerosis lesions. *Proc. Natl. Acad. Sci. USA* **89:** 4588–4592.

71. Poggi, A. *et al.* 2007. Adhesion molecules and kinases involved in gammadelta T cells migratory pathways: implications for viral and autoimmune diseases. *Curr. Med. Chem.* **14:** 3166–3170.

72. Rinaldi, L. *et al.* 2006. Longitudinal analysis of immune cell phenotypes in early stage multiple sclerosis: distinctive patterns characterize MRI-active patients. *Brain* **129:** 1993–2007.

73. Wohler, J.E. *et al.* 2009. Gammadelta T cells in EAE: early trafficking events and cytokine requirements. *Eur. J. Immunol.* **39:** 1516–1526.

74. Rajan, A.J. *et al.* 1996. A pathogenic role for gamma delta T cells in relapsing-remitting experimental allergic encephalomyelitis in the SJL mouse. *J. Immunol.* **157:** 941–949.

75. Spahn, T.W. *et al.* 1999. Decreased severity of myelin oligodendrocyte glycoprotein peptide 33–35-induced experimental autoimmune encephalomyelitis in mice with a disrupted TCR delta chain gene. *Eur. J. Immunol.* **29:** 4060–4071.

76. Odyniec, A. *et al.* 2004. Gammadelta T cells enhance the expression of experimental autoimmune encephalomyelitis by promoting antigen presentation and IL-12 production. *J. Immunol.* **173:** 682–694.

77. Ito, Y. *et al.* 2009. Gamma/delta T cells are the predominant source of interleukin-17 in affected joints in collagen-induced arthritis, but not in rheumatoid arthritis. *Arthritis Rheum.* **60:** 2294–2303.

78. Roark, C.L. *et al.* 2007. Exacerbation of collagen-induced arthritis by oligoclonal, IL-17-producing gamma delta T cells. *J. Immunol.* **179:** 5576–5583.

79. Rajan, A.J. *et al.* 2000. Experimental autoimmune encephalomyelitis on the SJL mouse: effect of gamma delta T cell depletion on chemokine and chemokine receptor expression in the central nervous system. *J. Immunol.* **164:** 2120–2130.

80. Rajan, A.J., J.D. Klein & C.F. Brosnan. 1998. The effect of gammadelta T cell depletion on cytokine gene expression in experimental allergic encephalomyelitis. *J. Immunol.* **160:** 5955–5962.

81. Kobayashi, Y. *et al.* 1997. Aggravation of murine experimental allergic encephalomyelitis by administration of T-cell receptor gammadelta-specific antibody. *J. Neuroimmunol.* **73:** 169–174.

82. Koenecke, C. *et al.* 2009. In vivo application of mAb directed against the gammadelta TCR does not deplete but generates "invisible" gammadelta T cells. *Eur. J. Immunol.* **39:** 372–379.

83. Cheng, L. *et al.* 2008. Mouse gammadelta T cells are capable of expressing MHC class II molecules, and of functioning as antigen-presenting cells. *J. Neuroimmunol.* **203:** 3–11.

84. Ponomarev, E.D. & B.N. Dittel. 2005. Gamma delta T cells regulate the extent and duration of inflammation in the central nervous system by a Fas ligand-dependent mechanism. *J. Immunol.* **174:** 4678–4687.

85. Lockhart, E., A.M. Green & J.L. Flynn. 2006. IL-17 production is dominated by gammadelta T cells rather than CD4 T cells during Mycobacterium tuberculosis infection. *J. Immunol.* **177:** 4662–4669.

86. Hirota, K. *et al.* 2011. Fate mapping of IL-17-producing T cells in inflammatory responses. *Nat. Immunol.* **12:** 255–263.

87. Hayday, A.C. 2009. Gamma delta T cells and the lymphoid stress-surveillance response. *Immunity* **31:** 184–196.

88. Hayday, A.C. 2000. [Gamma][delta] cells: a right time and a right place for a conserved third way of protection. *Annu. Rev. Immunol.* **18:** 975–1026.

89. Nedellec, S., M. Bonneville & E. Scotet. 2010. Human Vgamma9Vdelta2 T cells: from signals to functions. *Semin. Immunol.* **22:** 199–206.

90. Ness-Schwickerath, K.J., C. Jin & C.T. Morita. 2010. Cytokine requirements for the differentiation and expansion of IL-17A- and IL-22-producing human Vgamma2Vdelta2 T cells. *J. Immunol.* **184:** 7268–7280.

91. Caccamo, N. *et al.* 2011. Differentiation, phenotype and function of interleukin-17-producing human V{gamma}9V{delta}2 T cells. *Blood* **118:** 129–138.

92. Bettelli, E. *et al.* 2006. Reciprocal developmental pathways for the generation of pathogenic effector TH17 and regulatory T cells. *Nature* **441:** 235–238.

93. Veldhoen, M. *et al.* 2006. TGFbeta in the context of an inflammatory cytokine milieu supports de novo differentiation of IL-17-producing T cells. *Immunity* **24:** 179–189.

94. Fenoglio, D. *et al.* 2009. Vdelta1 T lymphocytes producing IFN-gamma and IL-17 are expanded in HIV-1-infected patients and respond to Candida albicans. *Blood* **113:** 6611–6618.

95. Peng, M.Y. *et al.* 2008. Interleukin 17-producing gamma delta T cells increased in patients with active pulmonary tuberculosis. *Cell. Mol. Immunol.* **5:** 203–208.

96. Cosmi, L. *et al.* 2008. Human interleukin 17-producing cells originate from a CD161+CD4+ T cell precursor. *J. Exp. Med.* **205:** 1903–1916.

97. Annibali, V. *et al.* 2011. CD161 (high) CD8+T cells bear pathogenetic potential in multiple sclerosis. *Brain* **134:** 542–554.

98. Maggi, L. *et al.* 2010. CD161 is a marker of all human IL-17-producing T-cell subsets and is induced by RORC. *Eur. J. Immunol.* **40:** 2174–2181.

99. Brandes, M., K. Willimann & B. Moser. 2005. Professional antigen-presentation function by human gammadelta T Cells. *Science* **309:** 264–268.

100. Vincent, M.S. *et al.* 1996. Apoptosis of Fashigh CD4+synovial T cells by borrelia-reactive Fas-ligand (high) gamma delta T cells in Lyme arthritis. *J. Exp. Med.* **184:** 2109–2117.

Ann. N.Y. Acad. Sci. ISSN 0077-8923

ANNALS OF THE NEW YORK ACADEMY OF SCIENCES

Issue: *The Year in Immunology*

# Lymphocyte signaling: regulation of FoxO transcription factors by microRNAs

Claudia Haftmann,[1] Anna-Barbara Stittrich,[1] Evridiki Sgouroudis,[1] Mareen Matz,[2] Hyun-Dong Chang,[1] Andreas Radbruch,[1] and Mir-Farzin Mashreghi[1]

[1]Deutsches Rheuma-Forschungszentrum Berlin, Berlin, Germany. [2]Department of Nephrology, Universitätsmedizin Charité Campus Mitte, Berlin, Germany

Address for correspondence: Mir-Farzin Mashreghi, Deutsches Rheuma Forschungszentrum Berlin, Charitéplatz 1, 10117 Berlin, Germany. mashreghi@drfz.de

The Forkhead box O (FoxO) family of transcription factors is important for the maintenance of immunological homeostasis and tolerance by controlling the development and function of B and T lymphocytes. Because dysregulation in FoxO activity can result in chronic inflammation and autoimmunity, the transcriptional activity of FoxO proteins is tightly controlled and generally dependent on complex posttranslational modifications that lead either to their nuclear entry and subsequent activation or, alternatively, to their nuclear export. The phosphatidylinositol 3-kinase (PI3K)–protein kinase B (PKB/Akt) axis represents the major pathway phosphorylating and thereby inactivating FoxO proteins. However, recent results have revealed an additional posttranscriptional mechanism of FoxO inactivation by microRNAs. The discovery of this molecular pathway may provide a new therapeutic avenue for the modulation of FoxO activity in immune-mediated diseases using either microRNA targeting antagomirs or synthetic microRNA mimics, a topic that is addressed in this review.

Keywords: Forkhead transcription factors; microRNA; lymphocytes; miR-182; FoxO1; FoxO3

## Introduction

The Forkhead box O (FoxO) family of transcription factors are mammalian homologs of *Caenorhabditis elegans* longevity dauer arrest gene DAF-16, which consists of four members: FoxO1, FoxO3, FoxO4, and FoxO6 (reviewed in Ref. 1). They act as transcriptional activators, by binding to the consensus core recognition motif TTGTTTAC[2,3] and control various cellular functions, including cell cycle arrest, detoxification of reactive oxygen species, autophagy, apoptosis, energy metabolism, and cell differentiation (reviewed in Ref. 4). These functions are strictly regulated and are mainly determined by the ability of FoxO proteins to interact with a variety of different transcription factors in response to a multitude of external stimuli, such as cytokine stimulation, B cell receptor (BCR), T cell receptor (TCR), and/or CD28 ligation-induced signals (reviewed in Refs. 1, 5–7).

Posttranslational modifications, including phosphorylation, acetylation, and mono- and polyubiquitination, control the activity of FoxO transcription factors. These kinds of modifications regulate FoxO protein levels, subcellular localization, and the ability to interact with other protein partners.[4,5] The best-studied signaling pathway that negatively regulates FoxO transcription factors is the phosphatidylinositol 3-kinase (PI3K)–protein kinase B (PKB/Akt) pathway. Following activation by external stimuli, Akt phosphorylates three conserved sites common to FoxO1, FoxO3, and FoxO4, resulting in diminished DNA-binding activity and nuclear exclusion of the FoxO transcription factors through the formation of a complex with the chaperone protein 14-3-3. In contrast, phosphorylation of FoxO transcription factors by MST1 (mammalian Ste20-like kinase) at conserved sites within the DNA-binding domain interrupts complex formation with the 14-3-3 protein and thus facilitates

doi: 10.1111/j.1749-6632.2011.06264.x

the retranslocation of FoxO proteins to the nucleus. This MST1-mediated modification overrides the effects of PI3K–Akt-mediated phosphorylation and allows a rapid response of FoxO transcription factors to oxidative stress. Thus, the activity of FoxO transcription factors and their subcellular localization can be either positively or negatively modulated depending on the site of phosphorylation (reviewed in Ref. 4).

In addition, the total levels of FoxO protein may also have dramatic effects on cellular functions. Several mechanisms controlling FoxO protein levels have been demonstrated. For example, in response to growth factors/cytokines and subsequent phosphorylation by Akt, FoxO transcription factors are subsequently polyubiquitinated and degraded by the proteasome.[8,9] However, it is still elusive how the balance between cytoplasmic sequestration and degradation is regulated (as discussed in Ref. 4). In contrast, acetylation or methylation can increase FoxO protein stability.[10,11] Acetylation inhibits polyubiquitination upon oxidative stress.[10] Methylation prevents the Akt-mediated phosphorylation of FoxO transcription factors and subsequent proteosomal degradation.[11]

On the transcriptional level, E2F-1 and STAT3 have been shown to bind to the promoters of *FoxO1* and *FoxO3* and induce their expression.[12,13] A global screening approach using chromatin immunoprecipitation combined with deep DNA sequencing (ChIP–Seq) demonstrated that E2A and EBF1 bind to the FoxO1 gene locus and determine B cell fate.[14] Furthermore, FoxO transcription factors can drive their own transcription in a positive feedback loop with FoxO3, and to a lesser extent FoxO1, which can induce the expression of FoxO1 via a conserved consensus binding site in the *FoxO1* promoter.[15,16] Furthermore, FoxC1, another member of the Forkhead box transcription factor family, binds to three conserved sites at the *FoxO1* promoter and induces the expression of FoxO1.[17]

Until recently it has remained unclear whether changes in FoxO protein levels are also mediated at the posttranscriptional level as a consequence of changes in messenger RNA (mRNA) stability.[4] However, within the last three years several groups have demonstrated that there is microRNA (miRNA)-mediated regulation of FoxO transcription factors.[18–23] Remarkably, the miRNA-182 has been shown to specifically target FoxO transcrip-

tion factors, irrespective of cell type.[18–20] In 2009, one study demonstrated that FoxO1 is coordinately targeted by three miRNAs, namely miR-27a, miR-96, and miR-182, in breast cancer cells,[18] whereas in another study miR-182 was shown to target FoxO3 in melanoma cells.[19] Our group has identified a role of miR-182 in targeting FoxO1 in activated helper T (Th) lymphocytes,[20] which will be discussed in this review.

## FoxO transcription factors in the immune system

The emerging immunological roles of FoxO transcription factors have been recently elucidated using cell type-specific deletion of FoxO1 and/or FoxO3 in mice[24–30] (reviewed in Refs. 6 and 7). Taken together, these genetic deletion approaches have demonstrated that FoxO transcription factors play an important role in regulating immunological homeostasis and tolerance by controlling the function and development of B and T lymphocytes.

It is known that the PI3K–Akt-mediated inactivation of FoxO1 is essential for the optimal proliferation of B cells. Indeed, ectopic expression of PI3K-independent variants of FoxO1 or FoxO3 in B cells resulted in cell cycle arrest and increased cell death.[31] In a similar approach, the overexpression of a FoxO3 mutant, lacking the residues normally phosphorylated by Akt, led to cell cycle arrest and light chain expression in pre-B cells as a result of inducing the expression of recombination activating gene (Rag)-1 and Rag-2.[32] Using shRNA technology to attenuate FoxO1 expression, Amin *et al.* demonstrated that FoxO1 can also induce Rag-1 and Rag-2 expression.[33] Moreover, Dangler *et al.* showed that loss of FoxO1 in the late pro-B cell stage caused lower expression of Rag-1 and Rag-2.[29] Furthermore, early deletion of FoxO1-blocked B cell differentiation at the pro-B cell stage due to a defect in interleukin 7 (IL-7) receptor alpha (IL-7Rα, CD127) expression. Deletion of FoxO1 in peripheral B cells was associated with defective expression of both L-selection (CD62L) and activation-induced cytidine deaminase (AID), which led to a failure in class-switch recombination and reduced IgG production upon immunization.[29] Together, these data strongly suggest that FoxO1 and FoxO3 are essential transcription factors involved in early B cell development and peripheral B cell function, with some redundancy in their activity.

The evidence that FoxO transcription factors are involved in T cell proliferation and survival soon followed. The first such study showed that IL-2 deprivation-dependent cell cycle arrest and apoptosis of T cells results from the activation of FoxO3 and subsequent induction of p27[Kip1] and Bim expression.[34] In accordance with this study, the ectopic expression of a constitutively active form of FoxO1 in human T cells inhibited proliferation, suggesting a cell-intrinsic mechanism regulating T cell quiescence.[35] FoxO3[Trap] mice, which express disabled *FoxO3* alleles resulting in FoxO3 deficiency, subsequently developed spontaneous lymphoproliferation and mild multiorgan autoimmune inflammation.[36] The absence of FoxO3 resulted in overactivation of NF-κB in Th cells of these mice, resulting in increased proliferation and effector cytokine production. In contrast, another study using two different FoxO3-deficient mouse models did not report any signs of spontaneous inflammation.[24] Instead, they observed increased expansion of T cell numbers after viral infection due to the enhanced capacity of FoxO3-deficient dendritic cells (DC) to sustain T cell viability by IL-6 production.

Recent studies have described the functional consequence of FoxO1 deficiency in T cells. FoxO1 is required for naive T cell maintenance in lymphoid tissues, as T cell-specific deletion of FoxO1 resulted in increased numbers of T cells with an activated phenotype (CD44[high]CD62L[low]).[25,27] After five to six months of age, mice developed a mild lymphoadenopathy and increased titers of dsDNA and nuclear antibody.[25] FoxO1-deficient T cells showed reduced expression of the chemokine receptor CCR7, the adhesion molecule CD62L, and sphingosine 1-phosphate receptor 1 (S1P1), which consequently led to impaired T cell homing to the lymph nodes.[25,27,28,37] Furthermore, it was shown that the marked reduction of naive T cell numbers in mice with T cell-specific ablation of FoxO1 could be attributed to impaired IL-7R expression.[25,27] Reconstitution of IL-7R in these cells largely restored the number of naive FoxO1-deficient T cells, revealing that diminished IL-7R and antiapoptotic Bcl-2 expression is responsible for the observed defects in naive T cell homeostasis.[25,28] Radiation bone marrow chimera experiments using FoxO1-deficient bone marrow-derived cells resulted in the development of severe colitis associated with a higher proportion of activated T cells and a concomitant reduction of regulatory T (T$_{reg}$) cell frequency.[25] In contrast, mixed radiation chimeric mice reconstituted with equal numbers of wild-type (WT) and FoxO1 knockout bone marrow cells did not develop colitis. In these chimeric mice there were greater numbers of WT T cells relative to FoxO1-deficient T cells owing to the competitive advantage of the former.[25] In addition, FoxO1 was essential to prevent systemic T cell activation. Purified FoxO1-deficient Th cells activated *in vitro* produced more effector cytokines, and the cells were biased toward Th1 differentiation.[28] The deletion of FoxO1 led to increased appearance of follicular Th cells and development of autoimmunity. Notably, *Bcl6* and *Il21* expression were significantly increased in FoxO1-deficient T cells, whereas *Prdm1* (gene encoding for the transcription factor Blimp1) expression was not altered. This prominent effect of T cell activation was not due to impaired homeostasis of naive T cells but rather to systemic T cell activation.[28] These findings demonstrate that in addition to lymph node homing and homeostasis, FoxO1 plays a role in the suppression of activation of at least naive T cells.

Another prominent function of FoxO transcription factors that has recently been described is their involvement in mediating the differentiation and function of T$_{reg}$ cells.[26,28] Although FoxO1 deficiency in mice alone yields a mild form of autoimmunity,[25,27,28] mice with T cell-specific deficiency of both FoxO1 and FoxO3 develope a severe lethal inflammatory disease.[26,28] This is in part due to a defect in thymic T$_{reg}$ cell development, resulting in reduced numbers of thymic and splenic T$_{reg}$ cells as well as impaired induction of T$_{reg}$ cells *in vitro*.[26,28] The transfer of WT T$_{reg}$ cells could correct the inflammatory disorder of the FoxO1/3a double-deficient mice.[26] Furthermore, the FoxO1/3a double-deficient T$_{reg}$ cells were functionally compromised, as they were unable to correct either Scurfy T cell-triggered systemic inflammation or naive T cell-induced transfer colitis.[26] It remains to be shown how FoxO transcription factors control the suppressive function of T$_{reg}$ cells. The observed functional defect of FoxO1/3a-deficient T$_{reg}$ cells may be due in part to the expression of inflammatory cytokines in such cells.[26,28] In addition, FoxO1/3a double-deficient T$_{reg}$ cells displayed diminished levels of both Foxp3 and a subset of T$_{reg}$-specific signature genes, including CTLA-4, GITR, and CD25 (IL-2 receptor alpha chain).[26]

Interestingly, FoxO1 and FoxO3 bind to conserved binding motifs in the *Foxp3* gene promoter and in intronic regulatory regions, further supporting the notion that *Foxp3* is a direct target of FoxO.[26,30]

## MicroRNA function in adaptive immunity

miRNAs are a class of small, endogenous, noncoding RNAs that regulate gene expression, principally at the posttranscriptional level. Like coding genes, miRNAs are mainly transcribed by RNA polymerase II. The resulting primary form of the miRNA (pri-miRNA) is cleaved by an enzyme complex containing Drosha into a precursor miRNA (pre-miRNA) and then transported by Exportin-5 into the cytoplasm. In a second step, the pre-miRNA is further processed by the RNAse III endonuclease Dicer into the mature form of the miRNA.[38] This 20–25 base pair long, double-stranded RNA molecule is incorporated into the RNA-induced silencing complex (RISC) and binds to mRNA $3'$-untranslated regions (UTR) that partially exhibit sequence complementarity to the miRNA. This interaction leads either to an inhibition of translation or cleavage and degradation of the mRNA (reviewed in Ref. 38). As a result, the quantity of the specific protein is reduced. By this mechanism, miRNAs can fine-tune gene expression and are involved in virtually all the cellular processes.

The central involvement of miRNAs in the development of a functional adaptive immune system was shown in studies in which the global miRNA biosynthesis was blocked by the conditional knockout of either Dicer or Drosha in B and T lymphocytes (reviewed in Ref. 38). In thymocytes, the subsequent attenuation of miRNA biosynthesis reduced the number and differentiation of mature T cells and the development of $T_{reg}$ cells.[39–43] Genetic ablation of the miRNA biosynthesis pathway altered the suppressive activity of $T_{reg}$ cells and triggered a severe inflammatory autoimmune disease.[41–43] The depletion of Dicer in early B lymphocytes or miR-17–92 cluster deficiency prevented the transition from pro- to pre-B cell stage and reduced antibody diversity.[44,45] In contrast, the elimination of the miRNA synthesis in late B cell stages resulted in an accumulation of self-reactive antibodies and autoimmunity.[46] In the meantime, many individual miRNAs and their function in B or T lymphocytes have been identified (reviewed in Refs. 38, 47, and 48).

## Posttranscriptional control of FoxO transcription factors by miRNAs in lymphocytes

In 2009, two independent groups originally described that FoxO transcription factors can be targeted by miRNAs.[18,19] In breast cancer cells, FoxO1 was coordinately targeted by miR-27a, miR-96, and miR-182. The inhibition of each miRNA resulted in induced levels of FoxO1 and reduced breast cancer cell survival.[18] In melanoma cells, the expression of FoxO3 and microphthalmia-associated transcription factor (MITF) was dependent on miR-182. The inhibition of miR-182 by anti-miRs (blocking antisense oligonucleotides) hindered melanoma cell migration and triggered their apoptosis.[19] MiRNA-182 was initially described as an organ sensory-specific miRNA expressed in a polycistronic cluster together with miR-96 and miR-183. Notably, the expression of the miRNA cluster could not be detected in spleen or thymus of healthy mice.[49] However, in different mouse models of systemic lupus erythematosus (SLE), the expression of the miR-182-96-183 cluster was dramatically induced in whole splenocytes.[50] These data suggest an important role for these miRNAs in the breakdown of immunological tolerance and the manifestation of chronic autoimmune inflammation.

Recently, our lab has elucidated the function of miR-182 in activated Th cells. Upon antigenic stimulation and costimulation via the coreceptor CD28, T cells start to proliferate and produce IL-2.[51,52] After this initial TCR/CD28–driven proliferation, the clonal expansion of activated T cells becomes independent of antigen and is promoted by IL-2.[53] In order to allow proliferation, T cell activation via TCR/CD28 and IL-2R signaling must inhibit FoxO1, which would otherwise block cell cycle progression by inducing the cell cycle inhibitor p27$^{Kip1}$.[1] In the early antigen-dependent phase of activation, FoxO1 is rapidly phosphorylated and excluded from the nucleus. However, signaling via TCR/CD28 and IL-2R is transient, and it remained unclear how FoxO1 was regulated in the late phase of clonal expansion. We demonstrated that in this phase FoxO1 is regulated posttranscriptionally by miRNA-182. Murine naive Th cells and human CD45RA$^+$ or CD45RO$^+$ Th cells expressed low basal levels of miR-182, which were markedly upregulated upon two days of activation. The induction of miR-182 was IL-2 dependent, as demonstrated by IL-2 neutralization in combination with CD25 blockade or by STAT5 inhibition. Furthermore, we observed enhanced STAT5 binding to a conserved STAT binding motif downstream of the miR-182 locus. Computational target prediction with the PicTar[54] and TargetScan[55] algorithm showed *FoxO1* to be a putative target for all members of the miR-182-96-183 cluster. In contrast to the overlapping binding sites for miR-96 and miR-182, the predicted miR-183 binding site in the *FoxO1* 3′UTR did not confer suppression to a reporter gene in activated Th cells. However, miR-96 does not seem to have a role in regulating *FoxO1*, as its expression was not detectable in either naive or activated Th cells.[20] In addition, using loss-of-function experiments, we could validate *FoxO1* as a major target of miR-182 in activated Th cells. The inhibition of miR-182 with antagomirs (chemically modified, cholesterol-coupled single-stranded RNA analogues complementary to miRNAs[56]) increased the levels of FoxO1 mRNA and protein, and limited population expansion of activated Th cells *in vitro* and *in vivo*. This effect was due to increased cell death and reduced proliferative capacity of antagomir-182–treated Th cells. Treatment of Th cells with miR-182–specific antagomirs attenuated the exuberant inflammatory response in an antigen-specific model of arthritis.[20] Our results demonstrate an important role of miR-182 in regulating the IL-2–driven clonal expansion of activated naive Th cells in part by targeting FoxO1. However, whether the expansion of effector and memory Th cells is affected by miR-182 remains unclear,[20,57] as they express little or no IL-2.[58] Because Th cell population expansion occurs in IL-2–deficient mice (reviewed in Ref. 59), we cannot exclude the possibility that common gamma chain cytokines, such as IL-7 and IL-15, induce miR-182 and promote the expansion of effector and memory Th cells.

Although the importance of IL-2 in $T_{reg}$ cell differentiation and survival is well established, it remains unclear whether the IL-2/STAT5/miR-182/FoxO axis is involved. The commitment of the Foxp3$^+$ $T_{reg}$ cell lineage comprises a two-step process in which the TCR/CD28 stimulation leads to the generation of $T_{reg}$ cell precursors with enhanced responsiveness to cytokine signals—for example, by inducing CD25. In the second step, IL-2 or, to a lesser extent, other common gamma chain cytokines activate STAT5, which in turn mediates the induction

of Foxp3.[60–62] In this context, the prolonged activation of the Akt-mammalian target of rapamycin (mTOR) pathway by TCR/CD28 stimulation has been demonstrated to substantially interfere with the differentiation and function of $T_{reg}$ cells,[63–65] presumably by inactivating FoxO transcription factors.[7,26,28,30] As it has been shown that miRNAs contribute to the development and maintenance of $T_{reg}$ cells,[40–43] it stands to reason that IL-2–induced miR-182 may target at least *FoxO1*, thus interfering with the differentiation and function of $T_{reg}$ cells.

In addition to miR-182, miR-155 has recently been shown to target FoxO3 in T cells.[66] Experiments with miR-155–deficient mice revealed that this miRNA plays a central role in the activation and function of B and T lymphocytes.[38,67] The expression of miR-155 is highly induced in mature activated T and B cells[68,69] and in $T_{reg}$ cells.[70] The elimination of miR-155 resulted in a reduction in the number of germinal center B cells, inhibited the formation of plasma cells, and repressed affinity maturation.[67,69,71,72] In Th cells, miR-155 deficiency promoted Th differentiation toward IL-4–producing Th2 cells and hindered Th1 and Th17 differentiation.[67,68,73] Therefore, miR-155 knockout mice were highly resistant to autoimmune encephalomyelitis (EAE). Furthermore, miR-155 was essential for IL-2–mediated proliferation of $T_{reg}$ cells.[70] So far, several immune-relevant targets have been reported for miR-155, including the transcription factors PU.1 and c-maf, as well as the enzyme AID, the suppressor of cytokine signaling 1 (SOCS1), src homology 2 domain-containing inositol-5-phosphate 1 (SHIP1), and interferon $\gamma$ (IFN-$\gamma$).[67,69–72,74,75] Yet, whether the newly discovered miR-155 target FoxO3 contributes to the observed phenotypes in B and T lymphocytes remains to be shown.

## FoxO transcription factors in immune-mediated diseases

Recently, it became evident that interfering with the PI3K–Akt pathway, which deactivates FoxO transcription factors, may be a promising approach for the treatment of chronic inflammation.[76] In mouse models of SLE and rheumatoid arthritis (RA), selective blockade of PI3K isoforms resulted in attenuated disease severity.[77–79] The inhibition of mTOR in a mouse model of SLE resulted in reduced Akt activation, ameliorated pathogenesis, and prolonged survival.[80] Furthermore, in a proof of concept study, the treatment of patients suffering from RA with everolimus (mTOR inhibitor) in combination with methotrexate showed clinical benefit.[81] However, the use of mTOR inhibitors, for example as an immunosuppressive regimen in transplantation, did not fulfill the high expectations based on strong therapeutic effects observed in animal models.[82] The highly divergent anti-inflammatory or pro-inflammatory functions of mTOR in immune cells might be responsible for the weak efficiency of everolimus in transplant patients.[83,84]

As discussed earlier, FoxO1 and/or FoxO3 deficiency can lead to chronic autoimmune inflammation by spontaneous T cell activation and increased effector differentiation, as well as impaired $T_{reg}$ cell function and differentiation.[25–28,30,36] In line with these observations, *FoxO1* transcript and FoxO1 protein levels in peripheral blood mononuclear cells (PBMCs) from patients with RA or SLE were significantly lower relative to healthy donors and inversely correlated with disease activity.[85] Similar results were observed in mouse models of SLE, in which FoxO1 and FoxO3 protein levels were decreased in splenocytes from MRL-lpr mice compared to MRL mice.[47] Notably, this reduction of FoxO protein levels inversely correlated with miR-182 expression.[47,50] Osteopontin, which is found to be highly expressed in various autoimmune diseases,[86] promoted pathogenesis in mouse models of experimental EAE by inactivating FoxO3, thereby enhancing the survival of activated T cells.[87] Therefore, it becomes attractive to consider treatments that restore the expression/activity of FoxO transcription factors in the context of chronic autoimmune inflammation. For example, in a mouse model of SLE, the peptide hCDR1 inhibited IFN-γ secretion and NF-κB activity in T cells, presumably by inducing the expression of FoxO3.[88] The hCDR1 peptide was also able to induce FoxO3 in PBMCs from lupus patients, which correlated with induced levels of TGF-β and Foxp3$^+$ $T_{reg}$ cells.[89] Treatment of lupus patients with hCDR1 peptide-ameliorated clinical symptoms.[90,91]

However, the function of FoxO transcription factors is highly cell- and context-dependent (reviewed in Ref. 92). For example, FoxO3-deficient mice are resistant to neutrophilic inflammation, with FoxO3-mediated suppression of Fas ligand (FasL) expression being required for neutrophil viability. Thus,

FoxO3-deficient neutrophils upregulated FasL expression and were more susceptible to TNF-α- and IL-1–induced apoptosis.[93] In contrast, the inactivation of FoxO3 by small interfering RNAs (siRNAs) led to increased survival of central memory and effector memory T cells, by reducing their susceptibility to Fas-mediated apoptosis and enhancing their proliferative capacity.[94–96] In line with these observations, HIV Tat-induced activation of FoxO3 activity promoted T cell and macrophage death.[97,98] These results provide at least for chronic HIV infection or neutrophilic inflammation the rationale for the development of specific FoxO inhibitors.[92]

## miRNA-based therapies for the modulation of FoxO activity in immune-mediated diseases

The manipulation of FoxO transcription factor expression represents an intriguing and sophisticated approach for the treatment of inflammatory diseases. With the discovery of miRNAs targeting FoxO transcription factors, it might now be possible to develop strategies to modulate FoxO expression. For example, in Th cell-mediated autoimmune diseases, antagomir-mediated inhibition of miR-182[56] could efficiently induce the expression of FoxO1 (presumably also FoxO3[19]) in effector Th cells, limiting their expansion thus reducing inflammation.[20] Conversely, the use of miRNA-182 mimics (chemically modified synthetic miRNAs)[99] could be useful to enhance the survival of neutrophils in neutrophilic inflammation[93] or to preserve central and effector memory CD4$^+$ Th cells and macrophages in chronic HIV infection.[94–98] However, the miRNA-based therapeutic manipulation of FoxO transcription factors bears some difficulties. The biggest challenge in this context is the specific delivery of the miRNA modulators into the target cell in order to avoid adverse effects in other cell types or tissues. For example, the delivery of miR-182 mimics could induce lymphoproliferative disease or other forms of cancer by systemic repression of FoxO transcription factors.[6,7,18,19,36] Because a single miRNA may target hundreds of genes, the therapeutic manipulation of a specific miRNA could have unanticipated adverse effects by influencing whole gene networks while having only moderate effects on the desired target.

However, progress is being made in the development and delivery of miRNA modulators as well as siRNAs (reviewed in Ref. 100). In 2010, Davis *et al.* were able to achieve gene silencing in humans after systemic administration of siRNA containing nanoparticles.[101] The inhibition of apolipoprotein B by an antisense oligonucleotide was effective for the treatment of patients with homozygous familial hypercholesterolemia.[102] The antagonism of the liver-specific miR-122 by a locked nucleic acid (LNA) oligonucleotide (SPC3649 or miravirsen) led to long-lasting suppression of hepatitis C virus (HCV) viremia and improved HCV-induced liver pathology in primates.[103] This was the first study demonstrating the therapeutic feasibility and safety of miRNA inhibition. Recently, miravirsen became the first miRNA-targeted drug to enter phase IIa clinical trials for the treatment of HCV-infected patients.[a] *In vivo* miRNA-based therapies for chronic autoimmune inflammatory disease are limited to studies in mice (reviewed in Ref. 104). For example, the delivery of double-stranded miR-15a mimic directly into the joints of arthritic mice-induced cell apoptosis in a Bcl-2–dependent manner.[105]

In addition to miR-182,[50] many other dysregulated disease-associated miRNAs have been identified and shown to be critical for the pathogenesis of autoimmune diseases by repressing various different immune related target genes (reviewed in Refs. 47, 100). Therefore, we assume that miRNA modulators will become a highly relevant and novel class of therapeutics for the treatment of immune-related diseases.

## Acknowledgments

This work was supported by the Deutsche Forschungsgemeinschaft (GRK1121 for A.-B.S.; SFB 618, SFB 650, SFB 633, and SFB TR52), the International Max Planck Research School for Infectious Diseases and Immunology (C.H.), and the FORSYS (Forschungseinheiten zur Systembiologie) program of the Federal Ministry of Education. The authors thank Dr. Mairi McGrath for a critical reading of the manuscript.

## Conflicts of interest

The authors declare no conflicts of interest.

---

[a] http://www.santaris.com/news/2010/09/23/santaris-pharma-advances-miravirsen-first-microrna-targeted-drug-enter-clinical-tria

## References

1. Peng, S.L. 2008. Foxo in the immune system. *Oncogene* **27:** 2337–2344.
2. Furuyama, T. *et al.* 2000. Identification of the differential distribution patterns of mRNAs and consensus binding sequences for mouse DAF-16 homologues. *Biochem. J.* **349:** 629–634.
3. Biggs, W.H., 3rd, W.K. Cavenee & K.C. Arden. 2001. Identification and characterization of members of the FKHR (FOX O) subclass of winged-helix transcription factors in the mouse. *Mamm. Genome.* **12:** 416–425.
4. Calnan, D.R. & A. Brunet. 2008. The FoxO code. *Oncogene* **27:** 2276–2288.
5. van der Vos, K.E. & P.J. Coffer. 2008. FOXO-binding partners: it takes two to tango. *Oncogene* **27:** 2289–2299.
6. Dejean, A.S., S.M. Hedrick & Y.M. Kerdiles. 2011. Highly specialized role of Forkhead box O transcription factors in the immune system. *Antioxid. Redox Signal.* **14:** 663–674.
7. Ouyang, W. & M.O. Li. 2011. Foxo: in command of T lymphocyte homeostasis and tolerance. *Trends Immunol.* **32:** 26–33.
8. Huang, H. *et al.* 2005. Skp2 inhibits FOXO1 in tumor suppression through ubiquitin-mediated degradation. *Proc. Natl. Acad. Sci. USA* **102:** 1649–1654.
9. Plas, D.R. & C.B. Thompson. 2003. Akt activation promotes degradation of tuberin and FOXO3a via the proteasome. *J. Biol. Chem.* **278:** 12361–12366.
10. Kitamura, Y.I. *et al.* 2005. FoxO1 protects against pancreatic beta cell failure through NeuroD and MafA induction. *Cell Metab.* **2:** 153–163.
11. Yamagata, K. *et al.* 2008. Arginine methylation of FOXO transcription factors inhibits their phosphorylation by Akt. *Mol. Cell* **32:** 221–231.
12. Nowak, K. *et al.* 2007. E2F-1 regulates expression of FOXO1 and FOXO3a. *Biochim. Biophys. Acta* **1769:** 244–252.
13. Oh, H.M. *et al.* 2011. STAT3 protein promotes T-cell survival and inhibits interleukin-2 production through up-regulation of Class O Forkhead transcription factors. *J. Biol. Chem* **286:** 30888–30897.
14. Lin, Y.C. *et al.* 2010. A global network of transcription factors, involving E2A, EBF1 and Foxo1, that orchestrates B cell fate. *Nat. Immunol.* **11:** 635–643.
15. Essaghir, A. *et al.* 2009. The transcription of FOXO genes is stimulated by FOXO3 and repressed by growth factors. *J. Biol. Chem.* **284:** 10334–10342.
16. Al-Mubarak, B., F.X. Soriano & G.E. Hardingham. 2009. Synaptic NMDAR activity suppresses FOXO1 expression via a cis-acting FOXO binding site: FOXO1 is a FOXO target gene. *Channels (Austin)* **3:** 233–238.
17. Berry, F.B. *et al.* 2008. FOXC1 is required for cell viability and resistance to oxidative stress in the eye through the transcriptional regulation of FOXO1A. *Hum. Mol. Genet.* **17:** 490–505.
18. Guttilla, I.K. & B.A. White. 2009. Coordinate regulation of FOXO1 by miR-27a, miR-96, and miR-182 in breast cancer cells. *J. Biol. Chem.* **284:** 23204–23216.
19. Segura, M.F. *et al.* 2009. Aberrant miR-182 expression promotes melanoma metastasis by repressing FOXO3 and

microphthalmia-associated transcription factor. *Proc. Natl. Acad. Sci. USA* **106:** 1814–1819.

20. Stittrich, A.B. *et al.* 2010. The microRNA miR-182 is induced by IL-2 and promotes clonal expansion of activated helper T lymphocytes. *Nat. Immunol.* **11:** 1057–1062.

21. Kong, W. *et al.* 2010. MicroRNA-155 regulates cell survival, growth, and chemosensitivity by targeting FOXO3a in breast cancer. *J. Biol. Chem.* **285:** 17869–17879.

22. Lin, H. *et al.* 2010. Unregulated miR-96 induces cell proliferation in human breast cancer by downregulating transcriptional factor FOXO3a. *PLoS One* **5:** e15797.

23. Hasseine, L.K. *et al.* 2009. miR-139 impacts FoxO1 action by decreasing FoxO1 protein in mouse hepatocytes. *Biochem. Biophys. Res. Commun.* **390:** 1278–1282.

24. Dejean, A.S. *et al.* 2009. Transcription factor Foxo3 controls the magnitude of T cell immune responses by modulating the function of dendritic cells. *Nat. Immunol.* **10:** 504–513.

25. Ouyang, W. *et al.* 2009. An essential role of the Forkhead-box transcription factor Foxo1 in control of T cell homeostasis and tolerance. *Immunity* **30:** 358–371.

26. Ouyang, W. *et al.* 2010. Foxo proteins cooperatively control the differentiation of Foxp3+ regulatory T cells. *Nat. Immunol.* **11:** 618–627.

27. Kerdiles, Y.M. *et al.* 2009. Foxo1 links homing and survival of naive T cells by regulating L-selectin, CCR7 and interleukin 7 receptor. *Nat. Immunol.* **10:** 176–184.

28. Kerdiles, Y.M. *et al.* 2010. Foxo transcription factors control regulatory T cell development and function. *Immunity* **33:** 890–904.

29. Dengler, H.S. *et al.* 2008. Distinct functions for the transcription factor Foxo1 at various stages of B cell differentiation. *Nat. Immunol.* **9:** 1388–1398.

30. Harada, Y. *et al.* 2010. Transcription factors Foxo3a and Foxo1 couple the E3 ligase Cbl-b to the induction of Foxp3 expression in induced regulatory T cells. *J. Exp. Med.* **207:** 1381–1391.

31. Yusuf, I. *et al.* 2004. Optimal B-cell proliferation requires phosphoinositide 3-kinase-dependent inactivation of FOXO transcription factors. *Blood* **104:** 784–787.

32. Herzog, S. *et al.* 2008. SLP-65 regulates immunoglobulin light chain gene recombination through the PI(3)K-PKB-Foxo pathway. *Nat. Immunol.* **9:** 623–631.

33. Amin, R.H. & M.S. Schlissel. 2008. Foxo1 directly regulates the transcription of recombination-activating genes during B cell development. *Nat. Immunol.* **9:** 613–622.

34. Stahl, M. *et al.* 2002. The forkhead transcription factor FoxO regulates transcription of p27Kip1 and Bim in response to IL-2. *J. Immunol.* **168:** 5024–5031.

35. Fabre, S. *et al.* 2005. Stable activation of phosphatidylinositol 3-kinase in the T cell immunological synapse stimulates Akt signaling to FoxO1 nuclear exclusion and cell growth control. *J. Immunol.* **174:** 4161–4171.

36. Lin, L., J.D. Hron & S.L. Peng. 2004. Regulation of NF-kappaB, Th activation, and autoinflammation by the forkhead transcription factor Foxo3a. *Immunity* **21:** 203–213.

37. Gubbels Bupp, M.R. *et al.* 2009. T cells require Foxo1 to populate the peripheral lymphoid organs. *Eur. J. Immunol.* **39:** 2991–2999.

38. O'Connell, R.M. *et al.* 2010. Physiological and pathological roles for microRNAs in the immune system. *Nat. Rev. Immunol.* **10:** 111–122.

39. Muljo, S.A. *et al.* 2005. Aberrant T cell differentiation in the absence of Dicer. *J. Exp. Med.* **202:** 261–269.

40. Cobb, B.S. *et al.* 2006. A role for Dicer in immune regulation. *J. Exp. Med.* **203:** 2519–2527.

41. Liston, A. *et al.* 2008. Dicer-dependent microRNA pathway safeguards regulatory T cell function. *J. Exp. Med.* **205:** 1993–2004.

42. Chong, M.M. *et al.* 2008. The RNAseIII enzyme Drosha is critical in T cells for preventing lethal inflammatory disease. *J. Exp. Med.* **205:** 2005–2017.

43. Zhou, X. *et al.* 2008. Selective miRNA disruption in T reg cells leads to uncontrolled autoimmunity. *J. Exp. Med.* **205:** 1983–1991.

44. Koralov, S.B. *et al.* 2008. Dicer ablation affects antibody diversity and cell survival in the B lymphocyte lineage. *Cell* **132:** 860–874.

45. Ventura, A. *et al.* 2008. Targeted deletion reveals essential and overlapping functions of the miR-17 through 92 family of miRNA clusters. *Cell* **132:** 875–886.

46. Belver, L., V.G. de Yebenes & A.R. Ramiro. 2010. MicroRNAs prevent the generation of autoreactive antibodies. *Immunity* **33:** 713–722.

47. Dai, R. & S.A. Ahmed. 2011. MicroRNA, a new paradigm for understanding immunoregulation, inflammation, and autoimmune diseases. *Transl. Res.* **157:** 163–179.

48. Belver, L., F.N. Papavasiliou & A.R. Ramiro. 2011. MicroRNA control of lymphocyte differentiation and function. *Curr. Opin. Immunol.* **23:** 368–373.

49. Xu, S. *et al.* 2007. MicroRNA (miRNA) transcriptome of mouse retina and identification of a sensory organ-specific miRNA cluster. *J. Biol. Chem.* **282:** 25053–25066.

50. Dai, R. *et al.* 2010. Identification of a common lupus disease-associated microRNA expression pattern in three different murine models of lupus. *PLoS One* **5:** e14302.

51. Iezzi, G., K. Karjalainen & A. Lanzavecchia. 1998. The duration of antigenic stimulation determines the fate of naive and effector T cells. *Immunity* **8:** 89–95.

52. van Stipdonk, M.J., E.E. Lemmens & S.P. Schoenberger. 2001. Naive CTLs require a single brief period of antigenic stimulation for clonal expansion and differentiation. *Nat. Immunol.* **2:** 423–429.

53. Jelley-Gibbs, D.M. *et al.* 2000. Two distinct stages in the transition from naive CD4 T cells to effectors, early antigen-dependent and late cytokine-driven expansion and differentiation. *J. Immunol.* **165:** 5017–5026.

54. Krek, A. *et al.* 2005. Combinatorial microRNA target predictions. *Nat. Genet.* **37:** 495–500.

55. Lewis, B.P. *et al.* 2003. Prediction of mammalian microRNA targets. *Cell* **115:** 787–798.

56. Krutzfeldt, J. *et al.* 2005. Silencing of microRNAs in vivo with 'antagomirs'. *Nature* **438:** 685–689.

57. O'Neill, L.A. 2010. Outfoxing Foxo1 with miR-182. *Nat. Immunol.* **11:** 983–984.

58. Szabo, S.J. *et al.* 2000. A novel transcription factor, T-bet, directs Th1 lineage commitment. *Cell* **100:** 655–669.

59. Horak, I. *et al.* 1995. Interleukin-2 deficient mice: a new model to study autoimmunity and self-tolerance. *Immunol. Rev.* **148:** 35–44.

60. Lio, C.W. & C.S. Hsieh. 2008. A two-step process for thymic regulatory T cell development. *Immunity* **28:** 100–111.

61. Burchill, M.A. *et al.* 2008. Linked T cell receptor and cytokine signaling govern the development of the regulatory T cell repertoire. *Immunity* **28:** 112–121.

62. Merkenschlager, M. & H. von Boehmer. 2010. PI3 kinase signalling blocks Foxp3 expression by sequestering Foxo factors. *J. Exp. Med.* **207:** 1347–1350.

63. Sauer, S. *et al.* 2008. T cell receptor signaling controls Foxp3 expression via PI3K, Akt, and mTOR. *Proc. Natl. Acad. Sci. USA* **105:** 7797–7802.

64. Haxhinasto, S., D. Mathis & C. Benoist. 2008. The AKT-mTOR axis regulates de novo differentiation of CD4+Foxp3+ cells. *J. Exp. Med.* **205:** 565–574.

65. Liu, G. *et al.* 2009. The receptor S1P1 overrides regulatory T cell-mediated immune suppression through Akt-mTOR. *Nat. Immunol.* **10:** 769–777.

66. Yamamoto, M. *et al.* 2011. miR-155, a modulator of FOXO3a protein expression, is underexpressed and cannot be upregulated by stimulation of HOZOT, a line of multifunctional Treg. *PLoS One* **6:** e16841.

67. Thai, T.H. *et al.* 2007. Regulation of the germinal center response by microRNA-155. *Science* **316:** 604–608.

68. Rodriguez, A. *et al.* 2007. Requirement of bic/microRNA-155 for normal immune function. *Science* **316:** 608–611.

69. Dorsett, Y. *et al.* 2008. MicroRNA-155 suppresses activation-induced cytidine deaminase-mediated Myc-Igh translocation. *Immunity* **28:** 630–638.

70. Lu, L.F. *et al.* 2009. Foxp3-dependent microRNA155 confers competitive fitness to regulatory T cells by targeting SOCS1 protein. *Immunity* **30:** 80–91.

71. Teng, G. *et al.* 2008. MicroRNA-155 is a negative regulator of activation-induced cytidine deaminase. *Immunity* **28:** 621–629.

72. Vigorito, E. *et al.* 2007. microRNA-155 regulates the generation of immunoglobulin class-switched plasma cells. *Immunity* **27:** 847–859.

73. O'Connell, R.M. *et al.* 2010. MicroRNA-155 promotes autoimmune inflammation by enhancing inflammatory T cell development. *Immunity* **33:** 607–619.

74. Banerjee, A. *et al.* 2010. Micro-RNA-155 inhibits IFN-gamma signaling in CD4+ T cells. *Eur. J. Immunol.* **40:** 225–231.

75. O'Connell, R.M. *et al.* 2009. Inositol phosphatase SHIP1 is a primary target of miR-155. *Proc. Natl. Acad. Sci. USA* **106:** 7113–7118.

76. Ghigo, A. *et al.* 2010. PI3K inhibition in inflammation: toward tailored therapies for specific diseases. *Bioessays* **32:** 185–196.

77. Barber, D.F. *et al.* 2005. PI3Kgamma inhibition blocks glomerulonephritis and extends lifespan in a mouse model of systemic lupus. *Nat. Med.* **11:** 933–935.

78. Camps, M. *et al.* 2005. Blockade of PI3Kgamma suppresses joint inflammation and damage in mouse models of rheumatoid arthritis. *Nat. Med.* **11:** 936–943.

79. Randis, T.M. *et al.* 2008. Role of PI3Kdelta and PI3Kgamma in inflammatory arthritis and tissue localization of neutrophils. *Eur. J. Immunol.* **38:** 1215–1224.

80. Stylianou, K. *et al.* 2011. The PI3K/Akt/mTOR pathway is activated in murine lupus nephritis and downregulated by rapamycin. *Nephrol. Dial. Transplant.* **26:** 498–508.

81. Bruyn, G.A. *et al.* 2008. Everolimus in patients with rheumatoid arthritis receiving concomitant methotrexate: a 3-month, double-blind, randomised, placebo-controlled, parallel-group, proof-of-concept study. *Ann. Rheum. Dis.* **67:** 1090–1095.

82. Powell, J.D. & G.M. Delgoffe. 2010. The mammalian target of rapamycin: linking T cell differentiation, function, and metabolism. *Immunity* **33:** 301–311.

83. Saemann, M.D. *et al.* 2009. The multifunctional role of mTOR in innate immunity: implications for transplant immunity. *Am. J. Transplant.* **9:** 2655–2661.

84. Saemann, M.D. & G. Remuzzi. 2009. Transplantation: time to rethink immunosuppression by mTOR inhibitors? *Nat. Rev. Nephrol.* **5:** 611–612.

85. Kuo, C.C. & S.C. Lin. 2007. Altered FOXO1 transcript levels in peripheral blood mononuclear cells of systemic lupus erythematosus and rheumatoid arthritis patients. *Mol. Med.* **13:** 561–566.

86. Morimoto, J. *et al.* 2010. Osteopontin; as a target molecule for the treatment of inflammatory diseases. *Curr. Drug Targets* **11:** 494–505.

87. Hur, E.M. *et al.* 2007. Osteopontin-induced relapse and progression of autoimmune brain disease through enhanced survival of activated T cells. *Nat. Immunol.* **8:** 74–83.

88. Sela, U. *et al.* 2006. The negative regulators Foxj1 and Foxo3a are up-regulated by a peptide that inhibits systemic lupus erythematosus-associated T cell responses. *Eur. J. Immunol.* **36:** 2971–2980.

89. Sthoeger, Z.M. *et al.* 2009. The tolerogenic peptide hCDR1 downregulates pathogenic cytokines and apoptosis and up-regulates immunosuppressive molecules and regulatory T cells in peripheral blood mononuclear cells of lupus patients. *Hum. Immunol.* **70:** 139–145.

90. Sthoeger, Z.M. *et al.* 2009. Treatment of lupus patients with a tolerogenic peptide, hCDR1 (Edratide): immunomodulation of gene expression. *J. Autoimmun.* **33:** 77–82.

91. Mozes, E. & A. Sharabi. 2010. A novel tolerogenic peptide, hCDR1, for the specific treatment of systemic lupus erythematosus. *Autoimmun. Rev.* **10:** 22–26.

92. Peng, S.L. 2010. Forkhead transcription factors in chronic inflammation. *Int. J. Biochem. Cell Biol.* **42:** 482–485.

93. Jonsson, H., P. Allen & S.L. Peng. 2005. Inflammatory arthritis requires Foxo3a to prevent Fas ligand-induced neutrophil apoptosis. *Nat. Med.* **11:** 666–671.

94. Riou, C. *et al.* 2007. Convergence of TCR and cytokine signaling leads to FOXO3a phosphorylation and drives the survival of CD4+ central memory T cells. *J. Exp. Med.* **204:** 79–91.

95. van Grevenynghe, J., *et al.* 2008. Lymph node architecture collapse and consequent modulation of FOXO3a pathway on memory T- and B-cells during HIV infection. *Semin. Immunol.* **20:** 196–203.

96. van Grevenynghe, J., *et al.* 2008. Transcription factor FOXO3a controls the persistence of memory CD4(+) T cells during HIV infection. *Nat. Med.* **14:** 266–274.

97. Cui, M. *et al.* 2008. Transcription factor FOXO3a mediates apoptosis in HIV-1-infected macrophages. *J. Immunol.* **180:** 898–906.

98. Dabrowska, A., N. Kim & A. Aldovini. 2008. Tat-induced FOXO3a is a key mediator of apoptosis in HIV-1-infected human CD4+ T lymphocytes. *J. Immunol.* **181:** 8460–8477.

99. Wang, V. & W. Wu. 2009. MicroRNA-based therapeutics for cancer. *BioDrugs* **23:** 15–23.

100. Jackson, A. & P.S. Linsley. 2010. The therapeutic potential of microRNA modulation. *Discov. Med.* **9:** 311–318.

101. Davis, M.E. *et al.* 2010. Evidence of RNAi in humans from systemically administered siRNA via targeted nanoparticles. *Nature* **464:** 1067–1070.

102. Raal, F.J. *et al.* 2010. Mipomersen, an apolipoprotein B synthesis inhibitor, for lowering of LDL cholesterol concentrations in patients with homozygous familial hypercholesterolaemia: a randomised, double-blind, placebo-controlled trial. *Lancet* **375:** 998–1006.

103. Lanford, R.E. *et al.* 2010. Therapeutic silencing of microRNA-122 in primates with chronic hepatitis C virus infection. *Science* **327:** 198–201.

104. Wittmann, J. & H.M. Jack. 2011. microRNAs in rheumatoid arthritis: midget RNAs with a giant impact. *Ann. Rheum. Dis.* **70**(Suppl 1): i92–i96.

105. Nagata, Y. *et al.* 2009. Induction of apoptosis in the synovium of mice with autoantibody-mediated arthritis by the intraarticular injection of double-stranded MicroRNA-15a. *Arthritis Rheum.* **60:** 2677–2683.

Ann. N.Y. Acad. Sci. ISSN 0077-8923

ANNALS OF THE NEW YORK ACADEMY OF SCIENCES
Issue: *The Year in Immunology*

# From interleukin-9 to T helper 9 cells

Michael Stassen, Edgar Schmitt, and Tobias Bopp

Institute for Immunology, University Medical Center of the Johannes Gutenberg University Mainz, Mainz, Germany

Address for Correspondence: Dr. Tobias Bopp, Institute for Immunology, University Medical Center of the Johannes Gutenberg University Mainz, Building 708, Langenbeckstrasse 1 D-55131 Mainz, Germany. boppt@uni-mainz.de

Interleukin-9 (IL-9), cloned more than 20 years ago, was initially thought to be a Th2-specific cytokine. This assumption was initially confirmed by functional analyses showing that both IL-9 and Th2 cells play an important role in the pathogenesis of asthma, IgE class switch recombination, and resolution of parasitic infections. However, recently it was shown that IL-9–producing CD4$^+$ T cells represent the discrete T helper subset Th9 cells. Herein, we will review the cytokines and transcription factors known to promote the development of Th9 cells and their potential functional properties in relation to the biological activities of IL-9. In addition, we will discuss how Th9 cells are related to Th2, Th17, and $T_{reg}$ cells, as both an alternative source of IL-9 and in view of the fact that plasticity of CD4$^+$ T cell differentiation is currently a strong matter of debate in immunologic research.

Keywords: T helper cell; IL-9; Th9; transcription factor; asthma; mast cell

## Introduction

Initiation and regulation of adaptive immunity is based on the complex interaction of a still-growing number of members of the CD4$^+$ T cell family. Obviously, different pathogens require distinct adaptive immune responses that are regulated by specific CD4$^+$ T helper (Th) cell subsets. Originally, several types of Th cells (including Th1 and Th2) were described with distinct functional properties.[1–4] However, these Th cells were largely characterized by a lack of typical subset-specific molecules. In 1986, Mosmann published the hypothesis that distinguished two T cell subsets, Th1 and Th2, on the basis of distinct patterns of Th1- and Th2-specific cytokines.[5–7] The distinct cytokine expression resulted in unique functional properties of Th1 and Th2 cells, implicating Th1 cells as controlling antiviral, antibacterial, and antiparasitic immune responses and Th2 cells as controlling defense against extracellular parasites and supporting humoral immune responses. Subsequently, interferon-γ (IFN-γ) and interleukin-4 (IL-4) were identified as the subset-specific "signature" cytokines for Th1 and Th2 cells, respectively. Besides IL-4, IL-9 was also described to be a Th2-derived cytokine.[8]

IL-9 was originally cloned and described as "p40" and functionally characterized as a T cell growth factor for long-term T cell lines, but not for freshly isolated T cells.[9,10] Independently, the T cell growth factor TCGFIII was identified and was found to be identical with p40.[11] In parallel, a mast cell growth-enhancing activity (MEA) was found to be produced by the same CD4$^+$ T cells that secreted TCGFIII, and ultimately p40, TCGFIII, and MEA were shown to represent the same cytokine, then designated "IL-9."[12,13]

The protein encoded by the *Il9* gene is a 14 kd glycoprotein composed of 144 amino acids, with a typical signal peptide of 18 amino acids. IL-9 colocalizes with CD3$^+$ T cells in the bronchoalveolar lavage of asthmatic patients;[14] and in murine *in vivo* models, IL-9 is expressed upon infection with pathogens like *Leishmania major*, *Trichuris muris*, and *Schistosoma mansoni*.[15–17] Consistent with this, depletion of CD4$^+$ T cells *in vivo* resulted in a significant reduction of IL-9 upon administration of cognate protein antigen.[18] In addition, bone marrow–derived mucosal mast cells (BMMC) and eosinophils were also identified as sources of IL-9.[19–22] Analyses of IL-9 production in T cells and BMMC revealed that

doi: 10.1111/j.1749-6632.2011.06351.x

IL-1 strongly upregulated IL-9 secretion.[19,23] Further analyses of BMMC demonstrated that LPS, IL-10, and kit-ligand, in addition to IL-1, could synergistically enhance the production of IL-9.[20,24] At the transcriptional level, GATA-1 was found to be essential for BMMC-derived IL-9 production.[25] Concerning naive CD4$^+$ T cells, stimulation in the presence of TGF-β and IL-4 synergistically enhanced IL-2–dependent IL-9 production, while IFN-γ inhibited IL-9 production.[26] Collectively, at the time these studies were published, the data suggested that IL-9 could be produced by a T cell subset different from Th2 cells.

Yet it was not clear whether IL-9 was being secreted by IL-4–producing Th2 cells or by a unique T cell subset that produces IL-9, as no suitable anti-IL-9 antibodies were initially available to identify IL-9/IL-4 double-producing cells. Fifteen years later, two groups finally demonstrated that a combination of IL-4 and TGF-β, as growth and differentiation factors, promotes the development of a CD4$^+$ T cell subset that preferentially produces IL-9, the subset was therefore called *Th9* cells.[27,28] FACS staining with IL-4– and IL-9–specific mAbs demonstrated that residual IL-4–producing cells within the Th9 population did not produce IL-9, and IL-4/IL-9 double-producing cells could not be found.[28] These results suggested that IL-9 measured in supernatants from Th2 cells was produced by Th9-like cells but not by IL-4–producing Th2 cells (Fig. 1).

## Characterization of Th9 cells

The functional diversity of Th cell subsets is chiefly based on specific cytokines, and their development from naive CD4$^+$ T cells relies on distinct cytokine signals that initiate differentiation by either transactivation or repression of subset-specific transcription factors. Upon activation by antigen-presenting cells (APCs) in the presence of TGF-β and IL-4, naive CD4$^+$ T cells differentiate into Th9 cells that are characterized by expression of high amounts of IL-9, as well as IL-10. However, Th9 cells do not coexpress the cytokines IL-4, IL-5, IL-13 (Th2), IL-17a (Th17), or IFN-γ (Th1) upon activation.[27–30] And despite their ability to produce high amounts of IL-10, no regulatory properties of Th9 cells have been described thus far.[27]

IL-9 produced by Th9 cells can enhance the proliferative capacity of long-term cultured T cell lines and prolong their survival.[10,11,27,28] Furthermore,

Th9 cells seem to contribute to the expression of CCL17 and CCL22 in allergic diseases.[30] By using either FACS-based analyses or quantitative real-time polymerase chain reaction (PCR) to determine cytokines produced by Th9 cells, Dardalhon *et al.* and Veldhoen *et al.*, confirmed their previous claim that Th9 cells are a discrete Th cell subset distinct from Th1, Th2, Th17, and regulatory T (T$_{reg}$) cells.[27,28] Accordingly, Th9 cells do not express subset-determining transcription factors like T-bet (Th1), GATA-3 (Th2), RORγT (Th17), or FoxP3 (T$_{reg}$ cells) at levels comparable to the respective T cell subsets, indicating that Th9 cells are an autonomous Th cell subset.

## Cytokines promoting IL-9–producing Th cell development

Additional Th cell subsets seem to have the ability to produce IL-9 upon cognate antigen recognition. For example, IL-9 was found to be present in supernatants of stimulated Th2 cells.[8] Additional analyses demonstrated that CD4$^+$ T cells *in vivo* can also produce IL-9 in an IL-4–independent manner and that IL-1 family members, together with TGF-β, can substitute for IL-4 in generating Th9 cells *in vitro*.[18,31] Furthermore, there is a lack of reliable data identifying IL-4/IL-9 coexpressing Th2 cells by intracellular cytokine staining,[32] which supports the data that a distinct population of cells develops under Th2-promoting conditions that have the ability to produce IL-9.

Also, in a skin allograft transplantation model, CD4$^+$CD25$^+$ T$_{reg}$ cells have been identified as a potential source for IL-9.[33] In this study, the authors concluded that T$_{reg}$ cell-derived IL-9 is important for the recruitment and activation of mast cells that mediate allograft acceptance. However, this study lacked reliable FACS analyses demonstrating, on a single-cell level, that FoxP3/IL-9 coexpressing T cells exist. Later, Veldhoehn *et al.* demonstrated that both naturally occurring FoxP3$^+$ T$_{reg}$ cells isolated from thymus and induced T$_{reg}$ cells (iT$_{regs}$) generated *in vitro* (by the stimulation of naive CD4$^+$ T cells in the presence of TGF-β and IL-2) do not produce IL-9 upon T cell receptor (TCR)-mediated stimulation.[28] Furthermore, polarizing conditions favoring the expression of IL-9 by human and murine naive CD4$^+$ T cells were shown to inhibit TGF-β–induced FoxP3 expression.[27,34] These disparities could be explained by the

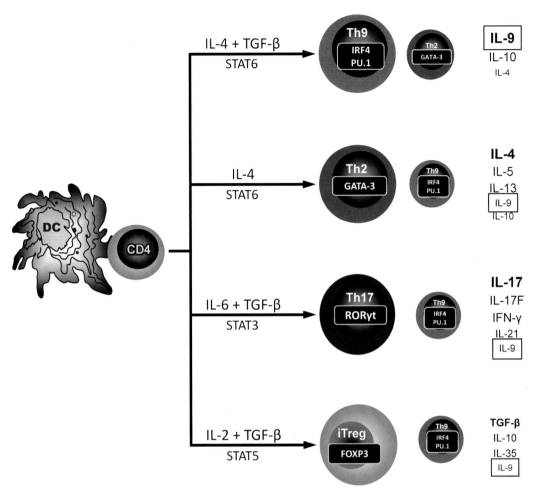

**Figure 1.** Multiple polarizing conditions permit Th9 development. Today, the classical monolithic view of T helper cell differentiation, in which stimulation of naive CD4$^+$ T cells in the presence of distinct polarizing conditions results in a homogenous and inflexible population of a distinct T helper cell subset, is called into question. For example, the ability to produce IL-9 was first linked to Th2 cells. However, recent studies reported that IL-9 can be additionally detected in the supernatants of Th9, Th17, and iT$_{reg}$ cells, all developing in the presence of TGF-β in combination with the indicated cytokines. However, detailed FACS analyses failed to identify IL-9/signature cytokine (Th2: IL-4, Th17: IL-17a) or master transcription factor (iT$_{reg}$: FoxP3) coexpressing T cells on a single-cell level. This allows the conclusion that under Th2 (IL-4), Th17 (TGF-β + IL-6) and iT$_{reg}$ (TGF-β + IL-2) polarizing conditions, a small proportion of T cells differentiates into IL-9–producing Th9 cells.

presence of IL-9–producing CD4$^+$CD25$^+$FoxP3$^-$ effector T cells within the CD4$^+$CD25$^+$FoxP3$^+$ T$_{reg}$ population. Supporting this conclusion, Soler *et al.* demonstrated that a small proportion of peripheral CD4$^+$CD25$^+$ T cells lacking FoxP3 expression additionally expresses CCR8 and is able to produce IL-9 upon CD3- and CD28-mediated activation.[35]

Interestingly, in combination with TGF-β, IL-9 promotes the development of another subset of Th cells, Th17 cells—so called because of their ability to produce high levels of IL-17a and IL-17f. It

was also shown that a Th population generated under Th17-promoting conditions comprises two major subsets of IL-17 (12.6%) and IL-9 (3.56%) single producers and a minor subset of IL-17/IL-9 (1.04%) double producers.[36] In addition, upon multiple rounds of polarization *in vitro* of human Th17 cells in the presence of TGF-β, IL-1β, IL-6, IL-21, and IL-23, IL-17/IL-9 coexpressing T cells, on a single-cell level, were detected.[34] In contrast, Putheti *et al.* demonstrated coexpression of GATA3 and RORC by human IL-9–producing T cells, but did not observe IL-9/IL-17–coproducing cells.[37] Furthermore, IL-23, a cytokine that is essentially involved in the maintenance of Th17 cells, opposes IL-9 production.[36,38] Additional analyses detected IL-9 in the supernatants of $CD4^+$ T cells stimulated under Th17-skewing conditions but failed to identify IL-17/IL-9–coexpressing $CD4^+$ T cells on a single-cell level.[32] Taken together, the polarization conditions used *in vitro* favor differentiation of Th2, Th17, or $iT_{reg}$ cells, but at the same time allow the concurrent development of small populations of IL-9–producing Th9 cells (Fig. 1). Especially pertaining to human IL-9–producing T cells, additional work is required to identify conditions that elicit Th9 cells with characteristics comparable to murine Th9 cells. Obviously, the *in vitro* polarization of naive $CD4^+$ T cells into T helper cells provides a simplified picture compared to the *in vivo* situation.

Given the vast diversity of microbial pathogens, a requirement for multiple, specialized T cell subsets, in combination with highly flexible transcriptional programs, is of vital importance. Indeed, multifunctional and versatile T helper cell populations can be detected during an adaptive immune response, and there is growing evidence that cytokine expression by Th cells *in vivo* is not as stable as was initially thought.[39–42] Hence, it is not surprising that, depending on the inflammatory conditions, Th9 cell populations appear to be flexible with respect to their ability to produce different cytokines. For example, murine asthma induced by the transfer of *in vitro*-generated Th9 cells but not by Th2 cells can be greatly ameliorated by the administration of neutralizing IL-9 antibodies, which indicates a "stability" of the IL-9–producing phenotype in allergic diseases.[29] On the other hand, *in vitro* restimulation of Th9 cells under Th1-, Th2-, or Th17-skewing conditions has little influence on the ability of the cells to produce IFN-γ or IL-17, but can result in strong induction of Th2-related cytokines.[32] In addition, adoptive transfer of myelin oligodendrocyte glycoprotein-specific Th9 cells has been shown to induce EAE symptoms concomitant with the ability to secrete IFN-γ.[38] In agreement with this, Lingnau *et al.* demonstrated that stimulation of naive $CD4^+$ T cells in the presence of TGF-β and IL-4 could lead to development of Th1-like cells independent of IL-12, a result that depends significantly on the concentrations of TGF-β and IL-4 used for polarization.[43] Thus, these variable outcomes strongly argue for a multilevel, hierarchical model of Th9 cell differentiation. The relative concentrations of the subset-directing cytokines TGF-β and IL-4 determine whether the majority of the resulting Th cells possess a Th2 (high IL-4/low TGF-β), Th9 (equal IL-4/TGF-β), or Th1 (low IL-4/ high TGF-β) phenotype. This basic response pattern of naive $CD4^+$ T cells to IL-4 and TGF-β can be further modified in the presence of other cytokines, as outlined below.

## Secondary cytokine signals that enhance IL-9 production

In addition to IL-4 and TGF-β, several cytokines seem to enhance IL-9 production by T cells. For example, IL-9 production by naive $CD4^+$ T cells after stimulation with ConA can be substantially enhanced in the presence of APCs.[23] Neutralization of IL-1α and IL-1β in this setting revealed that these cytokines can potentiate IL-9 production.[23] Interestingly, the production of IL-4 was only marginally enhanced in the presence of IL-1, indicating that IL-9 is regulated differently from Th2-derived cytokines.

IL-10 has also been suggested to promote IL-9 production in mice; such IL-10–dependence was demonstrated by impaired IL-9 production in IL-10–deficient mice upon immunization with keyhole limpet hemocyanin.[18] Yet blockade of IL-10 receptor by monoclonal antibodies on T cells has only marginal effects on their production of IL-9 *in vitro*.[28] For mast cells, on the contrary, IL-10 has a costimulatory function on IL-9 production in the presence of IL-1.[20] These data suggest that in contrast to the situation in mast cells, IL-10 receptor-mediated signal transduction may not directly modulate *Il9* gene expression in T cells. One possible explanation for this discrepancy is that enhanced IFN-γ production in IL-10–deficient mice attenuates IL-9 production by naive $CD4^+$ T cells.

Finally, a recent publication suggested a prominent role for IL-25 in enhancing IL-9 production by Th9 cells.[44] Angkasekwinai *et al.* demonstrated that IL-25–deficient mice show reduced airway inflammation in a model of asthma due to decreased IL-9 production.

## Physiological and pathophysiological relevance of IL-9

Because the definitive contribution of Th9 cells to IL-9–driven pathologies like allergic asthma, inflammatory gut diseases, microbial infections, autoimmunity, and tolerance is lacking, the following will, in most cases, discuss the role of IL-9 in these pathophysiologies without further addressing the definite source of this cytokine. However, we will highlight a potential role for Th9 cells when appropriate.

## IL-9 and allergic asthma

Human chromosome 5q31-q33 contains several genes that play important roles for the development of atopy and airway hyperresponsiveness (AHR). The *Il9* gene is located in this chromosomal region and was initially suggested to be a candidate gene for atopy and AHR due to the association of a distinct *Il9* allelic variant with increased serum total IgE levels in randomly selected individuals.[45] In mice, the *Il9* gene is located on the corresponding syntenic chromosome 13, and synteny and linkage homology implicate the *Il9* locus as a candidate for bronchial responsiveness in mice. In addition, the expression of *Il9* was found to be reduced in bronchial hyporesponsive mice,[46] and intratrachial administration of IL-9 induces asthmatic-like responses in naive mice, including lung eosinophilia, increased serum total IgE levels, and AHR.[47,48] These findings, suggesting a critical role for IL-9 in the pathogenesis of asthma, have been supported by transgenic approaches.

Lung-selective expression of IL-9 has been shown to cause airway inflammation, characterized by infiltrating eosinophils and lymphocytes, and pathologic changes, including epithelial cell hypertrophy, mucus production, and increased subepithelial deposition of collagen. In addition, *Il9*-expressing mice have increased AHR to inhaled bronchoconstrictors and the atypic presence of mast cells subepithelial and within the airway epithelium;[49] importantly, this phenotype developed without prior sensitization to allergen. Transgenic mice systemically over-expressing *Il9* display increased AHR to bronchoconstrictors, enhanced eosinophilic inflammation of the airways, and elevated serum IgE following senitization and challenge with the mold *Aspergillus fumigatus*.[50]

Further evidence for a crucial role of IL-9 in allergic airway disease is derived from experimental asthma studies in which antibody-mediated blockade of IL-9 during the sensitization phase attenuated lung eosinophilia, serum IgE, airway epithelial damage, and AHR.[51,52] Additional insight into underlying cellular mechanisms has come from studies using mice that inducibly express *Il9* in lungs.[53] In this setting, induced lung-specific expression of *Il9* mirrors the developing asthma-like phenotype seen in mice that constitutively expressed *Il9* in their lungs, as described above. After transgene induction in the lungs of these mice, expression of a panel of Th2-type cytokines was observed, including IL-13; importantly, blockade of IL-13 during *Il9* transgene expression prevented pathological changes in the lungs, such as cellular infiltration, epithelial cell hypertrophy, and mucus production, indicating that the function of IL-9 depends, at least in part, on IL-13.

Recently, Th9 cells were shown to be important contributors to the development of allergic airway disease.[29,30] Following adoptive transfer of *in vitro*-differentiated Th9 cells in RAG2-deficient mice, administration of neutralizing IL-9 antibody profoundly ameliorated Th9 cell-mediated asthma. In contrast, asthma severity only slightly improved upon IL-9 blockade in mice that received Th2 cells.[29]

Besides its roles in acute models of allergic airway disease, IL-9 has also been shown to be critical for the development of robust lung fibrosis—i.e., subepithelial deposition of collagen in chronic allergic lung inflammation.[54,55] In contrast to allergic fibrosis, however, injury-induced lung fibrosis in mice, in response to bleomycin or silica particles, was reduced in the presence of IL-9, which points to different underlying mechanisms of fibrotic pathogenesis.[56,57]

At the cellular level, IL-9 acts as a growth factor for mast cells,[13] increases the production of several cytokines in activated mast cells,[58] and, in the presence of stem cell factor (SCF), induces the expression of mast cell proteases.[59] Regarding B cells, IL-9 was reported to enhance IL-4–mediated production of IgE and IgG in human and murine B cells *in vitro*[60,61] and to promote the expansion of the B1 subset.[62] IL-9 also induces chemokine and mucus production in lung epithelial cells[63–65] and the expression of IL-5 receptor alpha-chain on eosinophils and airway smooth muscle cells.[22,48,66] In the latter, IL-9 was also reported to enhance the expression of chemokines by airway smooth muscle cells.[67] In this context, more recent findings indicate that the effects of IL-9 on lung epithelial cells, leading to mucus production and recruitment of eosinophils via

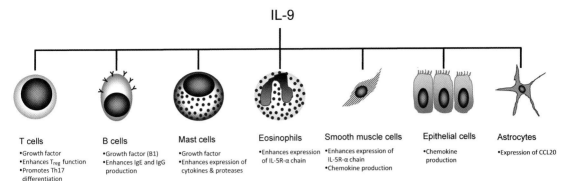

**Figure 2.** Effects of IL-9 on immune and nonimmune cells. IL-9 is a pleiotropic cytokine that affects multiple cell types. Potential sources for IL-9 include Th2, Th9, Th17, $T_{reg}$, and mast cells. Additional effects on lung epithelial cells leading to mucus production and recruitment of eosinophils via eotaxin are mediated through the induction of IL-13 production in hemopoietic cells. Recently, it was shown that IL-9 induces CCL20 production by astrocytes, presumably with the result that the infiltration of Th17 cells into the central nervous system is facilitated.

eotaxin, are mediated through the induction of IL-13 production in hemopoietic cells.[68] Taken together, the effects of IL-9 at the cellular level (summarized in Fig. 2) help to explain the role of IL-9 as an asthma-promoting cytokine through IL-13–dependent and IL-13–independent mechanisms.

In contrast to the findings described above, mice genetically deficient in *Il9* revealed that the absence of IL-9 did not affect the development of allergen-induced lung inflammation and AHR.[69] The discrepancy of this result with other work is at present unresolved, but it appears likely that in the extremely complex pathogenesis of experimental airway disease compensatory mechanisms act in the absence of IL-9. Unfortunately, the use of different mouse strains and different protocols to elicit airway disease in the publications cited above are also critical factors that render comparison of individual murine studies difficult.

Notwithstanding some contradictory results in mice, bronchial biopsy specimens from some human asthmatic patients show increased expression of *Il9* and of its receptor, compared to healthy controls.[14,70–72] Consequently, a humanized monoclonal antibody against IL-9 has recently been used in two phase II studies in asthmatics with some evidence of clinical activity.[73]

## IL-9 and inflammatory gut responses

Protective roles for IL-9 were shown in murine models for parasitic intestinal infections. IL-9 transgenic mice elicited a *Trichinella spiralis*-specific IgG1

response and developed intestinal mastocytosis—responsible for rapid parasite expulsion from the gut; similar results were also shown using the related nematode *Trichuris muris*.[16] In addition, active immunization against IL-9 inhibited expulsion of *T. muris*,[74] and transfer of IL-9–producing DC from IL-9 transgenic mice enhanced parasite-specific IgG1, intestinal mastocytosis, and elimination of *T. spiralis*.[75] Furthermore, it was also reported that IL-9 induces intestinal muscle hypercontractility, thereby facilitating worm expulsion.[76] Mast cells appear to be the main targets of IL-9 growth factor activity in these nematode infection models, and mast cell mediators critically contribute to eosinophilia, mucus production, and increased intestinal permeability and contractility, which leads to parasite expulsion.

However, gut-specific expression of *Il9* also is responsible for an intestinal anaphylaxis phenotype, as IL-9–deficient mice are unable to develop antigen-induced intestinal anaphylaxis, i.e., intestinal mastocytosis, mast cell activation, and diarrhea, in sensitized mice.[77] Investigations on the role of IL-9 in systemic anaphylaxis led to contradictory results. In one study it was reported that IL-9 given intravenously promotes systemic anaphylaxis in sensitized mice, although other publications have shown that this cytokine was not absolutely required for[78] or was even dispensable.[79]

Thus, IL-9 can promote pathogenesis in allergic reactions in lungs and the gut, and it appears that the ability of IL-9 to induce mastocytosis is also critical for the observations in anaphylaxis models.

## Microbial infections

Based on observations that infections with respiratory syncytial virus (RSV) are accompanied by high levels of IL-9 in bronchial secretions of patients, the role of IL-9 was investigated using a murine RSV model.[80] Depletion of IL-9 enhanced viral clearance from the lungs in general yet had complex effects on virus-induced immunopathogenesis, depending on the time point of depletion.

With regard to Gram-negative infections, prophylactic administration of IL-9 had a therapeutic activity in mice otherwise lethally infected with *Pseudomonas aeruginosa*.[81] The protective effect of IL-9 correlated with decreased production of proinflammatory mediators and the induction of the anti-inflammatory cytokine IL-10. In line with this finding is the observation that IL-9 inhibits release of TNF-α and oxidative burst in LPS-activated human monocytes expressing the IL-9 receptor, and thus might contribute to dampening fatal inflammatory responses.[82]

## IL-9 in autoimmunity and tolerance

Initially it was reported that T cells generated in the presence of IL-4 and TGF-β are able to produce IL-9 and IL-10 and induce the development of colitis and neuritis upon adoptive transfer in RAG-1–deficient recipients.[27]

IL-9 was also shown to be produced by Th17 cells that had been generated in the presence of IL-6 and TGF-β *in vitro* or were sorted as IL-17F reporter-positive T cells *ex vivo*. Importantly, neutralization of IL-9 delayed the onset of experimental autoimmune encephalomyelitis (EAE), a murine model for multiple sclerosis known to critically depend on the presence of Th17 cells. Using IL-9 receptor-deficient mice, not only were EAE symptoms delayed but disease severity was diminished.[83] Besides autoantigen-specific Th1 and Th17 T cell clones, it was also reported that Th9 cells are able to induce EAE pathology upon adoptive transfer, although with distinct histopathological characteristics.[38] In this context it was suggested that IL-9 promotes the development of autoantigen-specific T cells, as blockade of IL-9 suppressed both production of IL-17 by autoreactive T cells and their potency to initiate disease in adoptive transfer EAE.[84] Accordingly, induction of oral tolerance led to a reduction in Th17 cell numbers and production of IL-17 and

IL-9 that correlated with reduced overall inflammation in EAE mice.[85] In a recent study, it was shown that IL-9 induces CCL20 production by astrocytes *in vitro*, thereby establishing a link between IL-9 and the infiltration of Th17 cells into the central nervous system.[86] However, in contrast to these findings, one publication found a more severe course of EAE in mice lacking the IL-9 receptor.[36] Taken together, IL-9 is produced in autoimmune settings and serves proinflammatory roles, at least partly through its effects on Th17 cells.

With regard to immunological tolerance, IL-9 has been shown to link mast cells to $T_{reg}$ cell-dependent skin allograft tolerance.[33] In this model, $T_{reg}$ cell-derived IL-9 was important for the recruitment of mast cells that mediate tolerance—i.e., immunosuppression—without degranulation. Nevertheless, the physiological relevance of this finding is not clear, since mast cells can also be very potent proinflammatory cells, for example, IgE-mediated degranulation of mast cells breaks tolerance to established allocrafts.[87]

However, in a Th1- and Th17-dependent model of nephrotoxic serum nephritis (NTS), immune suppression by $T_{reg}$ cells depends on the recruitment of mast cells into kidney-draining lymph nodes. Using $T_{reg}$ cells derived from IL-9–deficient mice, it was demonstrated that $T_{reg}$ cell-mediated IL-9 is critical for mast cell recruitment and protection from NTS.[88] Thus, $T_{reg}$/mast cell interactions via IL-9 can be important for limiting inflammatory disease and allograft tolerance via protective mast cell responses. Yet, the nature of these protective mast cell functions remains elusive.

## Transcriptional regulation of *Il9* expression

Unlike the knowledge about the physiological and pathophysiological function of IL-9, knowledge of the transcriptional regulation of the *Il9* gene is rudimentary. As outlined above, stimulation of naive CD4$^+$ T cells with IL-4 and TGF-β selectively triggers IL-9 production; this highlights a prominent role for TGF-β receptor- and IL-4 receptor-mediated downstream signals, together with TCR-derived signals, for transcriptional regulation of Th9 cell development and function (Fig. 3). Consequently, altered IL-4 receptor signaling due, for example, to STAT6 deficiency results in a greatly reduced IL-9 production by Th9 cells.[28] Presumably this is due to reduced or no expression of

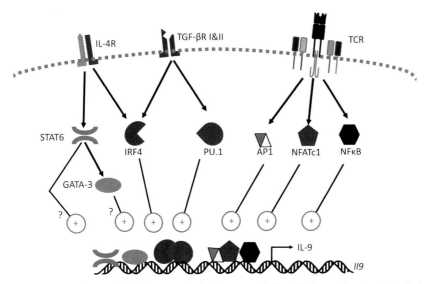

**Figure 3.** Transcriptional regulation of the *Il9* gene. The development of Th9 cells from naive CD4⁺ T cells is dependent on TCR-derived signals in the presence of TGF-β and IL-4. Hence, signals derived from the receptors for TGF-β and IL-4 as well leads to the expression and/or activation of transcription factors like IRF4, PU.1, and STAT6, essentially contributing to the initiation of *Il9* expression. In addition, downstream signals of the TCR leading to the expression of c-fos and c-jun (AP1), as well as NF-κB and NFAT translocation to the nucleus, contribute to the initiation of *Il9* transcription. Question marks indicate transcription factors, whose contribution to *Il9* expression needs further clarification. The displayed sequence of consensus binding sites does not reflect the actual order in the *Il9* promoter.

the gene *Gata3*, an important target for STAT6-dependent gene regulation. However, it can be assumed that other STAT6 target genes are involved in Th9 development and *Il9* expression as well, since GATA-3 directly regulates the expression of the Th2-associated genes *Il5* and *Il13*, which are repressed in Th9 cells.[28,89] In mast cells, we were able to show a crucial contribution of GATA-1 to the transcriptional regulation of the *Il9* gene.[24] Since T cells lack GATA-1 expression, GATA-3 could act in place of GATA-1 on the *Il9* promoter in Th9 cells. However, whether GATA-3 is only important in early developmental stages of Th9 cells or is, additionally, involved in the transcriptional regulation of *Il9* expression needs further clarification.

Obvious candidates acting downstream of TGF-β receptor kinases are Smad transcription factors. However, T cells deficient in Smad2 and Smad3 seem to have normal *Il9* expression, excluding a prominent role for these transcription factors in the regulation of *Il9* transcription.[90] Interestingly, Smad-independent TGF-β activity was reported to rely on the repression of eomesodermin (Eomes) expression, thereby promoting Th17 differentiation.[91] Initially, Eomes, a paralogue of T-bet, was shown to

promote IFN-γ production.[92–94] Since IFN-γ inhibits IL-9 production by CD4⁺ T cells, likely via induction of STAT1[95] (Fig. 4), it can be assumed that at least one function of TGF-β is to attenuate Th1 development and suppress IFN-γ production, possibly via inhibition of Eomes.

TCR-mediated signal transduction, ultimately leading to NFAT and NF-κB translocation to the nucleus, provides essential signals contributing to *Il9* transcription (Fig. 3). In this context, Gessner *et al.* demonstrated that IL-9 production indeed relies on the nuclear translocation of specific NFAT transcription factor family members, since calcineurin inhibition by cyclosporine A attenuates IL-9 production by T cells.[15] The positive effect of NFAT transcription factors on IL-9 production could be due either to a direct effect of NFAT on the *Il9* promoter or to an indirect effect of the more general role of NFAT in the regulation of *Il2* expression, which is a prerequisite for IL-9 production. In the latter case, a contribution of one of the three major isoforms of the inducible family member NFATc1/α has been implicated.[96]

With respect to the NF-κB pathway, it was demonstrated that IL-9 production by mast cells

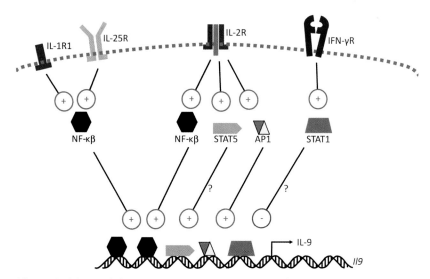

**Figure 4.** Amplifiers and inhibitors of *Il9* expression. Next to TGF-β and IL-4, IL-9 production by naive CD4$^+$ T cells relies on the presence of IL-2 and, hence, seems to be controlled by STAT5. Upon differentiation of naive CD4$^+$ T cells into Th9 cells, *Il9* expression can be further enhanced (+) or inhibited (−) by distinct cytokines. For example, IL-1 and IL-25 both induce NF-κB translocation to the nucleus and thus show an IL-9-enhancing capacity. The inhibitory effects of IFN-γ receptor signaling on *Il9* expression have been extensively demonstrated. Although the underlying molecular mechanisms are still elusive, IFN-γ most presumably exerts its inhibitory effect *via* the induction of STAT1. Question marks identify transcription factors whose contribution is arguable.

strictly relies on this transcription factor.[24] Notably, an NF-κB motif in the *Il9* promoter can be bound by the HTLV-I protein Tax, leading to an enhanced expression of *Il9* by adult T cell leukemia (ATL).[97] Consistent with this, it was shown that IL-1R1- and IL-25 receptor–mediated signals, which lead to NF-κB translocation to the nucleus, enhance IL-9 production (Fig. 4). In addition, IL-1α, IL-1β, IL-18, and IL-33 have analogous IL-9–inducing activities when interacting with TGF-β. However, these cytokines also stimulate IL-17 production,[31] excluding a unique role for NF-κB in the transcriptional regulation of the *Il9* gene in Th9 cells. Of course, members of the NFAT family of transcription factors and NF-κB contribute to the regulation of a great variety of cytokine genes, and hence lack specificity for Th9 development and IL-9 production. Recently, we and others were able to identify two transcription factors, interferon regulatory factor 4 (IRF4) and PU.1, that essentially contribute to IL-9 production by Th9 cells (Fig. 3).[29,30]

In 2010 IRF4 was demonstrated to be essential for the development and function of murine and human Th9 cells.[29] Using chromatin immunoprecipitation, these experiments showed binding of IRF4 to the *Il9* promoter in developing Th9 cells. In ad-

dition, deficiency in IRF4 precluded *Il9* expression and Th9 development, and siRNA-mediated silencing of IRF4 greatly diminished Th9 development, as well as IL-9 production in already established Th9 cells. Further work demonstrated that IRF4-deficient mice do not develop IL-9–dependent allergic inflammation in the lungs and have significantly reduced eosinophil recruitment due to a lack of Th9 cells. Together, these findings demonstrate the essential role of IRF4 in the development, maintenance, and effector function of Th9 cells.

Gene expression is tightly controlled by numerous *cis*-regulatory elements present within the promoter region of a given gene, in addition to *trans*-activating factors. A great variety of transcription factors form complexes to modulate transcriptional activity, and depending on their composition, these complexes can either promote or repress the expression of genes. Notably, IRF4 has also been shown to be involved in the development of Th2 and Th17 cells, underlining its essential role in Th cell differentiation more generally. Comparative analyses revealed that IRF4 is expressed in greater amount in T cells cultured under Th9-polarizing conditions, compared to Th2- or Th17-polarizing culture conditions.[29] Nonetheless, it has to be assumed that IRF4 regulates the development of different T cell subsets in concerted interactions with additional subset-determining transcription factors.

One possible partner for IRF4 in the regulation of Th9 development is the ETS transcription factor family member PU.1.[98] IRF4 was initially identified as PU.1-interacting protein. Like IRF4-deficient T cells, PU.1-deficient T cells show greatly diminished IL-9 production, compared to wild-type T cells, upon stimulation in the presence of TGF-β and IL-4.[30] In addition, PU.1-deficient mice show attenuated allergic pulmonary inflammation. On the other hand, ectopic expression of PU.1 not only represses Th2-associated cytokines—most likely by interfering with GATA-3 function—but also enhances IL-9 production in Th9 cells. However, PU.1 demonstrated only modest IL-9–enhancing activity upon transduction of Th cell subsets, whose development does not rely on the expression of IRF4. This result underestimates the essential role of IRF4 as a cooperation partner for PU.1 to drive *Il9* promoter activity. Moreover, PU.1 expression is transiently induced during Th2 development as well,[99] implying additional supplementary roles in the developmental programs of other T helper cells.

## Concluding remarks

The recent definition of a Th9 cell subset based on preferential production of IL-9 has stimulated efforts to identify a Th9 lineage-specific transcription factor. Results from recent studies have demonstrated that IRF4 and PU.1 are essentially involved in Th9 development and maintenance. However, IRF4 and PU.1 are also involved in the development of other Th subsets (e.g., Th2 and Th17). Thus knowledge about transcription factors and/or conditions that preferentially drive *Il9* expression and Th9 development is still relatively rudimentary and must be substantially improved. Nevertheless, the findings that Th9 cells serve as an important source of IL-9, which contributes fundamentally, for example to the development of asthma, has already put these cells into central focus of immune therapeutic strategies instrumental for the treatment of this and other allergic diseases.

## Acknowledgments

T.B. and E.S. are supported by the Deutsche Forschungsgemeinschaft (DFG), Grants SCHM 1014/5-1 (T.B. and E.S.), SFB TR52 TPA1 (T.B. and E.S.), GRK 1043: International Graduate School for Immunotherapy (E.S. and T.B.), the "Forschungszentrum Immunologie (FZI)," and The MAIFOR program of the University Medical Centre JGU Mainz (T.B. and E.S.). M.S. is supported by the DFG Grant STA984/1-2.

## Conflicts of interest

The authors declare no conflicts of interest.

## References

1. Tada, T., T. Takemori, K. Okumura, *et al.* 1978. Two distinct types of helper T cells involved in the secondary antibody response: independent and synergistic effects of Ia− and Ia+ helper T cells. *J. Exp. Med.* **147:** 446–458.

2. Swierkosz, J.E., K. Rock, P. Marrack, & J.W. Kappler. 1978. The role of H-2 linked genes in helper T-cell function: II. Isolation on antigen-pulsed macrophages of two separate populations of F1 helper T cells each specific for antigen and one set of parental H-2 products. *J. Exp. Med.* **147:** 554–570.

3. Imperiale, M.J., D.A. Faherty, J.F. Sproviero & M. Zauderer. 1982. Functionally distinct helper T cells enriched under different culture conditions cooperate with different B cells. *J. Immunol.* **129:** 1843–1848.

4. Kim, J., A. Woods, E. Becker-Dunn & K. Bottomly. 1985. Distinct functional phenotypes of cloned Ia-restricted helper T cells. *J. Exp. Med.* **162:** 188–201.

5. Mosmann, T.R., H. Cherwinski, M.W. Bond, *et al.* 1986. Two types of murine helper T cell clone: I. Definition according to profiles of lymphokine activities and secreted proteins. *J. Immunol.* **136:** 2348–2357.

6. Cherwinski, H., J. Schumacher, K. Brown & T. Mosmann. 1987. Two types of mouse helper T cell clone: III. Further differences in lymphokine synthesis between Th1 and Th2 clones revealed by RNA hybridization, functionally monospecific bioassays, and monoclonal antibodies. *J. Exp. Med.* **166:** 1229–1244.

7. Cher, D.J. & T.R. Mosmann. 1987. Two types of murine helper T cell clone: II. Delayed-type hypersensitivity is mediated by TH1 clones. *J. Immunol.* **138:** 3688–3694.

8. Schmitt, E., R. van Brandwijk, H.G. Fischer & E. Rude. 1990. Establishment of different T cell sublines using either interleukin 2 or interleukin 4 as growth factors. *Eur. J. Immunol.* **20:** 1709–1715.

9. Uyttenhove, C., R.J. Simpson & J. Van Snick. 1988. Functional and structural characterization of P40, a mouse glycoprotein with T-cell growth factor activity. *Proc. Natl. Acad. Sci. USA* **85:** 6934–6938.

10. Van Snick, J., A. Goethals, J.C. Renauld, *et al.* 1989. Cloning and characterization of a cDNA for a new mouse T cell growth factor (P40). *J. Exp. Med.* **169:** 363–368.

11. Schmitt, E., R. van Brandwijk, J. Van Snick, *et al.* 1989. TCGF III/P40 is produced by naive murine CD4+ T cells but is not a general T cell growth factor. *Eur. J. Immunol.* **19:** 2167–2170.

12. Moeller, J., L. Hültner, E. Schmitt, *et al.* 1990. Purification of MEA, a mast cell growth-enhancing activity, to apparent homogeneity and its partial amino acid sequencing. *J. Immunol.* **144:** 4231–4234.

13. Hultner, L., C. Druez, J. Moeller, *et al.* 1990. Mast cell growth-enhancing activity (MEA) is structurally related and functionally identical to the novel mouse T cell growth factor P40/TCGFIII (interleukin 9). *Eur. J. Immunol.* **20:** 1413–1416.

14. Shimbara, A., P. Christodoulopoulos, A. Soussi-Gounni, *et al.* 2000. IL-9 and its receptor in allergic and nonallergic lung disease: increased expression in asthma. *J. Allergy Clin. Immunol.* **105:** 108–115.

15. Gessner, A., H. Blum & M. Rollinghoff. 1993. Differential regulation of IL-9-expression after infection with Leishmania major in susceptible and resistant mice. *Immunobiology* **189:** 419–435.

16. Faulkner, H., J.C. Renauld, J. Van Snick & R.K. Grencis. 1998. Interleukin-9 enhances resistance to the intestinal nematode Trichuris muris. *Infect. Immun.* **66:** 3832–3840.

17. Fallon, P.G., P. Smith, E.J. Richardson, *et al.* 2000. Expression of interleukin-9 leads to Th2 cytokine-dominated responses and fatal enteropathy in mice with chronic Schistosoma mansoni infections. *Infect. Immun.* **68:** 6005–6011.

18. Monteyne, P., J.C. Renauld, J. Van Broeck, *et al.* 1997. IL-4-independent regulation of in vivo IL-9 expression. *J. Immunol.* **159:** 2616–2623.

19. Hültner, L., S. Koelsch, M. Stassen, *et al.* 2000. In activated mast cells, IL-1 up-regulates the production of several Th2-related cytokines including IL-9. *J. Immunol.* **164:** 5556–5563.

20. Stassen, M., M. Arnold, L. Hultner, *et al.* 2000. Murine bone marrow-derived mast cells as potent producers of IL-9: costimulatory function of IL-10 and kit ligand in the presence of IL-1. *J. Immunol.* **164:** 5549–5555.

21. Lorentz, A., S. Schwengberg, G. Sellge, *et al.* 2000. Human intestinal mast cells are capable of producing different cytokine profiles: role of IgE receptor cross-linking and IL-4. *J. Immunol.* **164:** 43–48.

22. Gounni, A.S., E. Nutku, L. Koussih, *et al.* 2000. IL-9 expression by human eosinophils: regulation by IL-1beta and TNF-alpha. *J. Allergy Clin. Immunol.* **106:** 460–466.

23. Schmitt, E., H.U. Beuscher, C. Huels, *et al.* 1991. IL-1 serves as a secondary signal for IL-9 expression. *J. Immunol.* **147:** 3848–3854.

24. Stassen, M., C. Muller, M. Arnold, *et al.* 2001. IL-9 and IL-13 production by activated mast cells is strongly enhanced in the presence of lipopolysaccharide: NF-kappa B is decisively involved in the expression of IL-9. *J. Immunol.* **166:** 4391–4398.

25. Stassen, M., M. Klein, M. Becker, *et al.* 2007. p38 MAP kinase drives the expression of mast cell-derived IL-9 via activation of the transcription factor GATA-1. *Mol. Immunol.* **44:** 926–933.

26. Schmitt, E., T. Germann, S. Goedert, *et al.* 1994. IL-9 production of naive CD4+ T cells depends on IL-2, is synergistically enhanced by a combination of TGF-beta and IL-4, and is inhibited by IFN-gamma. *J. Immunol.* **153:** 3989–3996.

27. Dardalhon, V., A. Awasthi, H. Kwon, *et al.* 2008. IL-4 inhibits TGF-β-induced Foxp3+ T cells and, together with TGF-β, generates IL-9+ IL-10+ Foxp3− effector T cells. *Nat. Immunol.* **9:** 1347–1355.

28. Veldhoen, M., C. Uyttenhove, J. Van Snick, *et al.* 2008. Transforming growth factor-β 'reprograms' the differentiation of T helper 2 cells and promotes an interleukin 9-producing subset. *Nat. Immunol.* **9:** 1341–1346.

29. Staudt, V., E. Bothur, M. Klein, *et al.* 2010. Interferon-regulatory factor 4 is essential for the developmental program of T helper 9 cells. *Immunity* **33:** 192–202.

30. Chang, H.-C., S. Sehra, R. Goswami, *et al.* 2010. The transcription factor PU.1 is required for the development of IL-9-producing T cells and allergic inflammation. *Nat. Immunol.* **9:** 527–534.

31. Uyttenhove, C., F. Brombacher & J. Van Snick. 2010. TGF-beta interactions with IL-1 family members trigger IL-4-independent IL-9 production by mouse CD4(+) T cells. *Eur. J. Immunol.* **40:** 2230–2235.

32. Tan, C., M.K. Aziz, J.D. Lovaas, *et al.* 2010. Antigen-specific Th9 cells exhibit uniqueness in their kinetics of cytokine production and short retention at the inflammatory site. *J. Immunol.* **185:** 6795–6801.

33. Lu, L.-F., E.F. Lind, D.C. Gondek, *et al.* 2006. Mast cells are essential intermediaries in regulatory T-cell tolerance. *Nature* **442:** 997–1002.

34. Beriou, G., E.M. Bradshaw, E. Lozano, *et al.* 2010. TGF-beta induces IL-9 production from human Th17 cells. *J. Immunol.* **185:** 46–54.

35. Soler, D., T.R. Chapman, L.R. Poisson, *et al.* 2006. CCR8 expression identifies CD4 memory T cells enriched for FOXP3+ regulatory and Th2 effector lymphocytes. *J. Immunol.* **177:** 6940–6951.

36. Elyaman, W., E.M. Bradshaw, C. Uyttenhove, *et al.* 2009. IL-9 induces differentiation of TH17 cells and enhances function of FoxP3+ natural regulatory T cells. *Proc. Natl. Acad. Sci. USA* **106:** 12885–12890.

37. Putheti, P., A. Awasthi, J. Popoola, *et al.* 2010. Human CD4 memory T cells can become CD4+IL-9+ T cells. *PLoS One* **5:**e8706.

38. Jager, A., V. Dardalhon, R.A. Sobel, *et al.* 2009. Th1, Th17, and Th9 effector cells induce experimental autoimmune encephalomyelitis with different pathological phenotypes. *J. Immunol.* **183:** 7169–7177.

39. Lee, Y.K., R. Mukasa, R.D. Hatton & C.T. Weaver. 2009. Developmental plasticity of Th17 and Treg cells. *Curr. Opin. Immunol.* **21:** 274–280.

40. Zhou, X., S. Bailey-Bucktrout, L.T. Jeker & J.A. Bluestone. 2009. Plasticity of CD4(+) FoxP3(+) T cells. *Curr. Opin. Immunol.* **21:** 281–285.

41. Zhou, L. & D.R. Littman. 2009. Transcriptional regulatory networks in Th17 cell differentiation. *Curr. Opin. Immunol.* **21:** 146–152.

42. Zhou, L., M.M. Chong & D.R. Littman. 2009. Plasticity of CD4+ T cell lineage differentiation. *Immunity* **30:** 646–655.

43. Lingnau, K., P. Hoehn, S. Kerdine, *et al.* 1998. IL-4 in combination with TGF-beta favors an alternative pathway of Th1 development independent of IL-12. *J. Immunol.* **161:** 4709–4718.

44. Angkasekwinai, P., S.H. Chang, M. Thapa, *et al.* 2010. Regulation of IL-9 expression by IL-25 signaling. *Nat. Immunol.* **11:** 250–256.

45. Doull, I.J., S. Lawrence, M. Watson, *et al.* 1996. Allelic association of gene markers on chromosomes 5q and 11q with atopy and bronchial hyperresponsiveness. *Am. J. Respir. Crit. Care Med.* **153:** 1280–1284.

46. Nicolaides, N.C., K.J. Holroyd, S.L. Ewart, *et al.* 1997. Interleukin 9: a candidate gene for asthma. *Proc. Natl. Acad. Sci. USA* **94:** 13175–13180.

47. Reader, J.R. 2003. Interleukin-9 induces mucous cell metaplasia independent of inflammation. *Am. J. Respir. Cell. Mol. Biol.* **28:** 664–672.

48. Levitt, R.C., M.P. McLane, D. MacDonald, *et al.* 1999. IL-9 pathway in asthma: new therapeutic targets for allergic inflammatory disorders. *J. Allergy Clin. Immunol.* **103:** S485–S491.

49. Temann, U.A., G.P. Geba, J.A. Rankin & R.A. Flavell. 1998. Expression of interleukin 9 in the lungs of transgenic mice causes airway inflammation, mast cell hyperplasia, and bronchial hyperresponsiveness. *J. Exp. Med.* **188:** 1307–1320.

50. McLane, M.P., A. Haczku, M. van de Rijn, *et al.* 1998. Interleukin-9 promotes allergen-induced eosinophilic inflammation and airway hyperresponsiveness in transgenic mice. *Am. J. Respir. Cell. Mol. Biol.* **19:** 713–720.

51. Kung, T.T., B. Luo, Y. Crawley, *et al.* 2001. Effect of anti-mIL-9 antibody on the development of pulmonary inflammation and airway hyperresponsiveness in allergic mice. *Am. J. Respir. Cell. Mol. Biol.* **25:** 600–605.

52. Cheng, G. 2002. Anti-interleukin-9 antibody treatment inhibits airway inflammation and hyperreactivity in mouse asthma model. *Am. J. Respir. Crit. Care Med.* **166:** 409–416.

53. Temann, U.-A. 2002. Pulmonary overexpression of IL-9 induces Th2 cytokine expression, leading to immune pathology. *J. Clin. Invest.* **109:** 29–39.

54. Van Den Brule, S., J. Heymans, X. Havaux, *et al.* 2007. Profibrotic effect of IL-9 overexpression in a model of airway remodeling. *Am. J. Respir. Cell. Mol. Biol.* **37:** 202–209.

55. Kearley, J., J.S. Erjefalt, C. Andersson, *et al.* 2010. IL-9 governs allergen-induced mast cell numbers in the lung and chronic remodeling of the airways. *Am. J. Respir. Crit. Care Med.* **183:** 865–875.

56. Arras, M., F. Huaux, A. Vink, *et al.* 2001. Interleukin-9 reduces lung fibrosis and type 2 immune polarization induced by silica particles in a murine model. *Am. J. Respir. Cell. Mol. Biol.* **24:** 368–375.

57. Arras, M., J. Louahed, J.-F. Heilier, *et al.* 2005. IL-9 protects against bleomycin-induced lung injury: involvement of prostaglandins. *Am. J. Pathol.* **166:** 107–115.

58. Wiener, Z., A. Falus, & S. Toth. 2004. IL-9 increases the expression of several cytokines in activated mast cells, while the IL-9-induced IL-9 production is inhibited in mast cells of histamine-free transgenic mice. *Cytokine* **26:** 122–130.

59. Eklund, K.K., N. Ghildyal, K.F. Austen & R.L. Stevens. 1993. Induction by IL-9 and suppression by IL-3 and IL-4 of the levels of chromosome 14-derived transcripts that encode late-expressed mouse mast cell proteases. *J. Immunol.* **151:** 4266–4273.

60. Petit-Frere, C., B. Dugas, P. Braquet & J.M. Mencia-Huerta. 1993. Interleukin-9 potentiates the interleukin-4-induced IgE and IgG1 release from murine B lymphocytes. *Immunology* **79:** 146–151.

61. Dugas, B., J.C. Renauld, J. Pene, *et al.* 1993. Interleukin-9 potentiates the interleukin-4-induced immunoglobulin (IgG, IgM and IgE) production by normal human B lymphocytes. *Eur. J. Immunol.* **23:** 1687–1692.

62. Vink, A., G. Warnier, F. Brombacher & J.C. Renauld. 1999. Interleukin 9-induced in vivo expansion of the B-1 lymphocyte population. *J. Exp. Med.* **189:** 1413–1423.

63. Dong, Q., J. Louahed, A. Vink, *et al.* 1999. IL-9 induces chemokine expression in lung epithelial cells and baseline airway eosinophilia in transgenic mice. *Eur. J. Immunol.* **29:** 2130–2139.

64. Longphre, M., D. Li, M. Gallup, *et al.* 1999. Allergen-induced IL-9 directly stimulates mucin transcription in respiratory epithelial cells. *J. Clin. Invest.* **104:** 1375–1382.

65. Louahed, J., M. Toda, J. Jen, *et al.* 2000. Interleukin-9 up-regulates mucus expression in the airways [see comments]. *Am. J. Respir. Cell. Mol. Biol.* **22:** 649–656.

66. Louahed, J. 2001. Interleukin 9 promotes influx and local maturation of eosinophils. *Blood* **97:** 1035–1042.

67. Baraldo, S., D.S. Faffe, P.E. Moore, *et al.* 2003. Interleukin-9 influences chemokine release in airway smooth muscle: role of ERK. *Am. J. Physiol. Lung Cell. Mol. Physiol.* **284:** L1093–L1102.

68. Steenwinckel, V., J. Louahed, C. Orabona, *et al.* 2007. IL-13 mediates in vivo IL-9 activities on lung epithelial cells but not on hematopoietic cells. *J. Immunol.* **178:** 3244–325.

69. McMillan, S.J., B. Bishop, M.J. Townsend, *et al.* 2002. The absence of interleukin 9 does not affect the development of allergen-induced pulmonary inflammation nor airway hyperreactivity. *J. Exp. Med.* **195:** 51–57.

70. Ying, S., Q. Meng, A.B. Kay & D.S. Robinson. 2002. Elevated expression of interleukin-9 mRNA in the bronchial mucosa of atopic asthmatics and allergen-induced cutaneous late-phase reaction: relationships to eosinophils, mast cells and T lymphocytes. *Clin. Exp. Allergy* **32:** 866–871.

71. Toda, M., M.K. Tulic, R.C. Levitt & Q. Hamid. 2002. A calcium-activated chloride channel (HCLCA1) is strongly related to IL-9 expression and mucus production in bronchial epithelium of patients with asthma. *J. Allergy Clin. Immunol.* **109:** 246–250.

72. Erpenbeck, V.J., J.M. Hohlfeld, B. Volkmann, *et al.* 2003. Segmental allergen challenge in patients with atopic asthma leads to increased IL-9 expression in bronchoalveolar lavage fluid lymphocytes. *J. Allergy Clin. Immunol.* **111:** 1319–1327.

73. Parker, J.M., C.K. Oh, C. Laforce, *et al.* 2011. Safety profile and clinical activity of multiple subcutaneous doses of MEDI-528, a humanized anti-interleukin-9 monoclonal antibody, in two randomized phase 2a studies in subjects with asthma. *BMC Pulmonary Med.* **28:** 11–14.

74. Richard, M., R. Grencis, N.E. Humphreys, *et al.* 2000. Anti-IL-9 vaccination prevents worm expulsion and blood eosinophilia in Trichuris muris-infected mice. *Proc. Natl. Acad. Sci. USA* **97:** 767–772.

75. Leech, M.D. & R. Grencis. 2006. Induction of enhanced immunity to intestinal nematodes using IL-9-producing dendritic cells. *J. Immunol.* **176:** 2505–2511.

76. Khan, W.I., M. Richard, H. Akiho, *et al.* 2003. Modulation of intestinal muscle contraction by interleukin-9 (IL-9) or IL-9 neutralization: correlation with worm expulsion in murine nematode infections. *Infect. Immun.* **71:** 2430–2438.

77. Forbes, E.E., K. Groschwitz, J.P. Abonia, *et al.* 2008. IL-9- and mast cell-mediated intestinal permeability predisposes to oral antigen hypersensitivity. *J. Exp. Med.* **205:** 897–913.

78. Knoops, L., J. Louahed, J. Van Snick & J.-C. Renauld. 2005. IL-9 promotes but is not necessary for systemic anaphylaxis. *J. Immunol.* **175:** 335–341.

79. Osterfeld, H., R. Ahrens, R. Strait, *et al.* 2010. Differential roles for the IL-9/IL-9 receptor & alpha-chain pathway in systemic and oral antigen-induced anaphylaxis. *J. Allergy Clin. Immunol.* **125:** 469–476.

80. Dodd, J.S., E. Lum, J. Goulding, *et al.* 2009. IL-9 regulates pathology during primary and memory responses to respiratory syncytial virus infection. *J. Immunol.* **183:** 7006–7013.

81. Grohmann, U., J. Van Snick, F. Campanile, *et al.* 2000. IL-9 protects mice from Gram-negative bacterial shock: suppression of TNF-alpha, IL-12, and IFN-gamma, and induction of IL-10. *J. Immunol.* **164:** 4197–4203.

82. Pilette, C., Y. Ouadrhiri, J. Van Snick, *et al.* 2002. IL-9 inhibits oxidative burst and TNF-alpha release in lipopolysaccharide-stimulated human monocytes through TGF-beta. *J. Immunol.* **168:** 4103–4111.

83. Nowak, E.C., C.T. Weaver, H. Turner, *et al.* 2009. IL-9 as a mediator of Th17-driven inflammatory disease. *J. Exp. Med.* **206:** 1653–1660.

84. Li, H., B. Nourbakhsh, B. Ciric, *et al.* 2010. Neutralization of IL-9 ameliorates experimental autoimmune encephalomyelitis by decreasing the effector T cell population. *J. Immunol.* **185:** 4095–4100.

85. Peron, J.P.S., K. Yang, M.-L. Chen, *et al.* 2010. Oral tolerance reduces Th17 cells as well as the overall inflammation in the central nervous system of EAE mice. *J. Neuroimmunol.* **227:** 10–17.

86. Zhou, Y., Y. Sonobe, T. Akahori, *et al.* 2011. IL-9 promotes Th17 cell migration into the central nervous system via CC chemokine ligand-20 produced by astrocytes. *J. Immunol.* **186:** 4415–4421.

87. De Vries, V.C., A. Wasiuk, K.A. Bennett, *et al.* 2009. Mast cell degranulation breaks peripheral tolerance. *Am. J. Transplant.* **9:** 1–11.

88. Eller, K., D. Wolf, J.M. Huber, *et al.* 2011. IL-9 production by regulatory T cells recruits mast cells that are essential for regulatory T cell-induced immune suppression. *J. Immunol.* **186:** 83–91.

89. Zhu, J., B. Min, J. Hu-Li, *et al.* 2004. Conditional deletion of Gata3 shows its essential function in T(H)1-T(H)2 responses. *Nat. Immunol.* **5:** 1157–1165.

90. Takimoto, T., Y. Wakabayashi, T. Sekiya, *et al.* 2010. Smad2 and Smad3 are redundantly essential for the TGF-beta-mediated regulation of regulatory T plasticity and Th1 development. *J. Immunol.* **185:** 842–855.

91. Ichiyama, K., T. Sekiya, N. Inoue, *et al.* 2011. Transcription factor Smad-independent T helper 17 cell induction by transforming-growth factor-beta is mediated by suppression of eomesodermin. *Immunity* **34:** 741–754.

92. Pearce, E.L., A.C. Mullen, G.A. Martins, *et al.* 2003. Control of effector CD8+ T cell function by the transcription factor eomesodermin. *Science* **302:** 1041–1043.

93. Suto, A., A.L. Wurster, S.L. Reiner & M.J. Grusby. 2006. IL-21 inhibits IFN-gamma production in developing Th1 cells through the repression of eomesodermin expression. *J. Immunol.* **177:** 3721–3727.

94. Yang, Y., J. Xu, Y. Niu, *et al.* 2008. T-bet and eomesodermin play critical roles in directing T cell differentiation to Th1 versus Th17. *J. Immunol.* **181:** 8700–8710.

95. Perumal, N.B. & M.H. Kaplan. 2011. Regulating Il9 transcription in T helper cells. *Trends Immunol.* **32:** 146–150.

96. Serfling, E., F. Berberich-Siebelt, S. Chuvpilo, *et al.* 2000. The role of NF-AT transcription factors in T cell activation and differentiation. *Biochim. Biophys. Acta* **1498:** 1–18.

97. Chen, J., M. Petrus, B.R. Bryant, *et al.* 2008. Induction of the IL-9 gene by HTLV-I Tax stimulates the spontaneous proliferation of primary adult T-cell leukemia cells by a paracrine mechanism. *Blood* **111:** 5163–5172.

98. Yee, A.A., P. Yin, D.P. Siderovski, *et al.* 1998. Cooperative interaction between the DNA-binding domains of PU.1 and IRF4. *J. Mol. Biol.* **279:** 1075–1083

99. Hadjur, S., L. Bruno, A. Hertweck, *et al.* 2009. IL4 blockade of inducible regulatory T cell differentiation: the role of Th2 cells, Gata3 and PU.1. *Immunol. Lett* **122:** 37–43.

Ann. N.Y. Acad. Sci. ISSN 0077-8923

ANNALS OF THE NEW YORK ACADEMY OF SCIENCES
Issue: *The Year in Immunology*

# Mechanisms of immunosenescence: lessons from models of accelerated immune aging

Sabine Le Saux, Cornelia M. Weyand, and Jörg J. Goronzy

Department of Medicine, Division of Immunology and Rheumatology, Stanford University School of Medicine, Stanford, California and Palo Alto Department of Veterans Affairs Health Care System, Palo Alto, California

Address for correspondence: Jörg J. Goronzy, M.D., Department of Medicine, Division of Immunology and Rheumatology, Stanford University School of Medicine CCSR Building, Room 2215, Mail Code 5166 269 Campus Drive West Stanford, CA 94305-5166 jgoronzy@stanford.edu

With increasing age, the ability of the adaptive immune system to respond to vaccines and to protect from infection declines. In parallel, the production of inflammatory mediators increases. While cross-sectional studies have been successful in defining age-dependent immunological phenotypes, studies of accelerated immune aging in human subpopulations have been instrumental in obtaining mechanistic insights. The immune system depends on its regenerative capacity; however, the T cell repertoire, once established, is relatively robust to aging and only decompensates when additionally stressed. Such stressors include chronic infections such as CMV and HIV, even when viral replication is controlled, and autoimmune diseases. Reduced regenerative capacity, chronic immune activation in the absence of cell exhaustion, T cell memory inflation, and accumulation of highly potent effector T cells in these patients synergize to develop an immune phenotype that is characteristic of the elderly. Studies of accelerated immune aging in autoimmune diseases have identified an unexpected link to chronic DNA damage responses that are known to be important in aging, but so far had not been implicated in immune aging.

Keywords: immune aging; thymic involution; HIV; CMV; autoimmunity; latency

## Introduction

The immune system is a dynamic system that is highly dependent on the regenerative power of hematopoietic precursor cells and that is constantly challenged by external and internal forces threatening the homeostasis of the system. It is not surprising that the immune system undergoes dramatic changes with age. In particular, the adaptive immune system is affected because it relies on complicated selection mechanisms, and it constantly has to find a balance between maintaining homeostasis and adapting to external stresses. Immune aging, therefore, includes the collective antigen experience of the organism stored as immune memory. At the same time, the major clinical manifestation of immune aging is an increased susceptibility to infections, both to new infections and also to some, but not all, chronic or latent infections. In immune aging research, it is, therefore, often difficult to decipher between adaptation, such as memory formation and cell differentiation, and defects such as cellular senescence. Frequently, age-associated changes reflect a combination of both. Most studies rely on comparison between cohorts of different ages. While these can reliably identify differences, the mechanism leading to these differences and their implications for immune health are not very well understood. Animal models are only partially helpful in providing mechanistic insights. In addition to the usual challenge that the murine differs substantially from the human system and that the environmental forces shaping the immune system in different species are fundamentally different,[1] animal models of immune aging face the additional challenge that for many questions it is not possible to telescope time. For example, it is not possible to extrapolate the consequences of thymic involution and homeostatic proliferation for cellular and organismal senescence from a species that has a life

doi: 10.1111/j.1749-6632.2011.06297.x

span of three years to humans living many decades.[2] Longitudinal studies in humans are very difficult because most immune changes associated with aging develop slowly. Longtime studies are not only costly, but also cannot incorporate the rapid technological progress that is being made in developing new immunometric tools.[3,4] Human models of accelerated immune aging have been increasingly explored in the last years to gain insights into the mechanisms and the consequences of the age-related changes in the human immune system. Studies of thymectomized individuals addressed the question of what the true contribution of thymic involution is for some of the phenotypes of immune aging.[5,6] Is it truly necessary to have an active thymus after the age of 20,[7,8] or is the involution of the thymus evolutionary?[9,10] Latent cytomegalovirus (CMV) infection appears to accelerate immune aging.[11,12] What are the mechanisms and what is the difference to other chronic infections that either induce lymphocyte exhaustion rather than immune aging[13] or that exhibit a fading T cell memory leading to reactivation of the latent viruses such as with varicella herpes zoster?[14] Human immunodeficiency virus (HIV) infection under highly active antiretroviral therapy (HAART) treatment has emerged as an interesting model to understand the influence of immune defects on morbidity and mortality of all causes.[15] Finally, accelerated immune aging is seen in some of the autoimmune diseases.[16–18] While it remains to be determined whether this accelerated immune aging is a cause or a consequence of the autoimmune disease, the elucidation of the mechanisms allows conclusions on the common pathway of immune aging in the healthy adult.

## Thymic involution accelerates immune aging

The thymus is known to undergo dramatic structural changes with age.[19,20] Relative thymic output is the highest during early life; absolute output starts to decline after puberty.[21,22] The structural changes are manyfold (Fig. 1). Thymopoietic niches disappear, while the thymic perivascular space increases. These changes are associated with a loss of thymic epithelial cells and thymocytes and the transformation of cells into adipocytes that infiltrate the perivascular space.[23] Given that thymic T cell production essentially ceases after organism growth has been completed, one could argue that

thymic involution is not a typical marker of aging, but rather that thymic production is a developmental step that is no longer needed when the peripheral T cell compartment is seeded with naive T lymphocytes.[8] Indeed, even shortly before and after birth, thymic T cell generation only contributes 50% of the newly generated T cell population in humans; the remainder is produced by peripheral homeostatic proliferation.[24] This initial clonal expansion may be necessary to develop clonal sizes of T lymphocytes sufficient to maintain a diverse repertoire in spite of stochastic loss and compensatory homeostatic proliferation.[25] Studies in DiGeorge syndrome patients in the first two years after thymic transplantation suggested that TCR independent are by far more important than TCR-dependent mechanisms in maintaining T cell compartment size under steady-state conditions.[26] The clonal sizes of naive T lymphocytes have been estimated to be in the order of 1,000–10,000 cells per clonotype.[27] Diversity is similar, but clonal sizes are much smaller in small species, such as the mouse,[28] where holes in the repertoire may develop.[29,30] Data in humans are not available, but acquired holes are unlikely to be the case in larger species. Consistent with this assessment, the diversity of the naive T cell repertoire is relatively stable with age up to 65 years in spite of only minimal influx of new thymocytes during adulthood.[31,32] Homeostatic proliferation, recruitment of naive cells into antigen-specific responses, and transition to the memory compartment may, therefore, increase the variance in clonal sizes, but is not sufficient to induce a significant contraction in repertoire diversity. Preliminary results using deep sequencing of T cell receptor genes are supportive of this interpretation;[33] formal and more detailed analyzes are still pending.

To address the question of whether early thymic demise accelerates immune aging, Appay *et al.* examined young adults thymectomized during early childhood as part of surgical corrections of life-threatening congenital heart defects.[6] Thymectomy during these surgical procedures has been common to improve access to the surgical field, although it is unlikely to be complete and may be quite variable in different individuals. Because there may be some residual tissue, the study provides a lower estimate of the effect of thymic depletion to accelerate immune aging over a 20+ year period. Consistent with other previous studies,[29,32] the authors showed

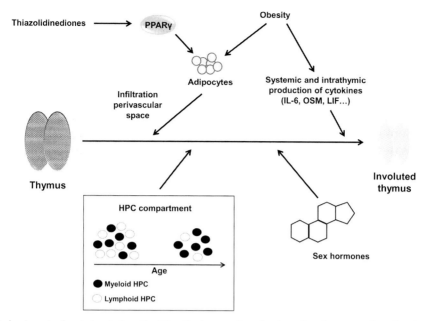

**Figure 1.** Mechanisms in thymic involution. Traditionally, increased production of sex hormones, intrathymic production of inflammatory mediators, and the age-dependent change in lineage commitment of hematopoietic stem cells have been associated with thymic involution. Recently identified accelerators of thymic involution are obesity and possibly PPARγ (peroxisome proliferator-activated receptor gamma) stimulators that are routinely used in the treatment of type II diabetes mellitus and that support adipocyte differentiation and invasion into the perivascular space.

that the absolute CD4$^+$ and CD8$^+$ T cell counts decline, mainly due to loss of naive T cells, and that oligoclonal expansions, mainly within memory CD8$^+$ T cells, emerge. These findings were quite variable in different individuals. A subgroup of individuals had a T cell repertoire characteristic of 50 years older than their biological age, including accumulation of end-differentiated and clonally expanded CD8$^+$ T cells with shortened telomeres.[6] This phenotype was highly associated with seropositivity for previous CMV infection, suggesting that thymic involution alone was not sufficient to destabilize the repertoire even when occurring in a young individual who at time of thymic removal had not established a full T cell repertoire. In synergy with chronic CMV infection, early thymus removal recapitulated the immune phenotype in young adults that is characteristic of the elderly (Fig. 2). In contrast, thymectomized CMV-negative young individuals had a normal T cell repertoire including a normal number of naive T cells. Intriguingly, the authors also found an increased production of inflammatory mediators in their cohort similar to elderly individuals. From their data, it remains undetermined whether this increased production requires

a coinfection with CMV or is also found in CMV-negative thymectomized individuals; nevertheless, the data support the notion that a T cell defect contributes to the activation of the innate immune system and the increased production of inflammatory cytokines in the elderly.

It is well established that aging of the hematopoietic stem cells, serological factors, as well as thymic microenvironment all contribute to thymic involution.[34–36] In spite of their ability to express telomerase, telomeres in hematopoietic stem cells erode with age. However, a shift in lineage commitment from lymphoid to myeloid potential appears to be more important for thymic dysfunction than classical senescence pathways induced by DNA damage accumulation or induction of tumor suppressor pathways in the stem cell.[37] Age-dependent genetic programming may in part account for this shift. Clonal expansion of intrinsically myeloid-based stem cells with robust renewal potential in the aging host may even be more important (Fig. 1). In further support of this interpretation, accelerated thymic involution in the telomere-dysfunctional mouse was conferred by the environment,

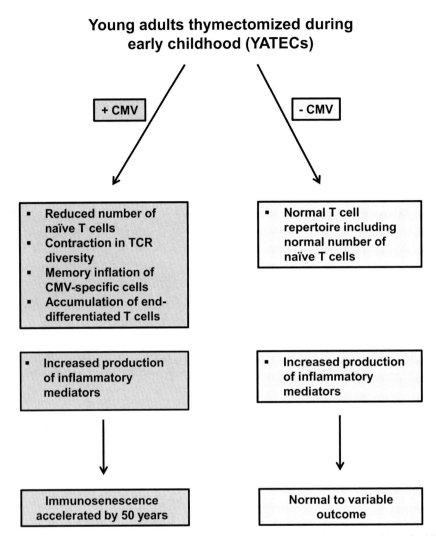

**Figure 2.** CMV infection accelerates immune aging after thymectomy. In individuals thymectomized in early childhood, T cell repertoire changes consistent with accelerated immune aging are mostly limited to those individuals who acquired a CMV infection. Increased production of inflammatory mediators is common in thymectomized individuals, supporting the notion that T cell defects contribute to age-associated inflammation. In the studies so far, the relationship between CMV infection and increased production of inflammatory factors was not examined.

but not by the stem cells expressing shortened telomeres. B and T cell development was only minimally impaired with mTERC$^{-/-}$ hematopoietic stem cells. Moreover, transplantation of dysfunctional thymi from mTERC$^{-/-}$ into wild-type mice restored thymic structure and rejuvenated its function.[38]

One major structural change in thymic organ involution is the infiltration of adipocytes into the perivascular space, which at least in part appears to be caused by a transformation of thymic resident cells into adipocytes.[35,39] Adipocyte development is under the control of peroxisome proliferator-activated receptor gamma (PPARγ) activity, which is targeted by thiazolidinediones, a class of compounds used in the treatment of diabetes mellitus.[40] Rosiglitazone, a member of this family, reduces thymic cellularity, lowered the frequency of T cell receptor excision circles (TREC)$^+$ and naive T cells, and reduced receptor diversity of the peripheral T cell repertoire in a murine model, consistent with the model that it accelerates T cell aging

(Fig. 1). Studies in human diabetic patients are not yet available. This action of rosiglitazone may be a concern for diabetic patients as well as an opportunity to better study the consequences for thymic involution for immune health and aging in an adult human population.

## Accelerated immune aging in CMV-infected individuals

The finding that CMV infection acts in concert with thymic involution to accelerate aging builds on cumulative evidence assembled over the last years.[41] One of the most striking features of immune aging is the shift in T cell subset distributions with a decline in naive T cell population and an increase in effector T cells. In particular, in the CD8 compartment, end-differentiated $CD45RA^+CD8^+CD28^-$ T cells accumulate with age.[42,43] Initial studies showed that this phenotype was characteristic for CMV-specific T cells, even in young individuals, drawing a comparison between the phenotypes found in immune aging and in chronic CMV infection.[44] Subsequent studies have provided evidence for a cross-relationship of CMV infection and immune aging converging into the hypothesis that chronic CMV infection accelerates immune aging (Fig. 3). This hypothesis was built on the following observations. The compartment of CMV-specific T cells in some individuals is huge and comprises a large proportion of the CD4, as well as the CD8, compartment, leading to the hypothesis that memory inflation during chronic infection outcompetes other specificities.[45] In support of this hypothesis, oligoclonal expansions in animal models were found to correlate with defective immune responses to third-party antigens.[46] Moreover, increased frequencies of the effector cell population lacking CD28 inversely correlated with vaccine responses to influenza antigen.[47,48] Inversion of the CD4:CD8 ratio, mainly induced by an expansion of $CD28^-CD8^+$ effector T cells, is the key determinant of an immune risk profile that has been shown to correlate with mortality and morbidity in a Swedish study of octogenarians.[49]

The prevailing hypothesis how chronic CMV infection may accelerate immune aging is that the virus induces an inflation in CMV-specific T cell memory. The first evidence for this hypothesis were HLA-A2 tetramer studies with the pp65 and eventually the IE-1 peptide of the CMV virus that showed $CD8^+$ T cell frequencies in the range of several percents of the total repertoire, significantly higher than for any other viral peptides.[44,50–53] In a more comprehensive study, Picker *et al.* characterized the CMV response using approximately 20,000 overlapping peptides and concluded that the CMV-specific response is very broad and can nearly comprise half of the total $CD8^+$ T cell repertoire in selected individuals.[54] In general, the $CD4^+$ T cell response to CMV is smaller; however, the Picker group also found a large percentage of the CD4 population being specific for CMV in selected individuals. In a study by Akbar *et al.*, expansion of $CD4^+CD28^-$ effector cell populations, either $CD45RA^+$ or $CD45RA^-$, were only found in anti-CMV antibody-positive individuals.[55] Moreover, many of these effector cell populations were specific for CMV antigens, suggesting that qualitatively $CD4^+$, as well as $CD8^+$, T cells are involved in the chronic CMV response, although the magnitude is higher for $CD8^+$ cells. The mechanism underlying these unopposed expansions of CMV-specific T cells to clonal sizes that may compromise the overall immune competence are unclear. Molecular profiling after initial CMV infection showed enhanced expression of genes associated with cell cycle and metabolic activity only in the acute phase, while at all later stages a gene expression signature consistent with a Th1 response, including the expression of Th1-associated transcription factors, eomesodermin, and T-bet, prevailed.[56] CMV-specific cells express high amounts of IFN-$\gamma$, perforin, and granzyme B as well as the fractalkine receptor that is frequently found on cytotoxic effector cells. Such an expression signature is not only limited to $CD8^+$ cells, but is also typical for CMV-specific $CD4^+$ T cell responses. The gene expression profile is completely different from that of exhausted T cells that usually develop in the presence of highly replicating tumors or viruses[57–59] and that are characterized by the expression of a number of inhibitory receptors, such as PD-1 or TIM-3, that impair T cell responses.[60,61] In contrast to exhausted T cells, the CMV-specific T cell response is fully functional, although CMV-specific effector cell populations also frequently express negative regulatory receptors, mostly of the MHC class I—recognizing receptor family such as KIR (killer-cell immunoglobulin-like receptor), KLR (killer-cell lectin-like receptor), and ILT (immunoglobulin-like transcript)[62] and not of the CD28 family, including

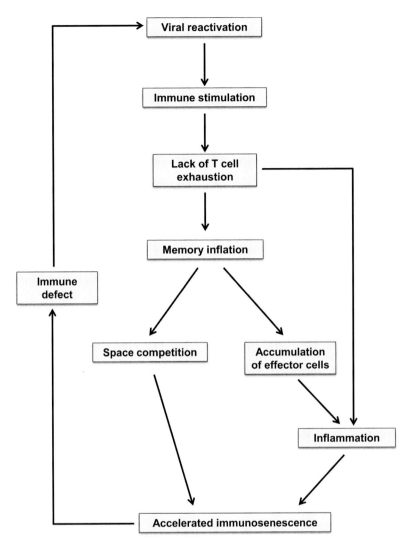

**Figure 3.** CMV-induced acceleration of immune aging. The current model of CMV-induced accelerated immune aging proposes that CMV infection induces T cell memory inflation over time due to chronic stimulation and lack of T cell exhaustion. In addition, increased production of inflammatory mediators due to innate immune stimulation as well as accumulation of T effector cells further compromises immune competence. Defects in the immune control mechanisms of viral latency will feed into a positive feedback loop of accelerated immune aging.

PD-1. This feature sets CMV-specific and age-associated T cell repertoire changes clearly apart from those of chronic active viral diseases.[63] In the latter case, CD8 T cells are getting increasingly dysfunctional, in part due to the expression of negative regulatory receptors PD-1 and TIM-3.[61] In the absence of chronic active infection with highly replicating viruses, PD-1 expression or other features of clonal exhaustion are not a typical marker for immune aging and do not explain the immune defects that are obvious with old age.

Mechanisms underlying the memory inflation to a latent virus are unclear. Memory inflation is not a typical finding for all herpes viruses; for example, T cell responses to varicella-zoster virus (VZV) tend to decline with age rather than to increase[64] and responses to Epstein–Barr virus (EBV) inversely correlate with the size of the CMV-specific compartment.[65] It is possible that the expansion of a highly competent CMV response is responsible for the lasting control of these viruses. Latent VZV infection tends to relapse in patients of old age who are at increased risk of shingles.[66] Animal models that would allow to further mechanistically examine this unique behavior of the CMV response do not exist. Murine gamma herpes viruses, such as gamma-HV68, establish latency, which is effectively controlled by the CD8[+] T cell response over time.[67] Gamma herpes virus-specific CD8[+] T cells remained functionally active, without evidence of clonal exhaustion, and also neither show a decrease nor an increase in frequency with age.[68]

Memory inflation of CMV-specific T cells is a finding of some, but not all, CMV-infected individuals. One of the epidemiological characteristics of CMV infection is that it can be acquired at any age.[69,70] The question whether the age at the time of primary CMV infection may determine the size and nature of the memory T cell response has not been studied. Nikolich-Zugich *et al.* have shown in mice that the global distinctive features of a primary CD8[+] T cell response to an immunodominant herpes simplex virus epitope, glycoprotein B 495–502, was highly conserved independent of what age at which the mice were first infected.[71] It remains to be seen whether this holds up for the CMV infection in humans.

While most studies at this time have focused on the hypothesis that chronic CMV infection accelerates aging and have tried to elucidate the mechanism of this acceleration, as well as the reasons for the variable contribution of CMV infection for immune aging in different individuals, the hypothesis cannot be excluded that memory inflation of the CMV-specific response is a consequence rather than the cause of age-related immune dysfunction. Studies in individuals of long-lived families in the Leiden longevity study have shown that, compared to the age-matched control group, the individuals who presumably carry longevity genes are less susceptible for the characteristic CMV-induced repertoire changes, including the accumulation of CMV-specific large effector cell populations.[72] While this initial finding was consistent with the hypothesis that CMV is an accelerator of immune aging, but only in genetic-susceptible individuals, subsequent studies yielded the surprising result that the incidence of CMV infection, as determined by a positive antibody titer, was much lower in members of long-lived families. These studies indicate that longevity genes protect from infection or allow for clearance of the infection. Consistent with this overall con-

cept, patients with chronic lymphocytic leukemia who are immunocompromised due to their disease have a markedly expanded CMV-specific CD4[+] T cell population, more than twice that of CMV-positive controls.[73] The magnitude of the CMV-specific CD4[+] T cell response correlated with disease stage and also with chemotherapy. Expansion of the CMV response was associated with the phenotypic marker profile that is also characteristic for the subset distribution in CMV-infected elderly individuals.[74] Possibly, immune defects in the innate or NK cell repertoire and their ability to control the CMV infection may lead to an expansion of the adaptive immune response to CMV. Alternatively, increased T cell death generating space may allow for the expansion of CMV-specific T cells. Such a concept would also be consistent with the findings that expansion of CMV-specific cells and intensity of the CMV-specific immune responses are correlated with overall increased morbidity in elderly individuals, such as in a recent study by Sansoni *et al.*, who found an inverse correlation of CD4 and of antibody responses to CMV with impaired health and physical and cognitive functional status.[75]

## Accelerated immune aging and HIV infection

Many of the T cell abnormalities associated with aging are similar to those observed in untreated HIV patients.[76–78] In fact, several of the biomarkers in T cell defects that are now considered as hallmarks of immunosenescence have been first and in more depth studied in the context of HIV infection.[79] Compared to age-matched controls, HIV-infected patients have reduced thymic function as determined by TREC frequencies,[80] a loss in naive T cells, a reduced T cell telomere length, an expansion of end-differentiated effector T cells that have lost the expression of CD28, and a contracted T cell repertoire.[78,79,81,82] All of these changes are also characteristic of the aging immune system in healthy individuals older than 70 years. Clinically, this accelerated immunosenescence in HIV patients has gained increasing relevance now that HIV-infected patients can be treated with antiretroviral therapy and their overall prognosis shifted from years to decades. Antiretroviral therapy can completely suppress viral replication and prevent acquired immune deficiency syndrome-related complications; nevertheless, HIV-infected patients age faster and

# HAART treated HIV patient

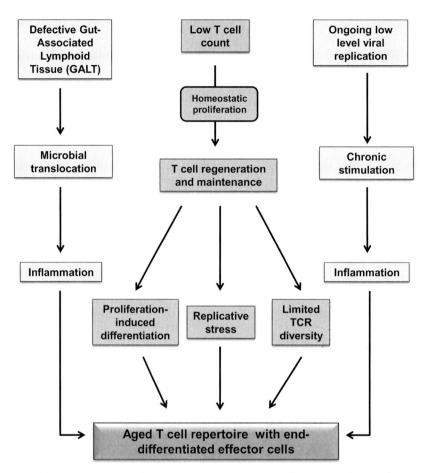

**Figure 4.** Accelerated immunosenescence in the HAART-treated HIV patient. The schematic diagram depicts possible defects and mechanisms that contribute to accelerated immune aging in HIV patients in whom viral replication is controlled on HAART treatment.

prematurely develop age-associated diseases ranging from frailty to cardiovascular disease, central nervous system complications, and renal disease.[83] The increased morbidity and mortality from all causes in HIV-infected patients has been proposed to be causally linked to accelerated immunosenescence. Although lymphocyte counts recover in many patients after the institution of antiretroviral therapy, not all HIV-associated immune defects can be restored.[84,85] Several lines of evidence suggest that the aging of the immune system continues to be accelerated even though viral replication is suppressed. Accelerated immune senescence features in treated HIV patients include

impaired hematopoiesis, impaired T cell generation and homeostasis, functional defects in vaccine responses, and increased constitutive production of inflammatory mediators comparable to what is observed in healthy elderly individuals.[76,78,86] Understanding immune aging in treated HIV-infected patients is, therefore, not only important to improve quality of life and life expectancy in these patients, but also provides a unique model to identify pathways that are central to normal immune aging (Fig. 4). Accelerated immune aging in HIV-infected patients is certainly not caused by a single mechanism. Obviously, the treated HIV patient needs to rebuild his or her T cell repertoire at an age when thymic function is compromised by age and even more so by the infection.[87] Even if normal lymphocyte numbers are being reached, T cell diversity and subset distribution may be compromised. Homeostatic proliferation to rebuild the repertoire will not only increase replicative stress to the system, but will also be associated with proliferation-induced differentiation even in the absence of antigen recognition, as shown in the murine system. Similar to the situation in the thymectomized children, cooccurrence with latent CMV infection in HIV-infected patients is likely a confounding cofactor that accelerates immune aging in a host who has a compromised T cell regenerative system and repertoire stability.[88] Restoring thymic activity for this rebuilding process will be more important than it is for normal immune aging, but similar needs can be envisioned for a number of medical conditions other than HIV infection, such as the condition after chemotherapeutic therapy. Strategies developed mostly in preclinical models to improve thymic output include sex hormone ablation; inhibition of c-kit; and administration of various growth factors, in particular growth hormone, keratinocyte growth factor, acetylated ghrelin, and interleukin (IL)-7.[89,90] In a clinical study of 22 HIV-infected patients with a mean age of 50 years and antiretroviral treatment of two years, daily subcutaneous injection of growth hormone increased thymic size, T cell output, and peripheral numbers of naive CD4[+] T cells.[91]

Accelerated aging in treated HIV patients provides an opportunity to understand how the senescent immune system contributes to major dysfunction in organ systems that are generally considered to not be dependent on immune function, such as the cardiovascular and nervous systems, lungs, and kidneys. Constitutively increased production of inflammatory mediators is likely an important link between immunosenescence and the accelerated dysfunction in several nonimmune organ systems. Deregulation of this inflammatory process in the treated HIV patients, as well as in the aging host, appears to be complex, and several pathways are currently being explored for their relevance. Expansion and activation of CD8 effector cell populations appear to contribute, in particular, when the immune system is not able to fully control latent viral infections and when features of T cell exhaustion are absent, as they are in the aging host. Cellular

senescence by itself induces the activation of gene regulatory pathways that control the production of inflammatory pathways not only in hematopoietic lineages, but also in nonimmune cells. Loss of the gut-associated lymphoid tissue is one of the hallmarks of HIV infection and is not easily reversible with antiretroviral therapy. Loss of gut mucosal integrity will lead to increased microbial translocation, which will stimulate the innate immune system and lead to the production of inflammatory mediators. How well the gut-associated lymphoid tissue is preserved in the healthy elderly host is not known.

## Accelerated immune aging and autoimmunity

Several autoimmune diseases have been associated with phenotypic changes that can be interpreted as accelerated immune aging. Many studies have focused on rheumatoid arthritis (RA), with a frequent disease onset in the second half of adult life. In initial studies, patients with RA have been found to have expanded effector CD4[+] and CD8[+] T cell populations that have lost the expression of CD28, a phenotypic marker that has been closely associated with immune aging.[92] Loss of CD28 was particularly evident in patients who had major organ complications in addition to the usual inflammation of small and large joints. Expansion of CD28[−] effector subpopulations has also been observed in other autoimmune diseases, such as Wegener's granulomatosis.[93] While the expansion of CD28[−] effector cell populations could be interpreted as a consequence of a chronic adaptive immune response to an autoantigen as part of the disease process, these clonal populations in the autoimmune disease have also been shown to correlate with CMV infection or even be CMV-specific, suggesting that the autoimmune-prone environment favors clonal expansions to CMV. Some other findings are also supportive of this concept. Telomeric erosion in hematopoietic lineages, including the hematopoietic stem cells, serves as a typical finding in immune senescence. Patients with RA have telomere lengths that are comparable to healthy individuals 20 years older in calendar age.[94] This telomeric erosion is not limited to memory and effector T cell populations, but also includes the naive CD4[+] T cell population, as well as the population of circulating hematopoietic precursor cells, clearly demonstrating that T cell erosion is not a consequence of the expansion

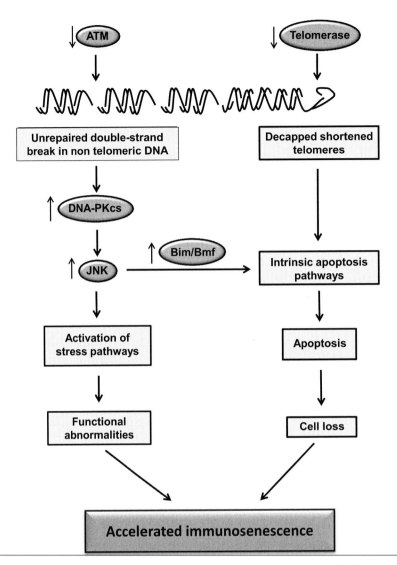

**Figure 5.** Defective DNA damage responses as a cause of accelerated immune aging in patients with rheumatoid arthritis. T cells from patients with RA exhibit shortened telomeres, increased number of DNA double-strand breaks, and chronic DNA damage responses due to defects in telomerase expression and ATM activity. As a consequence, cells undergo apoptosis or enter cellular senescence accelerating the aging process of the global immune system.

and increased replicative history of the T cell population responding to the recognition of autoantigen.[95,96] In part, this premature telomeric erosion in T cells is due to a reduced activation-induced expression of telomerase in naive T cells, consistent with the interpretation that telomeric erosion is not only the reflection of an increased replicative history.[97] Several lines of additional evidence suggest that T cell generation and T cell homeostasis are fundamentally disturbed in patients with RA. Patients with RA have a reduced number of TREC in their CD4 population, suggesting an age disproportional decline in thymic output and/or an increased peripheral replication and T cell loss.[94] Similarly, the repertoire of T cell receptor diversity in the naive T cell populations from patients with RA is contracted, and patients have a smaller number of different T cell receptor β-chain sequences with compensatory increase in clonal sizes, again a finding that could be induced by increased peripheral loss and compensatory homeostatic clonal expansion.[98]

If premature telomeric erosion and immune aging in RA are not consequences of increased replicative stress due to the inflammatory milieu or the increased proliferative activity of cells involved in the disease process, the underlying mechanism may be a primary defect and precede autoimmunity. Indeed, T lymphocytes from patients with RA have defects in their DNA repair machinery that result in increased susceptibility for apoptosis, in particular, in the naive T cell population (Fig. 5). Increased lymphocyte loss and the associated relative lymphopenia may be a risk factor for autoimmunity, as has been shown in several animal models.[16] In these models, lymphopenia induces IL-7– and/or IL-15–driven homeostatic proliferation, which lowered the level of T cell responsiveness and impaired tolerance to peripheral antigens. At least two mechanisms of accelerated cell loss have been described for naive T cells from patients with RA. First, naive RA T cells are compromised in expressing telomerase in the first days after antigen stimulation. The defective induction of telomerase not only accelerated telomere loss, but also rendered these cells more susceptible to undergo apoptosis. This increased apoptosis susceptibility was independent of telomeric erosion, but correlated with repressed transcription of Bcl-2.[99] Expression of Bcl-2, mainly induced by common gamma chain cytokines, such as IL-7, is important in preventing clonal downsizing after T cell activation and the transition into memory cells. Moreover, Bcl-2 expression is also important in determining T cell survival in homeostatic proliferation.

Telomerase deficiency, possibly independent of telomere elongation, is not the only defective DNA repair mechanism found in RA patients. RA T cells, both naive and memory cells, have an increased number of double-strand breaks in nontelomeric DNA. The underlying defect is a reduced production of the DNA damage-inducible protein kinase, ataxia telangiectasia mutated kinase (ATM).[100] The accumulation of fragmented DNA is associated with increased susceptibility to apoptosis. In parallel, and most likely as a compensatory mechanism to deal with the increased DNA damage, RA T cells show a robust induction of the DNA-dependent protein kinase catalytic subunit (DNA-PKcs).[101] The deficiency in ATM transcription and phosphorylation leads to the induction of p53-independent proapoptotic pathway. In parallel, chronic PKcs activation activates downstream signaling pathways including stress kinase pathways, as well as the inflammasome. The net effect of these changes is a reduced threshold to undergoing activation and increased susceptibility to enduring apoptosis, leading to increased attrition of peripheral T cells. Defective DNA maintenance is known to accelerate aging; in its most extreme forms, genetic polymorphisms of molecules involved in nuclear stability or DNA repair induce progeroid syndromes.[102,103] Similar mechanisms are likely to also contribute to the aging of cells of the immune system. In RA, the increased attrition of T cells accelerates immune aging and possibly also sets the stage for tolerance defects that eventually manifest in the form of peripheral arthritis and possibly also other autoimmune manifestations. This role of ATM defects in accelerating immune aging has been recently confirmed in patients with classical and mild variant ataxia telangiectasia.[104] Cellular phenotypes characteristic of an aged host were present disproportionate to the calendar age, in this model independent of the absence or presence of CMV infection.

## Synopsis

Immune aging is a multifaceted process that is obviously very heterogeneous in a population depending on genetic background and environmental factors. Identifying factors and pathways that accelerate or delay immune aging holds the promise to understand this process and to define interventions that influence the process. These may at least in part be different from interventions that delay the aging process in general. For example, while calorie restriction promotes longevity in all model systems including mammals, studies in nonhuman primates have shown its effects on immune aging to be very context dependent.[105] Rapamycin, which recently has been shown to mimic calorie restrictions in its effect and probably its mechanisms,[106,107] compromises the immune system at least as much as immune senescence does. We do not know much on how to prolong immune competence. Conversely, we have an increasing understanding of accelerated aging in models of chronic infections and autoimmunity. The mechanisms that drive immune aging in HIV-infected individuals certainly include the need to rebuild a functional CD4[+] T cell repertoire that has been destroyed by the viral infection, but appear to be more complex. CMV infection is a very instructive model different from most other viral infections based on its ability to induce memory inflation without much T cell exhaustion. The finding that defective DNA repair mechanisms accelerate immune aging in autoimmune diseases raises the question whether inflammation and autoimmunity drive DNA damage or whether DNA damage drives inflammation and autoimmunity, analogous to the Campisi model of cellular senescence associated production of inflammatory mediators.[108] Of particular interest, in all of these models, the accelerated aging process is not limited to the immune system, but involves other organ systems, in particular the cardiovascular system.

## Acknowledgments

This work was funded in part by grants from the National Institutes of Health, U19 AI57266, U19 AI090019, RC4 AG039014, R01 AR42527, R01 AI44142, R01 EY11916, and HL P01 HL58000.

## Conflicts of interest

The authors declare no conflicts of interest.

## References

1. Davis, M.M. 2008. A prescription for human immunology. *Immunity* **29**: 835–838.

2. Goronzy, J.J., W.W. Lee & C.M. Weyand. 2007. Aging and T-cell diversity. *Exp. Gerontol.* **42**: 400–406.

3. Bendall, S.C. *et al.* 2011. Single-cell mass cytometry of differential immune and drug responses across a human hematopoietic continuum. *Science* **332**: 687–696.

4. Nakaya, H.I. *et al.* 2011. Systems biology of vaccination for seasonal influenza in humans. *Nat. Immunol.* **12**: 786–795.

5. Prelog, M. *et al.* 2009. Thymectomy in early childhood: significant alterations of the CD4(+)CD45RA(+)CD62L(+) T cell compartment in later life. *Clin. Immunol.* **130**: 123–132.

6. Sauce, D. *et al.* 2009. Evidence of premature immune aging in patients thymectomized during early childhood. *J. Clin. Invest.* **119**: 3070–3078.

7. Aspinall, R. & D. Andrew. 2000. Thymic involution in aging. *J. Clin. Immunol.* **20**: 250–256.

8. Goldrath, A.W. & M.J. Bevan. 1999. Selecting and maintaining a diverse T-cell repertoire. *Nature* **402**: 255–262.

9. George, A.J. & M.A. Ritter. 1996. Thymic involution with ageing: obsolescence or good housekeeping? *Immunol. Today* **17**: 267–272.

10. Montecino-Rodriquez, E., H. Min & K. Dorshkind. 2005. Reevaluating current models of thymic involution. *Semin. Immunol.* **17**: 356–361.

11. Pawelec, G. *et al.* 2005. Human immunosenescence: is it infectious? *Immunol. Rev.* **205**: 257–268.

12. Akbar, A.N. & J.M. Fletcher. 2005. Memory T cell homeostasis and senescence during aging. *Curr. Opin. Immunol.* **17**: 480–485.

13. Kim, P.S. & R. Ahmed. 2010. Features of responding T cells in cancer and chronic infection. *Curr. Opin. Immunol.* **22**: 223–230.

14. Arvin, A. 2005. Aging, immunity, and the varicella-zoster virus. *N. Engl. J. Med.* **352**: 2266–2267.

15. Deeks, S.G. 2011. HIV infection, inflammation, immunosenescence, and aging. *Annu. Rev. Med.* **62**: 141–155.

16. Goronzy, J.J., L. Shao & C.M. Weyand. 2010. Immune aging and rheumatoid arthritis. *Rheum. Dis. Clin. North Am.* **36**: 297–310.

17. Weyand, C.M. & J.J. Goronzy. 2004. Stem cell aging and autoimmunity in rheumatoid arthritis. *Trends Mol. Med.* **10**: 426–433.

18. Goronzy, J.J. & C.M. Weyand. 2003. Aging, autoimmunity and arthritis: T-cell senescence and contraction of T-cell repertoire diversity—catalysts of autoimmunity and chronic inflammation. *Arthritis Res. Ther.* **5**: 225–234.

19. Steinmann, G.G. 1986. Changes in the human thymus during aging. *Curr. Top. Pathol.* **75**: 43–88.

20. Rodewald, H.R. 2008. Thymus organogenesis. *Annu. Rev. Immunol.* **26**: 355–388.

21. Lynch, H.E. *et al.* 2009. Thymic involution and immune reconstitution. *Trends Immunol.* **30**: 366–373.

22. Haynes, B.F. *et al.* 2000. The role of the thymus in immune reconstitution in aging, bone marrow transplantation, and HIV-1 infection. *Annu. Rev. Immunol.* **18**: 529–560.

23. Dixit, V.D. 2010. Thymic fatness and approaches to enhance thymopoietic fitness in aging. *Curr. Opin. Immunol.* **22**: 521–528.

24. Schonland, S.O. *et al.* 2003. Homeostatic control of T-cell generation in neonates. *Blood* **102**: 1428–1434.

25. Dowling, M.R. & P.D. Hodgkin. 2009. Modelling naive T-cell homeostasis: consequences of heritable cellular lifespan during ageing. *Immunol. Cell. Biol.* **87**: 445–456.

26. Ciupe, S.M. *et al.* 2009. The dynamics of T-cell receptor repertoire diversity following thymus transplantation for DiGeorge anomaly. *PLoS Comput. Biol.* **5**: e1000396.

27. Arstila, T.P. *et al.* 1999. A direct estimate of the human alphabeta T cell receptor diversity. *Science* **286**: 958–961.

28. Casrouge, A. *et al.* 2000. Size estimate of the alpha beta TCR repertoire of naive mouse splenocytes. *J. Immunol.* **164**: 5782–5787.

29. Yager, E.J. *et al.* 2008. Age-associated decline in T cell repertoire diversity leads to holes in the repertoire and impaired immunity to influenza virus. *J. Exp. Med.* **205**: 711–723.

30. Moon, J.J. *et al.* 2007. Naive CD4(+) T cell frequency varies for different epitopes and predicts repertoire diversity and responsivle magnitude. *Immunity* **27**: 203–213.

31. Goronzy, J.J. & C.M. Weyand. 2005. T cell development and receptor diversity during aging. *Curr. Opin. Immunol.* **17**: 468–475.

32. Naylor, K. *et al.* 2005. The influence of age on T cell generation and TCR diversity. *J. Immunol.* **174**: 7446–7452.

33. Robins, H.S. *et al.* 2009. Comprehensive assessment of T-cell receptor beta-chain diversity in alphabeta T cells. *Blood* **114**: 4099–4107.

34. Zoller, A.L. & G.J. Kersh. 2006. Estrogen induces thymic atrophy by eliminating early thymic progenitors and inhibiting proliferation of beta-selected thymocytes. *J. Immunol.* **176**: 7371–7378.

35. Manley, N.R. *et al.* 2011. Structure and function of the thymic microenvironment. *Front. Biosci.* **17:** 2461–2477.

36. Min, H., E. Montecino-Rodriguez & K. Dorshkind. 2004. Reduction in the developmental potential of intrathymic T cell progenitors with age. *J. Immunol.* **173:** 245–250.

37. Beerman, I. *et al.* 2010. Functionally distinct hematopoietic stem cells modulate hematopoietic lineage potential during aging by a mechanism of clonal expansion. *Proc. Natl. Acad. Sci. USA* **107:** 5465–5470.

38. Song, Z. *et al.* 2010. Alterations of the systemic environment are the primary cause of impaired B and T lymphopoiesis in telomere-dysfunctional mice. *Blood* **115:** 1481–1489.

39. Yang, H., Y.H. Youm & V.D. Dixit. 2009. Inhibition of thymic adipogenesis by caloric restriction is coupled with reduction in age-related thymic involution. *J. Immunol.* **183:** 3040–3052.

40. Youm, Y.H. *et al.* 2010. Thiazolidinedione treatment and constitutive-PPARgamma activation induces ectopic adipogenesis and promotes age-related thymic involution. *Aging Cell.* **9:** 478–489.

41. Derhovanessian, E., A. Larbi & G. Pawelec. 2009. Biomarkers of human immunosenescence: impact of Cytomegalovirus infection. *Curr. Opin. Immunol.* **21:** 440–445.

42. Kuijpers, T.W. *et al.* 2003. Frequencies of circulating cytolytic, CD45RA+CD27−, CD8+ T lymphocytes depend on infection with CMV. *J. Immunol.* **170:** 4342–4348.

43. Czesnikiewicz-Guzik, M. *et al.* 2008. T cell subset-specific susceptibility to aging. *Clin. Immunol.* **127:** 107–118.

44. Looney, R.J. *et al.* 1999. Role of cytomegalovirus in the T cell changes seen in elderly individuals. *Clin. Immunol.* **90:** 213–219.

45. Nikolich-Zugich, J. & B.D. Rudd. 2010. Immune memory and aging: an infinite or finite resource? *Curr. Opin. Immunol.* **22:** 535–540.

46. Brien, J.D. *et al.* 2009. Key role of T cell defects in age-related vulnerability to West Nile virus. *J. Exp. Med.* **206:** 2735–2745.

47. Goronzy, J.J. *et al.* 2001. Value of immunological markers in predicting responsiveness to influenza vaccination in elderly individuals. *J. Virol.* **75:** 12182–12187.

48. Saurwein-Teissl, M. *et al.* 2002. Lack of antibody production following immunization in old age: association with CD8(+)CD28(−) T cell clonal expansions and an imbalance in the production of Th1 and Th2 cytokines. *J. Immunol.* **168:** 5893–5899.

49. Wikby, A. *et al.* 1998. Changes in CD8 and CD4 lymphocyte subsets, T cell proliferation responses and non-survival in the very old: the Swedish longitudinal OCTO-immune study. *Mech. Ageing Dev.* **102:** 187–198.

50. Khan, N. *et al.* 2002. Cytomegalovirus seropositivity drives the CD8 T cell repertoire toward greater clonality in healthy elderly individuals. *J. Immunol.* **169:** 1984–1992.

51. Chidrawar, S. *et al.* 2009. Cytomegalovirus-seropositivity has a profound influence on the magnitude of major lymphoid subsets within healthy individuals. *Clin. Exp. Immunol.* **155:** 423–432.

52. van Leeuwen, E.M. *et al.* 2006. Human virus-specific CD8+ T cells: diversity specialists. *Immunol. Rev.* **211:** 225–235.

53. Palendira, U. *et al.* 2008. Selective accumulation of virus-specific CD8+ T cells with unique homing phenotype within the human bone marrow. *Blood* **112:** 3293–3302.

54. Sylwester, A.W. *et al.* 2005. Broadly targeted human cytomegalovirus-specific CD4 +and CD8+ T cells dominate the memory compartments of exposed subjects. *J. Exp. Med.* **202:** 673–685.

55. Fletcher, J.M. *et al.* 2005. Cytomegalovirus-specific CD4+ T cells in healthy carriers are continuously driven to replicative exhaustion. *J. Immunol.* **175:** 8218–8225.

56. Hertoghs, K.M. *et al.* 2010. Molecular profiling of cytomegalovirus-induced human CD8+ T cell differentiation. *J. Clin. Invest.* **120:** 4077–4090.

57. Fourcade, J. *et al.* 2010. Upregulation of Tim-3 and PD-1 expression is associated with tumor antigen-specific CD8+ T cell dysfunction in melanoma patients. *J. Exp. Med.* **207:** 2175–2186.

58. Sakuishi, K. *et al.* 2010. Targeting Tim-3 and PD-1 pathways to reverse T cell exhaustion and restore anti-tumor immunity. *J. Exp. Med.* **207:** 2187–2194.

59. Mueller, S.N. & R. Ahmed. 2009. High antigen levels are the cause of T cell exhaustion during chronic viral infection. *Proc. Natl. Acad. Sci. USA* **106:** 8623–8628.

60. Wherry, E.J. *et al.* 2007. Molecular signature of CD8+ T cell exhaustion during chronic viral infection. *Immunity* **27:** 670–684.

61. Jin, H.T. *et al.* 2010. Cooperation of Tim-3 and PD-1 in CD8 T-cell exhaustion during chronic viral infection. *Proc. Natl. Acad. Sci. USA* **107:** 14733–14738.

62. Weng, N.P., A.N. Akbar & J. Goronzy. 2009. CD28(-) T cells: their role in the age-associated decline of immune function. *Trends Immunol.* **30:** 306–312.

63. Akbar, A.N. & S.M. Henson. 2011. Are senescence and exhaustion intertwined or unrelated processes that compromise immunity? *Nat. Rev. Immunol.* **11:** 289–295.

64. Levin, M.J. *et al.* 2003. Decline in varicella-zoster virus (VZV)-specific cell-mediated immunity with increasing age and boosting with a high-dose VZV vaccine. *J. Infect. Dis.* **188:** 1336–1344.

65. Khan, N. *et al.* 2004. Herpesvirus-specific CD8 T cell immunity in old age: cytomegalovirus impairs the response to a coresident EBV infection. *J. Immunol.* **173:** 7481–7489.

66. Gershon, A.A. *et al.* 2010. Advances in the understanding of the pathogenesis and epidemiology of herpes zoster. *J. Clin. Virol.* **48**(Suppl 1): S2–S7.

67. Freeman, M.L. *et al.* 2010. Two kinetic patterns of epitope-specific CD8 T-cell responses following murine gammaherpesvirus 68 infection. *J. Virol.* **84:** 2881–2892.

68. Yager, E.J. *et al.* 2010. Differential impact of ageing on cellular and humoral immunity to a persistent murine gammaherpesvirus. *Immun. Ageing* **7:** 3.

69. Staras, S.A. *et al.* 2006. Seroprevalence of cytomegalovirus infection in the United States, 1988–1994. *Clin. Infect. Dis.* **43:** 1143–1151.

70. Stadler, L.P. *et al.* 2010. Seroprevalence of cytomegalovirus (CMV) and risk factors for infection in adolescent males. *Clin. Infect. Dis.* **51:** e76–e81.

71. Rudd, B.D. *et al.* 2011. Evolution of the antigen-specific CD8+ TCR repertoire across the life span: evidence for

clonal homogenization of the old TCR repertoire. *J. Immunol.* **186:** 2056–2064.

72. Derhovanessian, E. *et al.* 2010. Hallmark features of immunosenescence are absent in familial longevity. *J. Immunol.* **185:** 4618–4624.

73. Pourgheysari, B. *et al.* 2010. The number of cytomegalovirus-specific CD4+ T cells is markedly expanded in patients with B-cell chronic lymphocytic leukemia and determines the total CD4+ T-cell repertoire. *Blood* **116:** 2968–2974.

74. Pita-Lopez, M.L. *et al.* 2009. Effect of ageing on CMV-specific CD8 T cells from CMV seropositive healthy donors. *Immun. Ageing* **6:** 11.

75. Vescovini, R. *et al.* 2010. Intense antiextracellular adaptive immune response to human cytomegalovirus in very old subjects with impaired health and cognitive and functional status. *J. Immunol.* **184:** 3242–3249.

76. Desai, S. & A. Landay. 2010. Early immune senescence in HIV disease. *Curr. HIV/AIDS Rep.* **7:** 4–10.

77. Justice, A.C. 2010. HIV and aging: time for a new paradigm. *Curr. HIV/AIDS Rep.* **7:** 69–76.

78. Appay, V. *et al.* 2007. Accelerated immune senescence and HIV-1 infection. *Exp. Gerontol.* **42:** 432–437.

79. Kalayjian, R.C. *et al.* 2003. Age-related immune dysfunction in health and in human immunodeficiency virus (HIV) disease: association of age and HIV infection with naive CD8+ cell depletion, reduced expression of CD28 on CD8+ cells, and reduced thymic volumes. *J. Infect. Dis.* **187:** 1924–1933.

80. Dion, M.L. *et al.* 2004. HIV infection rapidly induces and maintains a substantial suppression of thymocyte proliferation. *Immunity* **21:** 757–768.

81. Effros, R.B. 2011. Telomere/telomerase dynamics within the human immune system: effect of chronic infection and stress. *Exp. Gerontol.* **46:** 135–140.

82. Effros, R.B. *et al.* 2005. The role of CD8+ T-cell replicative senescence in human aging. *Immunol. Rev.* **205:** 147–157.

83. Rickabaugh, T.M. *et al.* 2011. The dual impact of HIV-1 infection and aging on naive CD4 T-cells: additive and distinct patterns of impairment. *PLoS One* **6:** e16459.

84. Douek, D.C. *et al.* 1998. Changes in thymic function with age and during the treatment of HIV infection. *Nature* **396:** 690–695.

85. Dion, M.L. *et al.* 2007. Slow disease progression and robust therapy-mediated CD4 +T-cell recovery are associated with efficient thymopoiesis during HIV-1 infection. *Blood* **109:** 2912–2920.

86. Sauce, D. *et al.* 2011. HIV disease progression despite suppression of viral replication is associated with exhaustion of lymphopoiesis. *Blood* **117:** 5142–5151.

87. Teixeira, L. *et al.* 2001. Poor CD4 T cell restoration after suppression of HIV-1 replication may reflect lower thymic function. *AIDS* **15:** 1749–1756.

88. Appay, V. *et al.* 2011. Old age and anti-cytomegalovirus immunity are associated with altered T-cell reconstitution in HIV-1-infected patients. *AIDS* **25:** 1813–1822.

89. Hollander, G.A., W. Krenger & B.R. Blazar. 2010. Emerging strategies to boost thymic function. *Curr. Opin. Pharmacol.* **10:** 443–453.

90. Taub, D.D., W.J. Murphy & D.L. Longo. 2010. Rejuvena-tion of the aging thymus: growth hormone-mediated and ghrelin-mediated signaling pathways. *Curr. Opin. Pharmacol.* **10:** 408–424.

91. Napolitano, L.A. *et al.* 2008. Growth hormone enhances thymic function in HIV-1-infected adults. *J. Clin. Invest.* **118:** 1085–1098.

92. Goronzy, J.J. & C.M. Weyand. 2001. Thymic function and peripheral T-cell homeostasis in rheumatoid arthritis. *Trends Immunol.* **22:** 251–255.

93. Morgan, M.D. *et al.* 2011. CD4+CD28- T cell expansion in granulomatosis with polyangiitis (Wegener's) is driven by latent cytomegalovirus infection and is associated with an increased risk of infection and mortality. *Arthritis Rheum.* **63:** 2127–2137.

94. Koetz, K. *et al.* 2000. T cell homeostasis in patients with rheumatoid arthritis. *Proc. Natl. Acad. Sci. USA* **97:** 9203–9208.

95. Colmegna, I. *et al.* 2008. Defective proliferative capacity and accelerated telomeric loss of hematopoietic progenitor cells in rheumatoid arthritis. *Arthritis Rheum.* **58:** 990–1000.

96. Schonland, S.O. *et al.* 2003. Premature telomeric loss in rheumatoid arthritis is genetically determined and involves both myeloid and lymphoid cell lineages. *Proc. Natl. Acad. Sci. USA* **100:** 13471–13476.

97. Andrews, N.P. *et al.* 2010. Telomeres and immunological diseases of aging. *Gerontology* **56:** 390–403.

98. Wagner, U.G. *et al.* 1998. Perturbation of the T cell repertoire in rheumatoid arthritis. *Proc. Natl. Acad. Sci. USA* **95:** 14447–14452.

99. Fujii, H. *et al.* 2009. Telomerase insufficiency in rheumatoid arthritis. *Proc. Natl. Acad. Sci. USA* **106:** 4360–4365.

100. Shao, L. *et al.* 2009. Deficiency of the DNA repair enzyme ATM in rheumatoid arthritis. *J. Exp. Med.* **206:** 1435–1449.

101. Shao, L., J.J. Goronzy & C.M. Weyand. 2010. DNA-dependent protein kinase catalytic subunit mediates T-cell loss in rheumatoid arthritis. *EMBO Mol. Med.* **2:** 415–427.

102. Liu, Y. *et al.* 2006. DNA damage responses in progeroid syndromes arise from defective maturation of prelamin A. *J. Cell Sci.* **119:** 4644–4649.

103. Chen, T. *et al.* 2010. A functional single nucleotide polymorphism in promoter of ATM is associated with longevity. *Mech. Ageing Dev.* **131:** 636–640.

104. Exley, A.R. *et al.* 2011. Premature ageing of the immune system underlies immunodeficiency in ataxia telangiectasia. *Clin. Immunol.* **140:** 26–36.

105. Messaoudi, I. *et al.* 2008. Optimal window of caloric restriction onset limits its beneficial impact on T-cell senescence in primates. *Aging Cell.* **7:** 908–919.

106. Harrison, D.E. *et al.* 2009. Rapamycin fed late in life extends lifespan in genetically heterogeneous mice. *Nature* **460:** 392–395.

107. Miller, R.A. *et al.* 2011. Rapamycin, but not resveratrol or simvastatin, extends life span of genetically heterogeneous mice. *J. Gerontol. A Biol. Sci. Med. Sci.* **66:** 191–201.

108. Rodier, F. & J. Campisi. 2011. Four faces of cellular senescence. *J. Cell Biol.* **192:** 547–556.

Ann. N.Y. Acad. Sci. ISSN 0077-8923

ANNALS OF THE NEW YORK ACADEMY OF SCIENCES

Issue: *The Year in Immunology*

# Helminth–host immunological interactions: prevention and control of immune-mediated diseases

## David E. Elliott[1] and Joel V. Weinstock[2]

[1]Division of Gastroenterology, University of Iowa, Iowa City, Iowa. [2]Division of Gastroenterology, Tufts Medical Center, Boston, Massachusetts.

Address for correspondence: Joel V. Weinstock, MD, Division of Gastroenterology (Box 233), Tufts Medical Center, 800 Washington St., Boston, MA 02111. jweinstock2@tuftsmedicalcenter.org

Exposure to commensal and pathogenic organisms strongly influences our immune system. Exposure to helminths was frequent before humans constructed their current highly hygienic environment. Today, in highly industrialized countries, contact between humans and helminths is rare. Congruent with the decline in helminth infections is an increase in the prevalence of autoimmune and inflammatory disease. It is possible that exclusion of helminths from the environment has permitted the emergence of immune-mediated disease. We review the protective effects of helminths on expression of inflammatory bowel disease, multiple sclerosis, and animal models of these and other inflammatory diseases. We also review the immune pathways altered by helminths that may afford protection from these illnesses. Helminth exposure tends to inhibit IFN-$\gamma$ and IL-17 production, promote IL-4, IL-10, and TGF-$\beta$ release, induce CD4$^+$ T cell Foxp3 expression, and generate regulatory macrophages, dendritic cells, and B cells. Helminths enable protective pathways that may vary by specific species and disease model. Helminths or their products likely have therapeutic potential to control or prevent immune-mediated illness.

Keywords: helminths; dendritic cells; IBD; T$_{reg}$; macrophage; autoimmunity

## Introduction

The 20th century brought demise to Paul Ehrlich's 1901 dictum of horror autotoxicus, that the body's immune system would never attack host tissues to cause disease. In its place grew identification of more than 80 autoimmune or immune-mediated diseases. Most of these diseases emerged in the later half of the 20th century to become epidemic in highly developed industrialized countries. The National Institutes of Health now estimates that over 23.5 million Americans are afflicted with an autoimmune illness. Autoimmune disease ranks in the top 10 causes of death for women younger than 65 years of age. The dramatic emergence of these illnesses within two generations suggests that an environmental change has driven or permitted the immune dysregulation that results in autoimmunity, allergy, and inflammatory disease.

There are many striking environmental changes that have come with industrialization, but one that has immediate immunologic impact is loss of exposure to parasitic worms (helminths). Indoor plumbing, flush toilets, cement sidewalks, and well-regulated food industries conspire to prevent acquisition and transmission of helminths. In the United States, the prevalence of hookworm in Georgia schoolchildren dropped from 65% in the 1910s to less than 2% (mostly in recent immigrants) in the 1980s.[1,2] Trichinosis, whipworm (*Trichuris trichiura*) and pinworm (*Enterobius vermicularis*) infections show similar declines in prevalence. Loss of helminth exposure also occurred in postwar Western Europe. In other regions, as socioeconomic conditions rise, the prevalence of helminth infection falls. Whipworm infections in South Korean schoolchildren fell from about 75% in 1969 to 0.02% in 2004.[3] During this time span, the incidence of ulcerative colitis in Seoul, South Korea increased nearly sixfold.[4] Prior to the 20th century, every individual was likely to have had a helminth infection. Now, a previously ubiquitous and universal exposure has become exceedingly rare.

doi: 10.1111/j.1749-6632.2011.06292.x

This lack of helminth exposure could have a profound affect on our immune system that was shaped by exposure to commensal and pathogenic organisms. Immunologically, humans have battled helminths for millennia.[5] This multigenerational, ubiquitous challenge has swayed genetic variation. Many of the polymorphisms in genetic loci associated with autoimmune diseases have been selected by parasite-driven adaptation.[6] Helminths are complex multicellular organisms that have also adapted to their hosts. Helminths produce immune regulatory products and induce regulatory circuits to help maintain their niche. Loss of chronic helminth infection removes an "external immune governor" and leads to pathologic autoimmune and excessive inflammatory responses.

A common theme among the various dissimilar helminth species includes their capacity to strengthen both innate and adaptive immune regulatory circuitry. In addition, different helminths may influence different pathways. In the following sections, we will discuss the evidence for helminth–host interactions that prevent or control immune-mediated disease. We will approach this evidence according to the various helminthic effects on specific autoimmune and inflammatory diseases.

## Helminths and inflammatory bowel disease

Ulcerative colitis and Crohn's disease are collectively called inflammatory bowel disease (IBD). They are chronic inflammatory conditions of the gut that usually begin when people are in the second to third decade of life. Although the causes of these inflammatory diseases remain unknown, they are assumed to result from inappropriately aggressive mucosal immune responses to luminal substances. Identified are various genetic alterations that impart risk for, or protection from, acquiring these conditions.[7–9] Many of these genes have a role in mucosal barrier defense, innate immune, immune responsiveness, or immunoregulation. Yet, these gene alterations appear to function as factors that affect disease susceptibility, as the majority of patients with IBD display no particular genetic predisposition, and most patients bearing these "IBD genes" will never develop this condition.

IBD emerged as a growing health problem in highly developed countries in the latter half of the 20th century. The frequency of IBD is currently about 1 in 250 persons in some regions.[10–12] Previ-ously, these diseases were exceeding rare. IBD is now emerging rapidly in many underdeveloped countries.[13–16] Poorly defined environmental factors are likely the cause for this rapid change in disease frequency worldwide. Hygiene associated with modern day living and causing alteration in intestinal flora and fauna is postulated to be a major risk factor.[17] The *IBD hygiene hypothesis* proposes that modification in exposure to living organisms negatively affects development and maintenance of immune regulatory circuits that normally would afford protection from these diseases. Helminth infections are exceedingly strong inducers of regulatory circuits. Thus, loss of these infections in children and adults, a consequence of hygiene and strong public health measures, may be an important factor in disease causation.[18] Several clinical and epidemiologic studies support this concept.[19,20] Research exploring the use of helminths to treat Crohn's disease and ulcerative colitis suggests that these agents may be useful therapeutic agents both to treat and prevent IBD.[21–25]

## Animal models

Laboratories study various animal models that simulate human IBD[26] to identify potential mechanisms through which helminths suppress disease. In one model, trinitrobenzene sulfonic acid (TNBS) is administered intrarectally into healthy mice to induce colitis. Another model is the IL-10–KO mouse, which develops chronic colitis spontaneously. In this model, brief exposure to a nonsteroidal anti-inflammatory drug (NSAID) triggers the disease quickly and more uniformly throughout the colon making the model more useful for experimentation.

In a variant of the IL-10–KO mouse model of IBD, Rag mice (T and B cell deficient) are reconstituted with IL-10–KO T cells, and the mice are fed an NSAID orally to induce severe Th1/Th17-type colitis.[27] Human IBD is presumed to result from inappropriate T cell activation, in the gut lining, to luminal antigens. It is hard to study antigen-specific immunity in the intestines, since many poorly defined antigens provided by luminal organisms and orally consumed organic matter drive mucosal immune responses. To overcome this barrier, Rag mice also may receive, simultaneously with the IL-10–KO T cells, transgenic OT2 T cells bearing MHC class II-dependent TCR that recognize OVA. The OT2 cells subsequently appear in the gut allowing the study of

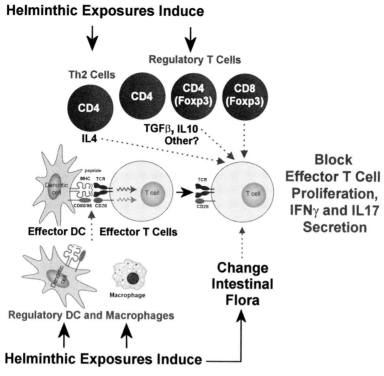

**Figure 1.** Helminth-induced regulatory circuits that limit inflammation.

how helminths work to regulation antigen-specific responses in the intestinal lamina propria.

Another valuable murine model of spontaneous IBD results from the reconstitution of Rag mice with CD25$^{lo}$ T cells. This model retains the capacity to make IL-10 and can be manipulated similarly to that of the IL-10–KO model to allow sophisticated analysis.

## Mechanisms of regulation

Helminths likely function to control IBD through induction of several independent regulatory pathways. They promote regulatory circuits involving cellular components of both innate and adaptive immunity, and stimulate release of several regulatory cytokines (Fig. 1).

### Regulatory dendritic cells

*Helmigmosomoides polygyrus bakeri* is a murine intestinal nematode with some genetic similarity to pinworm and hookworm (Fig. 2). T cell- and B cell-deficient Rag mice infected with *H. polygyrus bakeri* and then dewormed with a pharmaceutical agent before reconstitution with colitogenic IL-10–KO

T cells are protected from colitis.[27] This implies that *H. polygyrus bakeri* does not require direct interactions with T or B cells to render animals resistant to this disease.

IFN-$\gamma$ and IL-17 are proinflammatory cytokines implicated in driving colitis in both human and many murine models of IBD, including the ones described above.[28] The intestinal mucosa makes less IFN-$\gamma$ and IL-17 after *H. polygyrus bakeri* infection, whether the animals are primed for colitis or have been configured to remain free from disease. Thus, the decreased ability to produce these colitogenic cytokines is not simply secondary to the improvement in gut inflammation.

In the absence of adaptive immunity, exposing Rag mice to *H. polygyrus bakeri* greatly alters the function of the dendritic cells (DC) residing in the intestinal mucosa.[27] After *H. polygyrus bakeri* infection, intestinal DC only weakly support antigen-driven IFN-$\gamma$ secretion compared to DC from uninfected animals. More importantly, DC isolated from the MLN or intestines of *H. polygyrus bakeri*-infected Rag mice will block colitis and mucosal antigen-induced IFN-$\gamma$ and IL-17 responses when

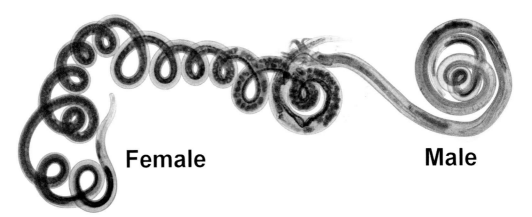

**Figure 2.** Male and female adult *Heligmosomoides polygyrus bakeri*. *H. polygyrus bakeri* is a nematode (round worm) that resides in the upper small intestine (duodenum and jejunum) of mice. The name of the parasite is changing from *H. polygyrus* to *H. bakeri*.

the DC are transferred into colitis-susceptible animals. Thus, without the aid of T or B cells, the process of helminth infection alters the function of the DC in the gut and MLN of Rag mice, rendering them highly regulatory.

How the DC work to silence mucosal antigenic stimulation is partly understood. T cells populate the gut and MLN normally after DC transfer, but the T cell response is quelled by the surrounding non-T cell elements of the lamina propria and MLN, which have become strongly regulatory. The regulatory DC block IFN-γ and IL-17 production by interfering with the interaction between proinflammatory DC and effector T cells that drive the inflammation. The regulatory DC must physically contact the other cellular components to control the response. This interaction does not promote IL-4 secretion and is not associated with enhanced IL-10 or TGF-β production, suggesting that the mechanism of regulation is not dependent on increased production of these cytokines (Weinstock, *et al.*, unpublished data).

There also are changes in expression of cell surface molecules on the intestinal DC.[27] This includes decreased expression of the costimulatory molecules CD80 and CD86; more widely expressed are PDCA-1, a marker of plasmacytoid DC,[29] and CD40. It is not yet determined if any of these changes in cell surface protein expression have importance for the capacity of these cells to block colitis or mucosal antigenic responses.

### Regulatory macrophages

Macrophages populate the intestines in abundance. Macrophages occur in one of several possible states

of cellular activation. Helminths induce the immune system of the host to produce IL-10 and Th2 cytokines like IL-4 and IL-5, which activate macrophages in ways distinct from macrophages exposed to Th1 cytokines. Such so-called *alternatively activated macrophages* display the mannose receptor and IL-4Ra on their outer membranes, and make some unique molecules like arginase-1, RELMa, Ym11, and some chitinases.[30] While they produce little IL-12, alternatively activated macrophages can make IL-10, TGF-β, and other immunomodulatory factors notable for limiting Th1-type inflammation.[31] Helminths may help protect from IBD through induction of alternatively activated macrophages.

Another frequently used model of IBD is dextran sodium sulfate (DSS)-induced enteritis. DSS administered orally to rodents damages the intestinal epithelial lining. This in turn induces gut inflammation that is relatively independent of adaptive immunity.

Infection of Balb/C mice with *Schistosoma mansoni* protects these animals from DSS-induced injury. In the DSS model of enteritis, it is the adult schistosome flukes living in the portal vein that shield the host from this inflammation, not their ova that lodge in the liver and intestinal wall. The mechanism of protection involves macrophages and functions independent of regulatory cytokines, such as IL-10 and TGF-β, and regulatory T cells.[32]

Cystatin, a secreted cysteine protease inhibitor of several species of filarial nematodes, protects mice from DSS colitis and an allergic-type airway hypersensitivity response. Macrophages and IL-10 are necessary for this protection,[33] although this has thus far only been demonstrated for the lung Th2-type inflammatory model. Cystatin induces macrophages to make IL-10 and IL-12 p40 through activation of intracellular signaling pathways like ERK and p38, which are MAP kinases.[34] This effect of cystatin on macrophages is the postulated mechanism of action.

In the IL-10–KO Rag model of IBD, exposure of Rag mice to *H. polygyrus bakeri* induces regulatory macrophages in the gut even before the mice are reconstituted with the colitogenic IL-10 deficient T cells. These intestinal macrophages inhibit antigen-induced, IL-17 and IFN-γ secretion, by a contact-dependent mechanism, when they are mixed with LPMC from mice with active colitis. The macrophages regulate with efficiency comparable to that of the *H. polygyrus bakeri*-induced intestinal regulatory DC described above. Also, when transferred into Rag mice along with the IL-10–KO T cells, they protect the mice from colitis and inhibit the intestinal antigenic response (Weinstock *et. al.*, unpublished data). Thus, *H. polygyrus bakeri* activates two distinct cells of innate immunity (macrophages and DC) both of which can quell mucosal antigenic responses and colitis. It is not yet established if these two cell types function interdependently or work separately to provide overlapping protection. Profiling these regulatory macrophages using real-time PCR technology suggests that these cells do not have the molecular profile of classical alternatively activated macrophages.

In another study using dinitrobenzene sulfonic acid (DNBS) instead of TNBS to induce IBD, infection with the intestinal tapeworm *H. diminuta* protects the mice from colitis through a macrophage-dependent mechanism. The infection induces within the colon increased expression of markers of alternatively activated macrophages. Alternatively activated macrophages transferred into mice will protect the animals from DNBS-induced injury, suggesting that alternatively activated macrophages induced by the natural infection are the critical protecting factor. Extracts from *H. diminuta* adult worms injected intraperitoneally also provides disease protection and selectively suppresses macrophage function *in vitro*.[35] Thus, this model, as well as the IL-10 transfer model of IBD, suggest that macrophages activated by helminth infection are sufficient to protect animals from IBD.[36]

Moreover, it is possible that some helminths make soluble factors that can mediate this process and substitute for the live agent.

## Regulatory type T cells and cytokines

Various animal models of IBD suggest that regulatory-type T cells are important for maintaining mucosal immune homeostasis and for controlling enteritis.[37] T cells that regulate immune responses are plentiful in the gut; most are Foxp3+ $T_{regs}$ that express CD4. In the colon, more than 50% of the Foxp3+ T cells also make IL-10. There also are T cells that do not express Foxp3, but which are also major sources for immune regulatory molecules like IL-10 and/or TGF-β.

Helminths induce expansion of regulatory T cell subsets within the intestinal mucosa and mesenteric lymph nodes of their hosts. After *H. polygyrus bakeri* infection lamina propria T cells have a greater capacity to make IL-10 and TGF-β.[38] A diverse array of helminths, such as *H. polygyrus bakeri* and *Schistosoma mansoni*, and the tapeworm *Hymenolepis diminuta* induce IL-10 secretion, which helps limit the colitogenic Th1 response and colitis in several animal models of IBD.[39,40] However, helminths also prevent colitis or suppress ongoing disease in IL-10–KO mice, suggesting that IL-10 is not essential for this control.[27,41]

*H. polygyrus bakeri* infection stimulates Foxp3 mRNA expression in T cells [41] and expands the number of Foxp3+ T cells in the mesenteric lymph nodes [42] and intestinal lamina propria. T cells from the MLN of *H. polygyrus bakeri*–infected IL-10–deficient mice can be transferred into worm-naive animals and stop ongoing colitis, attesting to the importance of T cells in helping to control colitis.[41] Also, colonic Foxp3+ CD4+ T cells, induced in the colon by *H. polygyrus bakeri*-infection, will prevent colitis when transferred into Rag mice reconstituted with CD25− T cells to make them susceptible to IBD. While most of the induced regulatory T cells are CD4+, some express CD8+ and can inhibit T lymphocyte proliferation via class I MHC interactions and cellular contact without the aid of IL-10 or TGF-β.[43] CD8+ $T_{regs}$ are implicated in the control of several diseases featuring immune dysregulation.[44,45]

Helminths can stimulate T cells, and other immune cell types, to make cytokines that impede development or function of T cell subtypes incriminated in IBD pathogenesis. Helminths, like *H. polygyrus bakeri* and *Schistosoma mansoni*, help protect mice from TNBS colitis by restraining the colonic Th1 IFN-γ response as well as IL-12 p40 secretion. Helminths promote the growth of IL-4–producing, Th2 cells. Abrogation of the Th2 pathway promotes persistence of disease and Th1 cell differentiation, showing the importance of Th2 cytokines for disease control in this murine model of IBD.[39] IL-17 frequently comes from Th17 cells and often has an important role in driving colitis. *H. polygyrus bakeri* blocks IL-17 secretion in part through stimulating IL-4 production and, to a lesser extent, IL-10 production, which affects Th17 cell function.[28] Disruption of Stat6 signaling specifically in T cells negates the ability of *H. polygyrus bakeri* infection to reverse established CD25[lo] T cell transfer colitis and inhibit IL-17 production (Elliott, unpublished data).

TGF-β is a critical cytokine in many immune reactions. Transgenic mice with T cells that do not signal correctly after TGF-β engagement cannot properly limit Th1 or Th2 responses in the gut and in other tissues, and thus these mice spontaneously develop colitis. In such transgenic mice, infection with *H. polygyrus bakeri* cannot prevent colitis or dampen mucosal Th1 responsiveness. This shows that *H. polygyrus bakeri* prevention of mucosal inflammation may require signaling of TGF-β through mucosal T cells.[46]

### Overcoming the epithelial barrier

It is not entirely known how intestinal helminths bypass the intestinal barrier to interface with the gut mucosal immune system. Helminths like *H. polygyrus bakeri* live mostly in the proximal small bowel but reduce inflammation in the colon and distal terminal ileum. Transfer of protection using mesenteric lymph nodes from *H. polygyrus bakeri*-infected mice, however, emphasizes the importance of the immune system in this protective process.[41]

There are several possible mechanisms. DC extend dendrites across the epithelial barrier, which would permit sampling of molecules released from helminths living in the intestinal lumen. *H. polygyrus bakeri* and other helminths cultured *in vitro* release factors that can modify DC activation,[47,48] impair DC-induced antibody responses,[48] and promote regulatory T cell development. Thus,

helminths produce substances that may affect the function of the DC that are sampling luminal contents.

The intestinal epithelial lining interfaces with the underlying immunocytes through release of regulatory molecules and direct cell contact. Interaction between intestinal helminths and the intestinal epithelium requires further consideration.

While some helminths swim freely in the gut lumen, others either mildly disrupt the mucosal barrier (e.g., hookworm) or attach to the intestinal wall by placing their heads beneath the epithelial lining (e.g., whipworm). This affords a further potential avenue for direct communication, for instance, with T cells to induce $T_{regs}$,[42] or with other cells of host immunity to promote regulation.[47]

There is an enormous quantity of bacteria in the intestines. Intestinal bacteria are important for the health of the mucosal immune system and readily interact with intestinal DC and other cells.[49] *H. polygyrus bakeri* infection rapidly shifts the abundance and distribution of some intestinal bacteria. There is a prominent increase in a family of bacteria called Lactobacillaceae. Various bacterial species within this group of organisms decrease intestinal inflammation in murine models of colitis.[50]

Helminths also can perturb the location and function of receptors of innate immunity. Bacteria often interact with host TLR and other receptors of innate immunity through release of LPS and other molecules. T cells in the intestinal lamina propria express TLR4 after *H. polygyrus bakeri* infection.[51] LPS engagement with T cell TLR4 stimulates release of regulatory cytokines such as IL-10 and TGF-β, rather than the expected proinflammatory molecules. This may allow bacterial LPS to suppress adaptive immunity by provoking regulatory T cells that make IL-10 and TGF-β. Some helminth products also can bind to TLRs on DC to promote a Th2/regulatory T cell response.[52]

There also are helminth species that suppress colitis while living in the systemic circulation or regions of the host distant to the intestines. Their mode of communication with host immunity may be different than those discussed above.

## Helminths and other immune-mediated diseases

Shared with IBD are the temporal and geographic prevalence patterns of multiple sclerosis (MS),

**Table 1. Animal modules of human disease that show improvement with helminths**

| Animal model | Human disease | Helminth studied |
| --- | --- | --- |
| TNBS and DNBS induced colitis | Crohn's disease | *S. mansoni* |
| | | *H. polygyrus bakeri* |
| | | *T. spiralis* |
| | | *H. diminuta* |
| IL10$^{-/-}$ colitis | Crohn's disease | *H. polygyrus bakeri* |
| | | *S. mansoni* |
| | | *T. muris* |
| Transfer colitis | Crohn's disease | *H. polygyrus bakeri* |
| Autoimmune encephalitis (EAE) | Multiple sclerosis | *S. mansoni* |
| | | *T. spiralis* |
| | | *H. polygyrus bakeri* |
| | | *F. hepatica* |
| NOD mouse | Type 1 diabetes | *S. mansoni* |
| | | *T. spiralis* |
| | | *H. polygyrus bakeri* |
| Streptozotocin-induced diabetes | Type 1 diabetes | *T. crassiceps* |
| MRL/lpr arthritis | Rheumatoid arthritis | *H. polygyrus bakeri* |
| | | *N. brasiliensis* |
| Collagen-induced arthritis | Rheumatoid arthritis | *S. mansoni* |
| | | *S. japonicum* |
| CFA arthritis | Rheumatoid arthritis | *H. diminuta* |
| Reactive-airway disease | Asthma | *S. mansoni* |
| | | *H. polygyrus bakeri* |
| | | *T. spiralis* |

type 1 diabetes (T1D), rheumatoid arthritis (RA), asthma, and many other autoimmune inflammatory diseases. This suggests that environmental factors which increase the risk for IBD, such as loss of helminth infections, also increase the risk for other immune-mediated illnesses. Investigators are studying the effect of helminth infection on development and expression of these inflammatory diseases using animal models (Table 1).

### Multiple sclerosis

Patients with MS that have helminthic infections (e.g., *Trichuris trichiura* and/or, *Ascaris lumbricoides, Strongyloides stercoralis*, and others) have a milder disease course compared to MS patients without helminths.[53] Furthermore, in a case report of four patients, pharmacological eradication of helminthic infections resulted in worsening MS activity.[54] Associated with helminth eradication was an increase in the number of PBMC making IFN-γ

and IL-12, and a decrease in the number of cells producing IL-10 and TGF-β. There also was a decrease in circulating CD4$^+$CD25$^+$Foxp3$^+$ T cells.[54] An open label trial of therapeutic *Trichuris suis* exposure in five patients with relapsing-remitting MS showed that helminth exposure resulted in fewer neurological symptoms and development of fewer CNS lesions, as measured by magnetic resonance imaging.[55] Lesion development recurred after discontinuation of *T. suis* administration. A Danish study showed similar results (personal communication).

Mice or rats immunized with myelin-associated peptides develop autoimmune encephalitis (EAE), which serves as a model of MS. Exposure of mice to *Schistosoma mansoni*, or even just to their dead eggs, protects mice from EAE.[56,57] Schistosome exposure suppresses Th1-type cytokine (IL-12 p40, IFN-γ, and TNF-α) and augments regulatory and Th2-type cytokine (TGF-β, IL-10, and IL-4) production by splenocytes and CNS cells. *Trichinella spiralis* infection also affords protection in the agouti rat EAE animal model of MS.[58] Trichinosis suppresses lymph node cell IFN-γ and IL-17 secretion while promoting IL-10 and IL-4 production, and it increases the number of CD4+CD25+Foxp3+ T cells in the spleen. Adoptive transfer of T cells from helminth-infected rats into helminth-naive rats protects these animals from developing EAE.[58] This shows that the process of protection is immunologically-mediated, and that T cells are sufficient to control the disease. Infection with *H. polygyrus bakeri*[59] or *Fasciola hepatica*[60] also suppresses EAE. These studies show that helminths can suppress organ-specific inflammation beyond colitis through circuits likely similar to those that inhibit intestinal inflammation.

## Type 1 diabetes (T1D)

Therapeutic trials using helminth exposure in patients with T1D are planned but not yet completed. For several years, laboratories have studied the effect of helminths on T1D using animal models of autoimmune diabetes such as the nonobese diabetic (NOD) mouse. Helminth exposure with *Schistosoma mansoni, T. spiralis,* or *H. polygyrus bakeri*[61–64] protects NOD mice from insulitis. Protective schistosome exposure is associated with induction of IL-10 and expansion of NKT cells.[62]

Intraperitoneal injection of soluble proteins isolated from schistosome eggs (SEA) also protects NOD mice from diabetes and increases pancreatic mononuclear cell production of TGF-β, IL-4, and IL-10.[65] In addition, SEA treatment increases the number of pancreatic and splenic CD4+CD25+Foxp3+ T cells[65] and induces alternatively activated peritoneal macrophages that make TGF-β.[66] Transferring splenocytes from SEA-treated NOD mice into untreated NOD recipients protects these animals from disease. Splenocytes depleted of CD4+CD25+ T cells cannot provide this protection.[65]

The cytokine profile associated with a protective *T. spiralis* or *H. polygyrus bakeri* infection differs from that induced by schistosome worms or SEA. Characteristic of a protective, *T. spiralis* exposure increased splenic IL-4 secretion without inducing IL-10 production or inhibiting IFN-γ synthesis.[63] Protection afforded by *H. polygyrus bakeri* infection associates with induction of alternatively activated

macrophages, and IL-4 secretion and inhibition of IFN-γ production. However, this protection is independent of IL-10 and CD25+ T cells.[64]

Another murine model of T1D is low-dose streptozotocin-induced diabetes. Infection with *Taenia crassiceps* (a tape worm) decreases insulitis shielding Balb/C and C57BL/6 mice from streptozotocin-induced diabetes. Protection is associated with increase in IL-4 and alternatively activated macrophages, but not with induction of regulatory T cells.[67] Thus, all of the classes of helminths (nematodes, cestodes, and trematodes) can confer protection in murine models of T1D, but different helminths may do so by triggering somewhat different regulatory pathways.

## Rheumatoid arthritis

There are no published clinical trials of helminth exposure in patients with rheumatoid arthritis, but the effect of helminths on arthritis has been tested in animal models of this disease. Polyarticular arthritis develops spontaneously in MRL/lpr mice that have impaired Fas gene expression. Infection of these mice with bacteria aggravates arthritis, while infection with a helminth (*H. polygyrus bakeri or Nippostrongylus brasiliensis*) reduces the incidence of arthritis and the degree of synovial hyperplasia.[68]

A more commonly used and well-described model of rheumatoid arthritis is collagen-induced arthritis. Mice infected with *S. mansoni* two weeks before sensitization with collagen in Freund's complete adjuvant (FCA) do not develop the expected polyarticular arthritis.[69] The reduction in arthritic score correlates with the number of worms per mouse. In protected animals, mitogen-stimulated splenocytes produce less IFN-γ, TNF-α, and IL-17, but more IL-4 and IL-10 than do splenocytes from mice without *S. mansoni* infection.[69] *Schistosoma japonicum*, which is closely related to *S. mansoni*, also protects mice from collagen-induced arthritis. As with *S. mansoni*, this protection associates with inhibition of IFN-γ production and augmentation of IL-4 and IL-10 secretion by mitogen-stimulated splenocytes.[70] However, there is no significant change in TNF-α production. Also, in contrast to protection afforded by *S. mansoni* exposure, infection with *S. japonicum* needs to advance to a patent (egg laying) stage at the time of collagen sensitization to inhibit arthritis development.[70] If this difference is not due to technical artifacts, it suggests that timing of helminth exposure relative to disease challenge may be an important factor even for closely related worms.

The rodent filarial nematode *Acanthocheilonema viteae*, which resides in host lymphatics, secretes a 62 kD phosphocholine-containing glycoprotein (ES-62) that prevents and treats established collagen-induced arthritis.[71] In mice protected from arthritis, their draining lymph node cells make less IFN-γ and TNF-α, and more IL-10, after collagen stimulation *in vitro*. Arthritis is inhibited even when ES-62 is administered subcutaneously after onset of collagen-induced inflammation.[71] Recombinant ES-62 (expressed in yeast) does not inhibit arthritis because it lacks the phosphocholine moiety.[72] These studies show that at least one systemically administered helminth-derived product can modulate arthritic disease activity but the molecule may require posttranslational modification to make it bioactive.

Another model of arthritis is inflammation provoked by intra-articular injection of CFA. This model allows assessment of joint discomfort by comparing CFA with saline-injected joints in the same animal. Exposure of mice to the tapeworm *Hymenolepis diminuta* before challenge reduces CFA-induced peak joint swelling and hastens resolution of inflammation in Balb/C and C57BL/6 mice.[73] Exposure to the helminth after CFA injection does not ease peak swelling but continues to hasten recovery. CFA increases TNF-α mRNA expression in joints; *H. diminuta* infection blocks this induction and also alters splenocyte cytokine profiles, increasing IL-4 and IL-10 production. Infection of IL-10–deficient mice with the tapeworm does not afford protection from CFA arthritis.[73] These experiments demonstrate that infection with a helminth residing in the intestinal lumen (*H. diminuta*) can protect from joint inflammation similar to a helminth (*Schistosoma* sp.) living in the mesenteric vasculature.

## Allergy/asthma

IBD, MS, T1D, and rheumatoid arthritis likely result from dysregulated Th1/Th17 responses, while excessive Th2-type inflammation probably drives allergy and asthma. Helminth exposure stimulates strong Th2 responses and would be predicted to worsen allergic inflammation. However, helminths actually induce immune regulatory circuits that suppress Th2-driven atopic disease.

Helminth infection may influence the frequency of wheezing that is a sign of asthma. People with *A. lumbricoides* or hookworm (*Necator*) infections are less likely to experience wheezing than people without these infections.[74] Also, inhabitants in areas endemic for *S. mansoni* report less wheezing compared to individuals living in nonendemic regions.[75]

Many epidemiological studies support the hypothesis that helminth exposure suppresses atopy, as measured by skin reaction to injected allergens. A study in Gabon, Africa showed that fewer children have atopic skin reactions to dust-mite allergens if they are infected with *Schistosoma hematobium*, compared to children without the helminth.[76] Furthermore, children repeatedly treated for geohelminths (e.g., *T. trichiura*) have increased skin reactions compared to untreated children.[77–79] However, in other epidemiologic and interventional studies, helminthic infection either had no effect on, or increased the frequency of, atopic responses.[79,80] Intensity and timing of helminth infection may explain some of theses differences in outcome. Individuals with the earliest and most sustained exposure may be the most protected against allergic inflammation.[81] This requirement for prolonged exposure also may explain the limited results of a recent double-blind placebo-controlled therapeutic trial of *T. suis* for seasonal allergic rhinitis.[82,83]

A major model of allergic inflammation is airway hyper-responsiveness (AHR) induced by aerosol challenge with an antigen in previously sensitized mice. The model permits measurement of airway reactivity (respiratory resistance and compliance) and analysis of pulmonary inflammation. Colonization with *H. polygyrus bakeri* before or during antigen sensitization inhibits subsequent airway reactivity[84] and inflammation[84,85] upon aerosol antigen challenge. Helminth exposure decreases allergen-specific IL-5 production, an effect shown in people with *S. mansoni* infections.[75]

Exposure to other helminths, such as *S. mansoni*[86] or *T. spiralis*,[87] also affords protection from allergic airway reactivity and inflammation. In both of these models, helminth exposure is associated with decreased allergen-stimulated IL-5 release and increased IL-10 and TGF-β production.

Transfer of mesenteric lymph node cells or splenocytes from colonized mice into helminth naive animals inhibits airway inflammation, showing induction of regulatory cell activity.

| Nematodes (Roundworms) | Cestodes (Tapeworms) | Trematodes (Flukes) |
|---|---|---|
| *Helmigmosomoides polygyrus bakeri* | *Hymenolepis diminuta* | *Schistosoma sp.* |
| *Trichuris sp.* | *Taenia crassiceps* | *Fasciola hepatica* |
| *Trichinella spiralis* | | |
| *Nippostrongylus brasiliensis* | | |
| *Acanthocheilonema viteae* | | |
| *Necator americanus* | | |

**Figure 3.** Helminth types successfully used to control immunological diseases. Helminths are divided into two phyla. The Nemathelminthes phylum contains the roundworms (Nematodes). The Platyhelminthes phylum contains the tapeworms (Cestodes) and the flukes (Trematodes). Although they are all called worms, the genetic distance between Nemathelminthes and Platyhelminthes is vast. The ability to parasitize another organism developed independently within these groups.

*H. polygyrus bakeri* exposure increases the percentage of CD4$^+$ T cells in the mesenteric and thoracic lymph nodes that express CD25 and Foxp3,[84,85] raising the possibility that T$_{regs}$ mediate protection with cell transfer. In addition, *H. polygyrus bakeri* colonization induces a CD19$^+$CD23$^+$ regulatory B cell population that transfers suppression of allergen-kindled airway inflammation independent of IL-10 production.[59] Like *H. polygyrus bakeri*, exposure to *S. mansoni* induces a population of CD19$^+$CD23$^+$ regulatory B cells that transfer protection from AHR.[88] In this model the regulatory B cells express CD1d, require intact IL-10 production, and act in part by increasing the number of pulmonary CD4$^+$CD25$^+$Foxp3$^+$ regulatory T cells in the lungs.[88] These observations show that helminths activate multiple regulatory circuits that can work independently and at times in concert to inhibit aberrant inflammation.

## How helminths communicate with the host immune system

It is conceivable that these organisms modulate host immunity through release of immune regulatory products or by display of such molecules on their integument. The previous paragraphs already described several molecules proposed to mediate such functions. These include cystatin and ES-62 both derived from various filarial species. Cystatin interacts with macrophages, whereas ES-62 is reported to modulate B cell, macrophage, and dendritic cell functions.[89] Calreticulin is a secretory product of the murine helminth *H. polygyrus bakeri*[90] and the human hookworm Necator americanus.[91] It binds scavenger receptor type A on dendritic cells, prompting a Th2 response. Other molecules and various other "excretory/secretory" factors have been described.[47] To date, no one molecule has been ascribed to the majority of helminth species, and none display the broadly powerful immune regulatory properties shown by the whole organisms. This suggests that no single helminth molecule is responsible for the broad spectrum of immune regulatory activities of various helminth species.

It also remains possible that some helminths, like those which reside in the gut, release factors that indirectly modulate host immunity through altering the composition of our complex intestinal microflora[92] or through other indirect means.

## Summary

Until very recently, helminth infection was ubiquitous. Helminth infection created a strong selective pressure on the human genome that outstrips that driven by bacteria and viruses.[93] Indeed, many of the pathways identified by genome-wide association studies that confer risk for autoimmune and inflammatory disease show genetic variation influenced by helminths in the environment.[6] Thus, it should come as no surprise that eradicating helminths can result in expression of diseases influenced by these pathways.

There are now many animal models representing a diverse range of diseases for which helminths either prevent and/or reverse ongoing pathology. The various animal models and epidemiological data suggest that many helminth species can mediate protection (Fig. 3). In some cases, different helminths may evoke dissimilar mechanisms to quell inflammation. This is not surprising since helminths have diverse evolutionary origins and inhabit unique niches in their host, which influences their access to the host's immune system. The models also suggest that the mechanisms of action will not necessarily be the same for all diseases or mouse strains, or for outbred individuals. Immunological diseases are caused by a vast array of gene interactions, environmental factors, and aberrant host immune responses. Thus, for helminths to modulate disease activity in a large number of patients with a wide range of diseases, one would expect that helminths possess the capacity to simultaneously, selectively, and/or sequentially modulate various immune regulatory pathways. At least in some diseases, helminths interface both with cells of innate and adaptive immunity to exert control. Their powerful stimulatory effect on regulatory dendritic cells, macrophages, T cells, B cells, and/or cytokines is particular noteworthy. While the mouse models hint at some of the potentially important immunologic mechanisms that protect from disease, mostly lacking are human studies validating these observations. Helminths are complex, multicellular animals that modulate and, at times, completely evade host immunity. In most circumstances, little is know regarding the molecular signals exchanged between helminth and host to mediate this process. Even less is known about which helminth products influence disease and how they work.

Continued study of how helminths prevent and reverse inflammatory diseases should help should help elucidate the pathophysiology that led to the emergence of these illnesses in industrialized, highly hygienic countries and hopefully will identify targets for therapy. Furthermore, helminths or their products may prove useful as pharmaceutical agents to control or prevent immune-mediated illness.

## Acknowledgments

This work was supported by DK38327, DK058755, the Broad Foundation, VAMC, the Schneider family, the Friedman family, and the Gilman family.

## Conflicts of interest

The authors are named on patents held by the University of Iowa for the use of helminths in autoimmune and inflammatory disease.

## References

1. Kappus, K.D., R.G.J. Lundgren, D.D. Juranek, *et al*. 1994. Intestinal parasitism in the United States: update on a continuing problem. *Am. J. Trop. Med. Hyg.* **50:** 705–713.
2. Wright, W.H. 1955. Current status of parasitic diseases. *Pub. Health Rep.* **70:** 966–975.
3. Hong, S.T., J.Y. Chai, M.H. Choi, *et al*. 2006. A successful experience of soil-transmitted helminth control in the Republic of Korea. *Korean J. Parasitol.* **44:** 177–185.
4. Yang, S.K., W.S. Hong, Y.I. Min, *et al*. 2000. Incidence and prevalence of ulcerative colitis in the Songpa-Kangdong District, Seoul, Korea, 1986–1997. *J. Gastroenterol. Hepatol.* **15:** 1037–1042.
5. Goncalves, M.L., A. Araujo & L.F. Ferreira. 2003. Human intestinal parasites in the past: new findings and a review. *Memorias do Instituto Oswaldo Cruz.* **98**(Suppl 1): 103–118.
6. Fumagalli, M., U. Pozzoli, R. Cagliani, *et al*. 2010. The landscape of human genes involved in the immune response to parasitic worms. *BMC Evol. Biol.* **10:** 264: 264.
7. Renz, H., M.E. von, P. Brandtzaeg, *et al*. 2011. Gene-environment interactions in chronic inflammatory disease. *Nat. Immunol.* **12:** 273–277.
8. Kaser, A, S. Zeissig & R.S. Blumberg. 2010. Genes and environment: how will our concepts on the pathophysiology of IBD develop in the future? *Dig. Dis.* **28:** 395–405.
9. Rosenstiel, P., C. Sina, A. Franke & S. Schreiber. 2009. Towards a molecular risk map—recent advances on the etiology of inflammatory bowel disease. *Semin. Immunol.* **21:** 334–345.
10. Manninen, P., A.L. Karvonen, H. Huhtala, *et al*. 2010. The epidemiology of inflammatory bowel diseases in Finland. *Scand. J. Gastroenterol.* **45:** 1063–1067.
11. Kappelman, M.D., S.L. Rifas-Shiman, K. Kleinman, *et al*. 2007. The prevalence and geographic distribution of Crohn's disease and ulcerative colitis in the United States. *Clin. Gastroenterol. Hepatol.* **5:** 1424–1429.
12. Loftus, E.V., Jr. 2004. Clinical epidemiology of inflammatory bowel disease: incidence, prevalence, and environmental influences. *Gastroenterology* **126:** 1504–1517.
13. Shin, D.H, D.H. Sinn, Y.H. Kim, *et al*. 2011. Increasing incidence of inflammatory bowel disease among young men

in Korea between 2003 and 2008. *Dig. Dis. Sci.* **56:** 1154–1159.

14. Wang, Y.F., Q. Ouyang & R.W. Hu. 2010. Progression of inflammatory bowel disease in China. *J. Dig. Dis.* **11:** 76–82.

15. Lakatos, L., G. Mester, Z. Erdelyi, *et al.* 2004. Striking elevation in incidence and prevalence of inflammatory bowel disease in a province of western Hungary between 1977–2001. *World J. Gastroenterol.* **10:** 404–409.

16. Yang, S.K., W.S. Hong, Y.I. Min, *et al.* 2000. Incidence and prevalence of ulcerative colitis in the Songpa-Kangdong District, Seoul, Korea, 1986–1997. *J. Gastroenterol. Hepatol.* **15:** 1037–1042.

17. Elliott, D.E., J.F.J. Urban, C.K. Argo & J.V. Weinstock. 2000. Does the failure to acquire helminthic parasites predispose to Crohn's disease? *FASEB J.* **14:** 1848–1855.

18. Weinstock, J.V. & D.E. Elliott. 2009. Helminths and the IBD hygiene hypothesis. *Inflamm. Bowel Dis.* **15:** 128–133.

19. Büning, J., N. Homann, D. von Smolinski, *et al.* 2008. Helminths as governors of inflammatory bowel disease. *Gut* **57:** 1182–1183.

20. Broadhurst, M.J., J.M. Leung, V. Kashyap, *et al.* 2010. IL-22+ CD4+ T cells are associated with therapeutic trichuris trichiura infection in an ulcerative colitis patient. *Sci. Transl. Med.* **2:** 60ra88.

21. Summers, R.W., D.E. Elliott, K. Qadir, *et al.* 2003. Trichuris suis seems to be safe and possibly effective in the treatment of inflammatory bowel disease. *Am. J. Gastroenterol.* **98:** 2034–2041.

22. Summers, R.W., D.E. Elliott, J.F. Urban, Jr., *et al.* 2005. Trichuris suis therapy in Crohn's disease. *Gut* **54:** 87–90.

23. Summers, R.W., D.E. Elliott, J.F. Urban, Jr., *et al.* 2005. Trichuris suis therapy for active ulcerative colitis: a randomized controlled trial. *Gastroenterology* **128:** 825–832.

24. Summers, R.W., D.E. Elliott & J.V. Weinstock. 2005. Is there a role for helminths in the therapy of inflammatory bowel disease? *Nat. Clin. Pract. Gastroenterol. Hepatology* **2:** 62–63.

25. Croese, J., J. O'neil, J. Masson, *et al.* 2006. A proof of concept study establishing Necator americanus in Crohn's patients and reservoir donors. *Gut* **55:** 136–137.

26. Elson, C.O., R.B. Sartor, G.S. Tennyson & R.H. Riddell. 1995. Experimental models of inflammatory bowel disease. *Gastroenterology* **109:** 1344–1367.

27. Hang, L., T. Setiawan, A.M. Blum, *et al.* 2010. Heligmosomoides polygyrus infection can inhibit colitis through direct interaction with innate immunity. *J. Immunol.* **185:** 3184–3189.

28. Elliott, D.E., A. Metwali, J. Leung, *et al.* 2008. Colonization with Heligmosomoides polygyrus suppresses mucosal IL-17 production. *J. Immunol.* **181:** 2414–2419.

29. Matta, B.M., A. Castellaneta & A.W. Thomson. 2010. Tolerogenic plasmacytoid DC. *Eur. J. Immunol.* **40:** 2667–2676.

30. Kreider, T., R.M. Anthony, J.F. Urban, Jr. & W.C. Gause. 2007. Alternatively activated macrophages in helminth infections. *Curr. Opin. Immunol.* **19:** 448–453.

31. Reyes, J.L. & L.I. Terrazas. 2007. The divergent roles of alternatively activated macrophages in helminthic infections. *Parasite Immunol.* **29:** 609–619.

32. Smith, P., N.E. Mangan, C.M. Walsh, *et al.* 2007. Infection with a helminth parasite prevents experimental colitis via a macrophage-mediated mechanism. *J. Immunol.* **178:** 4557–4566.

33. Schnoeller, C., S. Rausch, S. Pillai, *et al.* 2008. A helminth immunomodulator reduces allergic and inflammatory responses by induction of IL-10-producing macrophages. *J. Immunol.* **180:** 4265–4272.

34. Klotz, C., T. Ziegler, A.S. Figueiredo, *et al.* 2011. A helminth immunomodulator exploits host signaling events to regulate cytokine production in macrophages. *PLoS Pathog.* **7:** e1001248.

35. Johnston, M.J., A. Wang, M.E. Catarino, *et al.* 2010. Extracts of the rat tapeworm, Hymenolepis diminuta, suppress macrophage activation in vitro and alleviate chemically induced colitis in mice. *Infect. Immun.* **78:** 1364–1375.

36. Hunter, M.M., A. Wang, K.S. Parhar, *et al.* 2010. In vitro-derived alternatively activated macrophages reduce colonic inflammation in mice. *Gastroenterology* **138:** 1395–1405.

37. Boden, E.K. & S.B. Snapper. 2008. Regulatory T cells in inflammatory bowel disease. *Curr. Opin. Gastroenterol.* **24:** 733–741.

38. Setiawan, T., A. Metwali, A.M. Blum, *et al.* 2007. Heligmosomoides polygyrus promotes regulatory T cell cytokine production in normal distal murine intestine. *Infect. Immun.* **75:** 4655–4663.

39. Elliott, D., J. Li, A. Blum, *et al.* 2003. Exposure to schistosome eggs protects mice from TNBS-induced colitis. *Am. J. Physiol.* **284:** G385–G391.

40. Hunter, M.M., A. Wang, C.L. Hirota & D.M. McKay. 2005. Neutralizing anti-IL-10 antibody blocks the protective effect of tapeworm infection in a murine model of chemically induced colitis. *J. Immunol.* **174:** 7368–7375.

41. Elliott, D.E., T. Setiawan, A. Metwali, *et al.* 2004. Heligmosomoides polygyrus inhibits established colitis in IL-10-deficient mice. *Eur. J. Immunol.* **34:** 2690–2698.

42. Grainger, J.R., K.A. Smith, J.P. Hewitson, *et al.* 2010. Helminth secretions induce de novo T cell Foxp3 expression and regulatory function through the TGF-beta pathway. *J. Exp. Med.* **207:** 2331–2341.

43. Metwali, A., T. Setiawan, A.M. Blum, *et al.* 2006. Induction of CD8+ regulatory T cells in the intestine by Heligmosomoides polygyrus infection. *Am. J. Physiol. Gastrointest. Liver Physiol.* **291:** G253-G259.

44. Costantino, C.M., C. Baecher-Allan & D.A. Hafler. 2008. Multiple sclerosis and regulatory T cells. *J. Clin. Immunol.* **28:** 697–706.

45. Smith, T.R. & V. Kumar. 2008. Revival of CD8+ Treg-mediated suppression. *Trends Immunol.* **29:** 337–342.

46. Ince, M.N., D.E. Elliott, T. Setiawan, *et al.* 2009. Role of T cell TGF-beta signaling in intestinal cytokine responses and helminthic immune modulation. *Eur. J. Immunol.* **39:** 1870–1878.

47. Hewitson, J.P., J.R. Grainger & R.M. Maizels. 2009. Helminth immunoregulation: the role of parasite secreted proteins in modulating host immunity. *Mol. Biochem. Parasitol.* **167:** 1–11.

48. Segura, M., Z. Su, C. Piccirillo & M.M. Stevenson. 2007. Impairment of dendritic cell function by excretory-secretory

products: a potential mechanism for nematode-induced immunosuppression. *Eur. J. Immunol.* **37:** 1887–1904.

49. Strober, W. 2009. The multifaceted influence of the mucosal microflora on mucosal dendritic cell responses. *Immunity* **31:** 377–388.

50. Walk, S.T., A.M. Blum, S.A. Ewing, *et al.* 2010. Alteration of the murine gut microbiota during infection with the parasitic helminth Heligmosomoides polygyrus. *Inflamm. Bowel Dis.* **16:** 1841–1849.

51. Ince, M.N., D.E. Elliott, T. Setiawan, *et al.* 2006. Heligmosomoides polygyrus induces TLR4 on murine mucosal T cells that produce TGFbeta after lipopolysaccharide stimulation. *J. Immunol.* **176:** 726–729.

52. Carvalho, L., J. Sun, C. Kane, F. Marshall, *et al.* 2009. Review series on helminths, immune modulation and the hygiene hypothesis: mechanisms underlying helminth modulation of dendritic cell function. *Immunology* **126:** 28–34.

53. Correale, J. & M. Farez. 2007. Association between parasite infection and immune responses in multiple sclerosis. *Ann. Neurol.* **61:** 97–108.

54. Correale, J. & M.F. Farez. 2011. The impact of parasite infections on the course of multiple sclerosis. *J. Neuroimmunol.* 6–11.

55. Fleming, J., A. Isaak, J. Lee, *et al.* 2011. Probiotic helminth administration in relapsing-remitting multiple sclerosis: a phase 1 study. *Multiple Sclerosis* **17:** 743–754.

56. Sewell, D., Z. Qing, E. Reinke, *et al.* 2003. Immunomodulation of experimental autoimmune encephalomyelitis by helminth ova immunization. *Int. Immunol.* **15:** 59–69.

57. La Flamme, A.C., K. Ruddenklau & B.T. Backstrom. 2003. Schistosomiasis decreases central nervous system inflammation and alters the progression of experimental autoimmune encephalomyelitis. *Infect. Immun.* **71:** 4996–5004.

58. Gruden-Movsesijan, A., N. Ilic, M. Mostarica-Stojkovic, *et al.* 2010. Mechanisms of modulation of experimental autoimmune encephalomyelitis by chronic Trichinella spiralis infection in Dark Agouti rats. *Parasite Immunol.* **32:** 450–459.

59. Wilson, M.S., M.D. Taylor, M.T. O'Gorman, *et al.* 2010. Helminth-induced CD19+CD23hi B cells modulate experimental allergic and autoimmune inflammation. *Eur. J. Immunol.* **40:** 1682–1696.

60. Walsh, K.P., M.T. Brady, C.M. Finlay, *et al.* 2009. Infection with a helminth parasite attenuates autoimmunity through TGF-beta-mediated suppression of Th17 and Th1 responses. *J. Immunol.* **183:** 1577–1586.

61. Cooke, A., P. Tonks, F.M. Jones, *et al.* 1999. Infection with Schistosoma mansoni prevents insulin dependent diabetes mellitus in non-obese diabetic mice. *Parasite Immunol.* **21:** 169–176.

62. Zaccone, P., Z. Fehervari, F.M. Jones, *et al.* 2003. Schistosoma mansoni antigens modulate the activity of the innate immune response and prevent onset of type 1 diabetes. *Eur. J. Immunol.* **33:** 1439–1449.

63. Saunders, K.A., T. Raine, A. Cooke & C.E. Lawrence. 2007. Inhibition of autoimmune type 1 diabetes by gastrointestinal helminth infection. *Infect. Immun.* **75:** 397–407.

64. Liu, Q., K. Sundar, P.K. Mishra, *et al.* 2009. Helminth infection can reduce insulitis and type 1 diabetes through CD25- and IL-10-independent mechanisms. *Infect. Immun.* **77:** 5347–5358.

65. Zaccone, P., O. Burton, N. Miller, *et al.* 2009. Schistosoma mansoni egg antigens induce Treg that participate in diabetes prevention in NOD mice. *Eur. J. Immunol.* **39:** 1098–1107.

66. Zaccone, P., O.T. Burton, S. Gibbs, *et al.* 2010. Immune modulation by Schistosoma mansoni antigens in NOD mice: effects on both innate and adaptive immune systems. *J. Biomed. Biotechnol.* 795210. Epub; 2010 Mar 1.:795210.

67. Espinoza-Jimenez, A., I. Rivera-Montoya, R. Cardenas-Arreola, *et al.* 2010. Taenia crassiceps infection attenuates multiple low-dose streptozotocin-induced diabetes. *J Biomed. Biotechnol.* 850541. Epub; 2010 Jan 4.:850541.

68. Salinas-Carmona, M.C., lC-G de, I. Perez-Rivera, *et al.* 2009. Spontaneous arthritis in MRL/lpr mice is aggravated by Staphylococcus aureus and ameliorated by Nippostrongylus brasiliensis infections. *Autoimmunity* **42:** 25–32.

69. Osada, Y., S. Shimizu, T. Kumagai, *et al.* 2009. Schistosoma mansoni infection reduces severity of collagen-induced arthritis via down-regulation of pro-inflammatory mediators. *Int. J. Parasitol.* **39:** 457–464.

70. He, Y., J. Li. W. Zhuang, *et al.* 2010. The inhibitory effect against collagen-induced arthritis by Schistosoma japonicum infection is infection stage-dependent. *BMC Immunol.* **11:** 28:28.

71. McInnes, I.B., B.P. Leung, M. Harnett, *et al.* 2003. A novel therapeutic approach targeting articular inflammation using the filarial nematode-derived phosphorylcholine-containing glycoprotein ES-62. *J. Immunol.* **171:** 2127–2133.

72. Harnett, M.M., D.E. Kean, A. Boitelle, *et al.* 2008. The phosphorycholine moiety of the filarial nematode immunomodulator ES-62 is responsible for its anti-inflammatory action in arthritis. *Ann. Rheum. Dis.* **67:** 518–523.

73. Shi, M., A. Wang, D. Prescott, *et al.* 2011. Infection with an intestinal helminth parasite reduces Freund's complete adjuvant-induced monoarthritis in mice. *Arthritis Rheum.* **63:** 434–444.

74. Scrivener, S., H. Yemaneberhan, M. Zebenigus, *et al.* 2001. Independent effects of intestinal parasite infection and domestic allergen exposure on risk of wheeze in Ethiopia: a nested case-control study. *Lancet* **358:** 1493–1499.

75. Araujo, M.I., B.S. Hoppe, M. Medeiros, Jr, E.M. Carvalho. 2004. Schistosoma mansoni infection modulates the immune response against allergic and auto-immune diseases. *Mem. Inst. Oswaldo Cruz* **99**(Suppl 1): 27–32.

76. van den Biggelaar, A.H., R. van Ree, L.C. Rodrigues, *et al.* 2000. Decreased atopy in children infected with Schistosoma haematobium: a role for parasite-induced interleukin-10. *Lancet* **356:** 1723–1727.

77. van den Biggelaar, A.H., L.C. Rodrigues, R. van Ree, *et al.* 2004 Long-term treatment of intestinal helminths increases mite skin-test reactivity in Gabonese schoolchildren. *J. Infect. Dis.* **189:** 892–900.

78. Endara, P., M. VacaVaca, M.E. Chico, *et al.* 2010. Long-term periodic anthelmintic treatments are associated with increased allergen skin reactivity. *Clin. Exp. Allergy.* **40:** 1669–1677.

79. Flohr, C., L.N. Tuyen, R.J. Quinnell, *et al.* 2010. Reduced helminth burden increases allergen skin sensitization but not clinical allergy: a randomized, double-blind, placebo-controlled trial in Vietnam. *Clin. Exp. Allergy.* **40:** 131–142.

80. Palmer, L.J., J.C. Celedon, S.T. Weiss, *et al.* 2002. Ascaris lumbricoides infection is associated with increased risk of childhood asthma and atopy in rural China. *Am. J. Respir. Crit. Care Med.* **165:** 1489–1493.

81. Smits, H.H., B. Everts, F.C. Hartgers & M. Yazdanbakhsh. 2010. Chronic helminth infections protect against allergic diseases by active regulatory processes. *Curr. Allergy Asthma Rep.* **10:** 3–12.

82. Bager, P., J. Arnved, S. Ronborg, *et al.* 2010. Trichuris suis ova therapy for allergic rhinitis: a randomized, double-blind, placebo-controlled clinical trial. *J. Allergy Clin. Immunol.* 125: 123–130.

83. Summers, R.W., D.E. Elliott & J.V. Weinstock. 2010. Trichuris suis might be effective in treating allergic rhinitis. *J. Allergy Clin. Immunol.* **125:** 766–767.

84. Kitagaki, K., T.R. Businga, D. Racila, *et al.* 2006. Intestinal helminths protect in a murine model of asthma. *J. Immunol.* **177:** 1628–1635.

85. Wilson, M.S., M.D. Taylor, A. Balic, *et al.* 2005. Suppression of allergic airway inflammation by helminth-induced regulatory T cells. *J. Exp. Med.* **202:** 1199–1212.

86. Mangan, N.E., R.N. van, A.N. McKenzie & P.G. Fallon. 2006. Helminth-modified pulmonary immune response protects mice from allergen-induced airway hyperresponsiveness. *J. Immunol.* **176:** 138–147.

87. Park, H.K., M.K. Cho, S.H. Choi, *et al.* 2011. Trichinella spiralis: infection reduces airway allergic inflammation in mice. *Exp. Parasitol.* **127:** 539–544.

88. Amu, S., S.P. Saunders, M. Kronenberg, *et al.* 2010. Regulatory B cells prevent and reverse allergic airway inflammation via FoxP3-positive T regulatory cells in a murine model. *J. Allergy Clin. Immunol.* **125:** 1114–1124.

89. Harnett, M.M., A.J. Melendez & W. Harnett. 2010. The therapeutic potential of the filarial nematode-derived immunomodulator, ES-62 in inflammatory disease. *Clin. Exp. Immunol.* **159:** 256–267.

90. Rzepecka, J., S. Rausch, C. Klotz, *et al.* 2009. Calreticulin from the intestinal nematode Heligmosomoides polygyrus is a Th2-skewing protein and interacts with murine scavenger receptor-A. *Mol. Immunol.* **46:** 1109–1119.

91. Kasper, G., A. Brown, M. Eberl, *et al.* 2001. A calreticulin-like molecule from the human hookworm Necator americanus interacts with C1q and the cytoplasmic signalling domains of some integrins. *Parasite Immunol.* **23:** 141–152.

92. Walk, S.T., A.M. Blum, S.A. Ewing, *et al.* 2010. Alteration of the murine gut microbiota during infection with the parasitic helminth Heligmosomoides polygyrus. *Inflamm. Bowel Dis.* **16:** 1841–1849.

93. Fumagalli, M., U. Pozzoli, R. Cagliani, *et al.* 2009. Parasites represent a major selective force for interleukin genes and shape the genetic predisposition to autoimmune conditions. *J. Exp. Med.* **206:** 1395–1408.

Ann. N.Y. Acad. Sci. ISSN 0077-8923

ANNALS OF THE NEW YORK ACADEMY OF SCIENCES

Issue: *The Year in Immunology*

# Induction of gut IgA production through T cell-dependent and T cell-independent pathways

Mats Bemark,[1] Preben Boysen,[2] and Nils Y. Lycke[1]

[1]Department of Microbiology and Immunology, Mucosal Immunobiology and Vaccine Center (MIVAC), Institute of Biomedicine, University of Gothenburg, Gothenburg, Sweden. [2]The Institute for Food Safety and Infection Biology, Norwegian School of Veterinary Sciences, Oslo, Norway

Address for correspondence: Mats Bemark, MIVAC, Department of Microbiology and Immunology, University of Gothenburg, P.O. Box 435, 40530 Gothenburg, Sweden. mats.bemark@immuno.gu.se

The gut immune system protects against mucosal pathogens, maintains a mutualistic relationship with the microbiota, and establishes tolerance against food antigens. This requires a balance between immune effector responses and induction of tolerance. Disturbances of this strictly regulated balance can lead to infections or the development inflammatory diseases and allergies. Production of secretory IgA is a unique effector function at mucosal surfaces, and basal mechanisms regulating IgA production have been the focus of much recent research. These investigations have aimed at understanding how long-term IgA-mediated mucosal immunity can best be achieved by oral or sublingual vaccination, or at analyzing the relationship between IgA production, the composition of the gut microbiota, and protection from allergies and autoimmunity. This research has lead to a better understanding of the IgA system; but at the same time seemingly conflicting data have been generated. Here, we discuss how gut IgA production is controlled, with special focus on how differences between T cell-dependent and T cell-independent IgA production may explain some of these discrepancies.

Keywords: IgA; commensal microbiota; B cell; class switch recombination; gut-associated lymphoid tissues

> *"What is there more kindly than the feeling between host and guest?"*
>
> Aeschylus,
> *The Libation Bearers*, 458 BC

## Introduction

A majority of disease-causing viruses and bacteria enter the body through the mucosa. In the gut, protective immunity is often observed following infection, and production of secretory IgA (SIgA) is an important mechanism that hinders pathogenic invasion.[1] Prophylactic mucosal vaccines are hence an attractive preventive measure that can influence global health.[2] Thus far, however, few vaccines with the ability to induce protective gut SIgA responses have been developed. This is partly due to an incomplete understanding of the requirements for long-term memory following mucosal immunization, in general, and IgA memory, in particular. Concomi-

tant with protection, the gut immune system must also prevent inadvertent reactions to the microbiota or to food antigens. Hence, nonresponsiveness or immune tolerance is a hallmark of the regulatory mechanisms that prevail at mucosal membranes. Erroneous activation of the mucosal immune system can result in chronic inflammation and the development of autoimmunity or allergy.[3] Thus, the mucosal immune system must maintain a finely tuned balance between tolerance and immune protection against pathogens. A better understanding of induction and maintenance of mucosal SIgA responses will facilitate the development of mucosal vaccines and novel strategies to suppress allergies and autoimmunity.

IgA-producing plasma cells are primarily situated within the lamina propria (LP) of the mucosa but are also present in the bone marrow and secondary lymphoid organs.[4] More IgA is produced than of all other antibody classes combined. Due

doi: 10.1111/j.1749-6632.2011.06378.x

**Table 1.** Open questions with regard to gut IgA production

· Which B cell lineages are involved in IgA production, and to which extent do they contribute during different types of responses?

· What is the significance of different supporting cell types?

· What is the relative importance of different signaling molecules?

· What cell types produce which B cell-activating signaling molecules *in vivo*?

· What is the phenotype of memory B cells generated after mucosal responses, and how long-lived are they?

· Are there short-lived and long-lived mucosal plasma cells?

· What is the difference between T cell-dependent and T cell-independent mucosal antigens?

· What differences are there in the mucosal response T cell-dependent and T cell-independent antigens?

· What is the relative importance of different IgA inductive sites?

· Can IgA class switch recombination take place in nonorganized tissue, that is, the lamina propria?

· Are specific naive B cells homing to gut-associated lymphoid tissues, or can any recirculating naive cells enter?

· What is the relative importance of different inductive sites in different types of responses?

· Why do mucosal memory B cells and plasma cells home to different mucosal inductive and effector sites?

· How and where are different homing molecules induced?

· Why are there constitutive germinal centers in gut-associated lymphoid tissues?

· Does immunization lead to the formation of new germinal centers or do activated B cells invade existing ones?

· To which extent do mucosal B cells pass germinal centers before becoming IgA-producing plasma cells?

· What is the relationship between IgA-producing plasma cells in the mucosa and plasma cells producing IgA and IgG in the bone marrow?

to its association with the joining (J)-chain, mucosal IgA is mostly polymeric, whereas IgA produced at other sites is monomeric.[5] After secretion from plasma cells mucosal IgA is transported across epithelial cells through polymeric Ig receptor (pIgR)-mediated transcytosis.[6] Additional complexity is found in humans that have two IgA subclasses, IgA1 and IgA2.[5] In humans, monomeric IgA1 antibodies dominate in serum, whereas both IgA1 and IgA2 are produced at mucosal sites.[7] Recent studies have focused on how B cells are induced to produce IgA. These investigations have increased our understanding of IgA production, but there are still many unanswered questions, and in some cases controversies remain within the field (Table 1). The aim of this review is to highlight some of these issues, with a special focus on how differences between T cell-dependent and T cell-independent gut IgA responses may explain some seemingly conflicting findings.

## IgA class switch recombination and somatic hypermutation

Class switch recombination (CSR) and somatic hypermutation (SHM) take place in activated B cells.[8,9] CSR is a process during which DNA is deleted from

the antibody heavy chain constant (C) region to allow the IgM C region to be exchanged for downstream regions, while keeping the antigen-binding variable (V) region (Fig. 1). SHM creates random mutations in V regions. SHM is crucial for affinity maturation in germinal centers (GC), a process that requires interactions between B cells, antigens on follicular dendritic cells (FDC), and follicular helper T cells (T$_{FH}$).[10] Both SHM and CSR are initiated through the activation induced cytosine deaminase (AID) protein.[8] The function of AID is controlled in multiple ways to ensure that its action is restricted to activated B cells. AID targets the antibody genes for CSR and SHM through deamination of cytosine in DNA to uracil. The current model for how the uracil residues are subsequently converted to mutations implies proliferative replication.[8] The model does not strictly rule out CSR in nonproliferating cells. However, this has never been observed, and, indeed, high AID expression was found not to be sufficient for activation of SHM or CSR in nonproliferating cells.[11,12] Notably, although SHM and CSR usually are linked, there are examples where one occurs in the absence of the other, suggesting that they require different AID modifications and supporting proteins.[9]

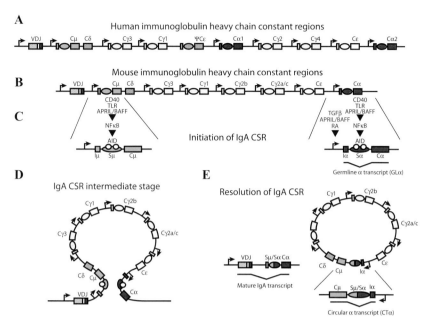

**Figure 1.** Human and mouse immunoglobulin heavy chain constant regions and class switch recombination to IgA. (A and B) Humans and mice have a similar organization of their constant regions, although they probably evolved through distinct processes. A large duplication created four IgG, two IgE, and two IgA regions in humans, but one IgE region is now a pseudogene ($\Psi$C$\epsilon$). In mice, only the constant regions for IgG expanded, leaving single downstream IgE and IgA regions. (C) Signals that induce AID expression (CD40, TLR, or APRIL/BAFF) and germline $\alpha$ transcripts (GL$\alpha$) from the I$\alpha$ promoter (TGF-$\beta$, APRIL/BAFF, RA) initiate IgA CSR by targeting the IgM and IgA switch regions. (D) This will bring the switch regions close to each other and will generate double stranded DNA breaks in them. (E) When the double stranded breaks are resolved, the recombination will create an antibody gene expressing IgA in the genome, and nonintegrated switch circle. For a short period, circular $\alpha$ transcripts (CT$\alpha$) are initiated from the I$\alpha$ promoter where the small I$\alpha$ exon is spliced to C$\mu$. The presence of CT$\alpha$ transcripts is the most conclusive evidence available for ongoing IgA CSR.

Mice have a single C$\alpha$, whereas humans have two (C$\alpha_1$ and C$\alpha_2$) (Fig. 1).[7] Upstream from C$\alpha$ is the IgA switch region (S$\alpha$). Germline (GL$\alpha$) transcription can be initiated from promoters attached to a small nontranslated exon (I$\alpha$) to target the S$\alpha$ region for CSR.[9] In addition to CSR from IgM to IgA, sequential switching has been described.[13] In this case, an already class-switched antibody gene rearranges to S$\alpha$. Expression of AID, GL$\alpha$ transcription, and proliferation of B cells are prerequisites for IgA CSR. They are, however, not sufficient, and other molecular markers are needed to experimentally demonstrate ongoing CSR.[9,11] During CSR, IgA switch circles and postswitch $\alpha$ circle transcripts (CT$\alpha$) occur, and as CT$\alpha$ are short lived after completing CSR, they are the best available proof of recent IgA CSR.[14,15]

## Signals inducing IgA CSR

A variety of signals promotes the formation of IgA-producing plasma cells. Among these are antigens binding to the B cell receptor (BCR), NF-$\kappa$B inducing signals, factors that induce transcription from the I$\alpha$ promoter, and cytokines that promote B cell differentiation and/or cell survival. BCR signals dictate the antigen-specificity of B cell responses. Antigen binding elicits a number of signals that activate the B cell, triggers antigen uptake, endosomal processing, and MHC II presentation. This signal, not unique for IgA CSR, is discussed in detail in recent reviews.[16,17] NF-$\kappa$B signals also promote CSR, possibly through the activation of AID.[18,19] The major trigger for NF-$\kappa$B during systemic T cell-dependent responses is CD40.[20] When T cell-independent antigens trigger CSR, extensive BCR cross-linking or Toll-like receptor (TLR) stimulation induces NF-$\kappa$B instead.[21] For IgA CSR, CD40 and TLR signals are important but not essential.[22–24] A third pathway that can activate NF-$\kappa$B and trigger IgA CSR is the binding of a proliferation-inducing ligand (APRIL) or B cell activating factor (BAFF; TNF family member) to the transmembrane activator and calcium modulator and cyclophilin ligand interactor (TACI).[25,26] In this case, APRIL or BAFF also induces GLα transcripts. Both TACI- and APRIL-deficient mice have lowered levels of serum IgA but not any changes in IgG levels, suggesting specific roles in supporting IgA production.[27–30] In APRIL-deficient mice, specific T cell-dependent IgA responses were also diminished after mucosal immunization, whereas IgG responses after systemic immunizations were unaffected compared to those in wild-type mice.[30]

Transforming growth factor (TGF)-β is arguably the most important factor directing B cells toward IgA differentiation.[31] TGF-β induces binding of SMAD3/4 and Runx3 to a TGF-β responsive element in the Iα promoter, thereby activating GLα transcription.[31] The *in vivo* importance of TGF-β for IgA CSR was elegantly demonstrated in mice that lack TGF-β receptors on B cells.[32,33] In these mice, the number of IgA-producing plasma cells is decreased 10–100 fold, and no antigen-specific IgA production is detected after immunization. IgA antibodies were still present, although at levels fivefold lower than in wild-type (WT) mice. Whether this was due to homeostatic expansion of rare B cells still expressing TGF-β receptors or to IgA CSR in the absence of TGF-β signals is not known. Other factors with the ability to induce Iα promoter transcription are BAFF, APRIL (discussed above), all-trans-retinoic acid (RA), vasoactive intestinal peptide (VIP), and IgA-inducing protein (IGIP). RA has many functions in the gut, the most noted being imprinting of gut homing through induction of $\alpha_4\beta_7$ integrins.[34] However, RA also supports IgA differentiation in concert with cytokines and other factors produced by dentritic cells (DC).[35,36] RA can enhance TGF-β–induced transcription through an RA response element in the Iα promoter.[37] Depletion of vitamin A (the RA precursor) impairs IgA production.[38] This supports a role in IgA CSR, but as vitamin A has many functions in the body, this might occur indirectly. VIP induces IgA CSR through increased expression of GLα transcripts, but the mechanism is unclear.[39] VIP stimulation also induces IGIP expression in DC, a factor that can further activate GLα transcription.[40] A variety of other cytokines also influence gut IgA production, probably through promoting survival and differentiation of plasma cells. The strongest cases have been presented for interleukin (IL)-4, IL-5, IL-6, IL-10,

IL-15, and, more recently, IL-21.[41] IL-21 supports plasma cell differentiation in GC, but recent studies have suggested specific roles in human IgA CSR, including AID induction, activation of Iα promoters, and imprinting of gut homing properties.[42,43] In mice, IL-21 inhibits TGF-β induced activation of GLγ2b transcription, suggesting that it ensures that IgA and not IgG2b is produced at mucosal sites.[44]

## Gut-associated lymphoid tissue

The mucosal humoral immune system consists of inductive sites, where B cells are activated and clonally expanded, and effector sites, where the cells terminally differentiate into IgA antibody-secreting cells.[4] Gut-proximal inductive sites are referred to as gut-associated lymphoid tissue (GALT; Fig. 2). Formation of Peyer's patches (PP) and colon patches (cP) is programmed during fetal development. Lymphoid tissue inducer cells (LTi) interact with stromal cells and attract lymphocytes.[45] Blocking lymphotoxin (LT) or IL-7 signaling during pregnancy prevents formation of PP and cP in the progeny.[46,47] The formation of isolated lymphoid follicles (ILF) is dependent on bacterial colonization in mice, but not in humans, in which they are present already at birth.[48,49] In mice, there seems to be a gradual differentiation of ILF starting from cryptopatches containing LTi-like cells, to immature ILF (iILF) structures with B cell follicles, to mature ILF (mILF) with GC.[50,51]

PP, cP, and mILF are covered with a follicle-associated epithelium (FAE) in which specialized M cells transport luminal antigens into the follicle through transcytosis.[52] On the basolateral side of the M cell, DC, macrophages, T cells, and B cells are present in the subepithelial dome (SED). Here, immature DC take up and process antigen and then migrate to the intrafollicular T cell areas. In ILF they end up close to B cell follicles, as ILF lack distinct T cell areas.[53,54] Mesenteric lymph node (MLN) B cell follicles occasionally contain GC, but PP invariably host GC in their B cell follicles.[4] Whereas GC within cP have been described, they seem to be less prevalent than in PP (Fig. 3). Around 100–200 ILF are present in each mouse small intestine, but only a small fraction of these are mILF with GC.[50,51]

Signals needed for formation of GALT GC are different than for systemic GC. In GALT they are constitutively present, whereas systemically they are only induced after immunization.[55] Both

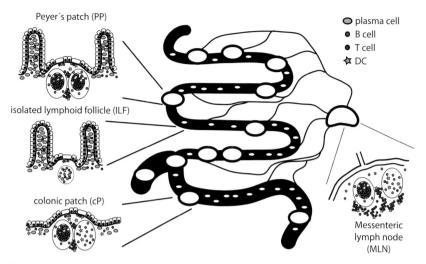

**Figure 2.** B cells in mouse GALT. Along the small and large intestine are larger (Peyers patches and colonic patches; PP and cP) and smaller (isolated lymphoid follicles; ILF) organized assemblies of lymphoid cells. B cell follicles in PP invariably contain germinal centers, whereas follicles in cP rarely do. T cell zones are situated between the follicles. Above the follicles is the subepithelial dome. Here, M cells deliver antigen from the lumen to B cells, T cells, and DC. Germinal centers are very rare in ILF, and no distinct T cell areas are present in ILF. PP, cP, and ILF are surrounded by a lamina propria filled with IgA-producing plasma cells, T lymphocytes, and DC, but rarely naive B cells. Lymphatics from gut tissue and GALT drain to mesenteric lymph nodes (MLN). These are organized as other lymph nodes, and B cell follicles in them may contain germinal centers.

require CD40 signals, but T cell subsets distinct from archetypical CD4[+] T cells can substitute in GALT.[22,56] PP GC can form without antigenic stimulation and are present in mice with monoclonal antigen receptors that do not react to known mucosal antigens, and in gene-targeted mice in which the viral protein LMP2 mimics the antibody heavy chain.[57,58] Bacterial signals are not strictly required for PP GC but play an important role in the formation of mouse ILF.[51,59,60] Similarly, bacterial stimulation can induce GC formation in cP; enlarged GCs are observed during DSS-induced colitis that disrupts the mucosal barrier in the colon.[61,62]

When discussing these prerequisites and signals involved in formation of GALT tissues in mice, it should be remembered that laboratory mice do not represent animals living under normal evolutionary pressure.[63] Lab mouse strains are inbred and carry genomes that differ substantially from wild mice. Laboratory-reared mice are also fed a controlled diet and breeding occurs under pathogen-free conditions. We determined if the organization of the GALT was different in wild-living compared to laboratory-reared mice and found that the general organization was similar, with perhaps slightly more IgA[+] cells present in villi from wild-living mice

(Fig. 4). PP and cP were well developed, with large GC areas, and, interestingly, ILF were relatively rare in the small intestines and did not host GC.

## Functions of IgA

Specific IgA antibodies protect against bacteria and viruses by inhibiting bacterial adherence, neutralizing viruses, and blocking toxins.[4] Other functions include binding of antigens before trancytosis, which leads to retrograde transport of antigens into the lumen, and activation of cells through binding to Fc receptors.[64,65] Although these functions of SIgA are well-defined, it has been difficult to assess which critical roles SIgA has in mouse models. IgA-deficient mice and humans produce increased levels of compensatory IgM antibodies that are transported into the lumen through the same pIgR-mediated transcytosis mechanism as IgA.[66,67] Moreover, pIgR- and J-chain deficient mice, although not capable of actively secreting SIgA, "leak" antibodies through the mucosa into the lumen, likely due to a perturbed mucosal barrier function.[68–72] Subsequently, the importance of SIgA may be underestimated using these models. Still, even in the presence of the compensatory mechanisms, these mouse models show increased susceptibility to

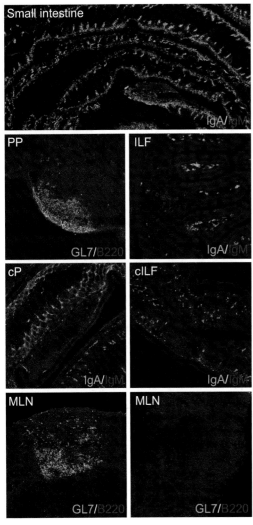

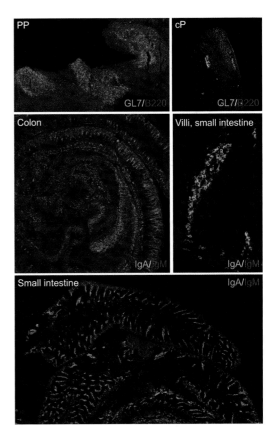

**Figure 4.** GALT in wild-caught mice. Wild-living mice were trapped in the Oslo area in Norway, and freeze sections were prepared as in Figure 3. PP are larger than in laboratory mice and contain larger germinal center areas. Germinal centers are also present in cP, although they are smaller than in the PP. The colon contains both cP and ILF, but no IgM+ cells outside of these areas. Small intestinal villi are filled with IgA-producing plasma cells, whereas IgM+ cells are only observed in PP. Of note, ILF are very rare, if at all present, in the small intestine, but are often observed in the colon.

**Figure 3.** GALT in laboratory mice. Freeze section prepared from gut and GALT of C57BL/6 mice were immunofluorescently labeled with anti-IgM (green) and anti-IgA (red) or GL7 (green) and B220 (red) before analysis by confocal microscopy. IgA-expressing plasma cells filled the villi of the small intestine, but no IgM+ cells are present there. IgM+ cells are instead situated in PP, one of which are present in the gut section, and ILF. A small ILF from the small intestines and a large from the colon are shown, as well as a larger cP. B cell follicles in PP invariably contain germinal centers, but cP rarely do. MLN contain B cell follicles with (left-hand side) or without (right-hand side) germinal centers.

infections, including rotavirus, influenza, *Salmonella typhimurium*, and *Giardia muris*.[1,4] The protective mucosal SIgA-response that has been studied in most detail in mice is, however, that against cholera toxin (CT). After mucosal immunization with CT, SIgA effectively prevents toxin-binding to epithelial cells and an ensuing diarrheal episode.[73,74] This feature was essential for the development of the drinkable cholera vaccine Dukoral® (Crucell, Leiden, the Netherlands), a vaccine based on killed cholera bacteria mixed with the nontoxic B subunit of CT.[2,75] Interestingly, effective protection against CT appears to be dependent on SHM to produce high-affinity antibodies.[76]

IgA reactive to commensal bacteria is present in gut secretions but not in serum, suggesting a specific involvement of SIgA in maintaining the microbiota.[77] This is supported by the observations that B cell-deficient mice are less effective in controlling lymphatic bacterial spread to MLN after colonization of new bacterial species, and that preimmunization of WT mice inhibits bacterial spreading.[78] In addition, IgA appears to tailor the composition of the microbiota; if IgA production is reintroduced into AID-deficient mice, disturbances in the intestinal microbiota associated with AID deficiency are reversed.[79] An experiment based on *Bacteroides thetaiotaomicron* mono-colonization showed that one specific antibody against a bacterial capsular polysaccharide was sometimes sufficient to diminish pathogenic activation of the innate immunity.[80] An anti-inflammatory effect of IgA is also evident after birth. Pups with mothers not producing milk IgA develop strong inflammation-induced IgA responses against microbiota when their mothers are still feeding them milk. However, if the mothers are IgA proficient, the pups do not develop inflammation-induced IgA responses until weaned.[81,82] This protection from inflammation can be maintained with a very limited IgA repertoire, arguing that high-affinity interactions with the microbiota may not be needed.[81]

## T cell-dependent and T cell-independent IgA production

Three types of antibodies are found in serum: natural, T cell-independent (TI), and T cell-dependent (TD). In mice, these are linked to different cell lineages, namely B1, marginal zone (MZ), and follicular B2 B cells.[83] Similar pathways have been identified for mucosal IgA production (Table 2). Some antigens require T cell help to induce SIgA responses, whereas others do not. In addition, IgA without any known antigen specificity is produced. Some is produced even in germ free (GF) mice fed antigen-free diets, but the term *natural IgA* in general refers to nonspecific SIgA produced in the absence of antigenic stimulation in normal colonized mice.[84,85] It is almost impossible to discriminate between the contribution of natural IgA versus specific TI IgA, and both forms are discussed under TI responses below.

### T cell-dependent responses
CT is the most powerful oral immunogen known, and more than 25% of all IgA-secreting plasma cells can be CT specific after repeated immunizations. In addition, CT has adjuvant activity when mixed with coadministered antigens. In addition to mucosal production of SIgA, oral immunization with CT also results in production of antigen-specific serum IgA and IgG.[86] Early studies using ligated intestinal loops for immunizations revealed that PP was the prime site for induction of anti-CT IgA responses in the gut.[87,88] More recently, the role of an intact and correctly organized GALT was confirmed as necessary for a strong anti-CT IgA response, because mice lacking MLN and PP as a consequence of LTβR-Ig and TNFR55-Ig treatment during fetal life failed to respond to CT.[89] What makes CT such a powerful mucosal antigen/adjuvant is still enigmatic, but targeting of DC and direct effects on B cells have been demonstrated.[90–93]

Production of specific antibodies after oral CT-immunization depends on CD40 signals and CD4[+] T cells, making it a typical TD response.[22,56] The roles for other molecules, cells, and organ structures in gut CT responses have been extensively investigated (Table 3). Notably, many gene-targeted mice do not respond to oral CT immunization, although they show SIgA production. Furthermore, in many gene-deficient strains, mucosal and systemic immunity are differentially regulated. The differences in IgA production observed between CD28-deficient mice and mice that express CTLA4-Ig to block CD28/B7 signals are particularly confounding. Transgenic CTLA4-Ig mice show impaired responses to oral CT immunization despite the presence of PP GC, serum IgA, and gut SIgA, whereas disruption of CD28 is associated with almost normal local SIgA CT responses despite a lack of GC in the PP and, instead, a loss of serum IgA.[99,100] A possible explanation for this is that CTLA4-Ig can inhibit inflammation and rejection through a non-CD28–dependent mechanism involving indoleamine 2,3-dioxygenase (IDO) and inducible nitric oxide synthase (iNOS).[106,107] Recent studies indeed provide links between both IDO and iNOS and IgA production; TNF-α– and iNOS–producing (Tip) DC have been shown to support IgA CSR, and IDO can trigger production of TGF-β in DC.[24,108]

### T cell-independent responses
Nude mice that lack a functional thymus produce some IgA despite lacking essentially all T cells and PP GC.[109] The fact that this IgA production is not due to TI T cell functions was subsequently confirmed in mice lacking TCRαβ and TCRγδ T cells.[110] T cell-deficient mice could indeed even initiate

**Table 2.** Comparison between TD and TI responses

| | Antibody class | Plasma cells | Longevity | Formation of memory cells | B cell type | Typical antigens |
|---|---|---|---|---|---|---|
| **Systemic responses** | | | | | | |
| Natural IgM | IgM | ? | +++ | – | B1 | – |
| TI response | IgM > IgG | Peripheral organs | + | – (+) | MZB | TLR ligands, Repeated epitopes |
| TD response | IgG > IgM | BM | ++ | ++ | B2 | Proteins |
| **Mucosal responses** | | | | | | |
| Natural IgA | IgA | LP | +++ | – | ? | – |
| TI response | IgA | LP | + | – (+) | B2 (B1?) | Commensal bacteria |
| TD responses | IgA > IgG, IgM[a] | LP/BM | ++ | ++/+ | B2 | Pathogens Toxins |

TI, T cell-independent; TD, T cell-dependent; BM, bone marrow; LP, lamina propria; B1, B1 B cells; MZB, marginal zone B cells; B2, follicular B2 cells.

[a]IgG- and IgM-producing cells are found in the bone marrow but rarely in GALT or LP.

rotavirus-specific SIgA responses following infection.[111] It was subsequently demonstrated that SIgA reactive to the commensal microbiota was produced through a TI mechanism.[77] TI IgA production did not require organized B cell follicles in PP or mILF, as it was observed in mice lacking TNFR1, but the absence of any IgA production in *aly/aly* and LTα-deficient mice indicated that other organized lymphoid tissues were still needed. The site for TI IgA induction is likely the SED or B cell follicles of PP or ILF, where TCRβ/δ-deficient mice host AID-expressing B cells in close contact with CD11c+ DC.[45] Notably, there is specificity in TI antibodies; after mono-colonization the SIgA produced is specific for that particular bacterial species.[59] Other groups have, however, argued that a majority of SIgA antibodies are nonspecific natural IgA and form in response to any bacterial colonization of GF mice.[85]

A third site suggested to be important for IgA CSR during TI responses is the LP.[14] This has subsequently become a rather controversial issue with regard to IgA B cell differentiation. Data supporting LP CSR comes from both mice and human studies (discussed later). The most important argument for CSR outside of GALT is that mice lacking LTi cells due to Id2 or RORγt deficiency, and therefore missing organized GALT structures, have been found to produce some IgA.[45,60,112] Low numbers of AID-expressing cells can indeed be detected in the mouse LP.[60] Importantly, however, CSR, requires cell proliferation, which, to our knowledge, has not been demonstrated in the mucosal LP of either humans or mice. Most cells expressing AID in the LP are indeed already IgA+, suggesting that AID-expressing cells in the LP could be postswitch cells.[113] Notably, IgA CSR in gut LP has never been confirmed by the presence of postswitch CTα in mice, whereas it has repeatedly been documented in gut tissues verified to contain lymphoid follicles.[22,114,115] It could be argued that this is due to low sensitivity of the CTα assays.[60,116,117] However, such an explanation seems unlikely, as studies that failed to detect postswitch CTα in nonorganized LP readily detected these in tissues harboring ILFs.[22,114,115]

### Lessons from CD40-deficient mice

CD40-deficient mice have a similar phenotype as mice that lack T cells, with no GC or systemic responses against TD antigens.[22] Both strains, however, have well organized PP containing SED and B cell follicles, and maintain ILF structures.[22,45] They also produce substantial, but subnormal, amounts of gut SIgA and serum IgA, cannot respond to TD-antigens, and fail to develop SIgA antibodies after immunizations with CT. Using the CD40-deficient mouse model, we sought to identify TI

**Table 3.** CT responses in mouse models

| Mouse model | Gut SIgA | Serum IgA | PP GC | Gut SIgA response | | Serum IgA response | | Systemic immunization | Ref. |
|---|---|---|---|---|---|---|---|---|---|
| | | | | CT | Antigen | CT | Antigen | | |
| IL-4[−/−] | ++ | ++ | − | ++ | − | − | ++ | ND | 94 |
| IL-6[−/−] | ++ | ++ | ++ | ++ | ++ | ++ | ++ | ++ | 95 |
| IL-17[−/−] | ND | ND | ND | ND | − | ND | − | ND | 96 |
| APRIL[−/−] | + | + | ND | ND | ND | ND | + | ++/+ | 30 |
| CD4[−/−] | ++ | | ++ | − | − | + | (+) | (+) | 56,97 |
| CD8[−/−] | ++ | ++ | ++ | ++ | +++ | ++ | ++ | ++ | 56,97 |
| CD19[−/−] | ++ | ++ | ++ | + | (+) | + | (+) | ++ | 98 |
| CD28[−/−] | ++ | − | − | ++ | ++ | − | ND | − | 99 |
| CD40[−/−] | ++ | ++ | − | − | − | − | − | − | 22 |
| CTLA4-Ig tg | ++ | ++ | ++ | + | + | − | (+) | + | 100 |
| TGF-βR-B | + | + | ++ | ND | ND | ND | − | ++/−[a] | 32,33 |
| IFN-γR[−/−] | ++ | ++ | ++ | ++ | + | ++ | + | ++ | 101 |
| CCR10[−/−] | ++ | ++ | ++ | −/+ | ND | ND | ND | ND | 102,103 |
| TNF/LTα[−/−] | − | ND | No PP/MLN | − | − | − | − | ++ | 104 |
| *In utero* LTβR-Ig | ++ | ND | No PP | + | + | + | + | ND | 104 |
| *In utero* LTβR-Ig TNFR55-Ig | ++ | ND | No PP/MLN | ND | − | ND | ND | ND | 89 |
| J-chain[−/−] | + | +++ | ++ | +/++[b] | ND | +++ | ND | ++ | 70 |
| pIgR[−/−] | (+) | +++ | ++ | +/++[b] | ND | ND | ND | ++ | 105 |
| AID[−/−] | − | − | +++ | −[c] | −[c] | −[c] | −[c] | −[c] | 76 |
| AID[G23S] | ++ | ++ | +++ | + | ND | ND | ND | ND | 76 |

The ability of the indicated mouse models to produce gut SIgA, serum IgA, host GC in PP, respond to CT or coadministered antigen with specific IgA in gut or serum after oral immunization, and to respond to systemic immunization with IgG are indicated. The mouse models were gene targeted (−/−), gene-deleted in B cells only (TGFβR-B), expressing a mutated gene (AID[G23S]), transgenic for a decoy receptor (CTLA4-Ig) or treated *in utero* with decoy receptors. AID[G23S] mice carry a point mutated AID gene that efficiently induce CSR but only support very limited SHM.

ND, not determined; −, undetectable or very low response; +, lowered response; ++, normal response; +++, enhanced response.

[a] A slightly increased responses for most classes, but no specific IgA produced.

[b] J-chain and pIgR deficient mice have plasma cells but cannot secrete SIgA antibodies.

[c] AID[−/−] B cells cannot switch and therefore do not produce any IgA but may still respond with IgM.

IgA-inductive sites using AID expression, GLα transcripts, and postswitch CTα as markers. We found that GLα, AID, and CTα were present in PP from CD40-deficient and WT mice.[22,114] We also found these markers expressed in cryosections of gut LP, but only when these sections contained ILFs; whereas carefully dissected gut tissues devoid of ILF never showed AID and CTα expression. Interestingly, as we identified B cells undergoing IgA CSR in PP, we found a population of proliferating GL7[int] cells in both CD40-deficient and WT mice. The GL7[int] population expressed AID and postswitch CTα, and had undergone no or very limited SHM. By contrast, in WT mice, GL7[high] GC B cells carried mutations and expressed AID but lacked CTα, suggesting that IgA CSR in PP normally occurs prior to that cells enter into GC reactions. We believe the GL7[int] B cells are identical to AID-expressing B cells present in PP of TCRβ/δ deficient mice.[45] Consistent with this concept of extensive pre-GC IgA CSR is the observation that the majority of IgA[+] B cells in PP express the GC markers AID and CD95.[113]

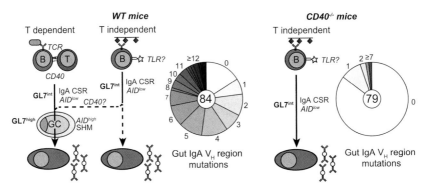

**Figure 5.** A comparison of IgA production in WT and CD40-deficient mice. In CD40-deficient mice, TD responses are absent. Although the IgA levels in serum and gut tissue reach levels approximately half that in WT mice, IgA V regions do not show sign of hypermutation. B cells expressing intermediate levels of GL7 express postswitch CTα, although they express relatively low levels of AID. In WT mice, CSR in PP is also restricted to unmutated GL7int cells, suggesting that these are the cells undergoing IgA CSR during both TD and TI responses. IgA in the gut lamina propria is mutated in WT mice, suggesting that most plasma cells derive from cells that had proliferated and mutated in GC after CSR. It is currently unclear if the low frequency of unmutated antibodies in WT mice is due to that antibodies generated in TI responses only make up a small proportion of plasma cells in WT mice, or if cells activated during TI responses enter into germinal centers and mutate.

Two important observations were made from randomly cloned LP IgA V regions.[114] First, clonally related cells were present in spatially separated gut regions in WT and CD40-deficent mice. Thus, B cells clonally expand before seeding the LP. Second, whereas more than 85% of all V regions carried mutations in WT mice, less than 15% had mutations in CD40-deficient mice. These observations suggested that B cells generated during TD responses class-switched to IgA at a GL7int stage prior to entering GC, and then proliferated and mutated in GC (Fig. 5). B cells can indeed enter into preformed GC during systemic responses, and recent work in our laboratory suggest that antigen-activated gut B cells can also enter preformed PP GC (Bergqvist *et al.* submitted).[118,119] According to our model, B cells activated by TI antigens switch to IgA during the GL7int stage, but what happens to the cells after CSR is less clear. In CD40-deficient mice they clearly seed the LP without entering a GC. As essentially all gut LP plasma cells in WT mice have gone through extensive SHM, it is possible that in this case TI activated B cells enter GC prior to migrating to the LP to mutate their V regions. Alternatively, TI activated B cells undergo IgA CSR at the GL7int stage and then directly migrate to the gut LP without acquiring mutations. Notably, in the latter case, the proportion of TI-generated IgA plasma cells in the gut LP is low compared to a dominant contribution of TD antigen-driven cells.

## Cells involved in IgA production

Few IgA-producing plasma cells are present at birth, and a massive induction is observed after weaning. Mice living under GF conditions produce little IgA even after weaning, only between 10% and 20% of IgA produced by WT mice.[77,84] IgA induction after weaning or after colonization of GF mice is associated with a rapid influx of IgA-producing cells into the GALT and increased size of PP.[59] Microbial colonization, therefore, plays a major role in establishing normal IgA production in mice. Monocolonization experiments have indicated that bacterial species differ in their ability to stimulate IgA production. In particular, noncultivable, intestinal, segmented filamentous bacteria are effective at triggering IgA production.[120] More recently, another type of noncultivable bacterium, *Alcaligenes*, was shown to drive IgA production after invading PP and ILF.[121]

Bacterial colonization may influence IgA production via induction of NF-κB through the TLR–MyD88 axis and the nucleotide-binding oligomerization domain (NOD) leucine-rich repeat receptors (NLR). These pathways have overlapping but nonredundant roles in GALT. For example, NOD1 triggers development of iILF, whereas TLR signals are needed for formation of mILF.[122] The role for NLR proteins in IgA production has been poorly studied. Normal levels of IgA were found in the serum of NOD1-deficient animals, and the inflammasome, but not NLRP3, were needed for influenza-specific nasal secretion of IgA.[123,124] With regard to TLR signals, there are conflicting data reporting that MyD88-deficient mice produce normal or decreased levels of IgA.[23,24,125,126] Moreover, it has been demonstrated that mice which simultaneously lack TLR2, 4, and 9 have decreased levels of IgA, and that GC in PP of MyD88-deficient mice are small and functionally deficient because of a lack of TLR signaling in the FDC network.[24,126]

In mice it is unclear to what extent different B cell lineages—namely follicular B2, MZ B cells, and B1 B cells—contribute to IgA responses.[4] In particular, the importance of B1 B cells has been debated.[127] B1 cells are mainly localized to the peritoneum and this population is, at least partly, self-renewing. The contribution of B1 cells to the population of SIgA-producing plasma cells has been estimated to be anywhere between <5% to 50% depending on which experimental model used. A possible explanation could be that some models rely on lymphopenic and/or irradiated animals for adoptive transfers of naive B cells.[128] In these models, homeostasis may lead to selective proliferation of self-renewing B1 cells, giving them an unnatural advantage. Furthermore, irradiation can disturb the integrity of the gut wall, leading to leakage of bacterial components. LPS injected into the peritoneal cavity can trigger egress of peritoneal B1 cells through the omentum, which then preferentially home back to the peritoneum or gut tissues.[129,130] It has also been suggested that precursors present in adult spleen seed the peritoneum, and that these subsequently enter the gut to produce most IgA.[131] However, a carefully performed experiment in which mice were treated to have different antibody allotypes in B1 and B2 cells suggested that self-renewing B1 cells contributed minimally to gut IgA production even though they still contributed to natural serum IgM.[128] We obtained similar results when GFP-expressing B cells were transferred into the peritoneum of WT mice. Long-term chimerism of GFP-expressing and GFP-nonexpressing B1 cells was achieved, but at best very limited numbers of IgA-producing gut plasma cells expressed GFP several weeks after transfer (Bergqvist and Bemark, unpublished). Thus, it seems that while B1 cells can reach the gut and produce IgA under some conditions, self-renewing B1 cells contribute very little to

IgA production under normal steady-state conditions.

Diverse T cells are present in GALT, including Th1, Th2, Th9, Th17, $T_{reg}$, Tr1, $T_{FH}$, CD8$^+$ α/β T cells, and γ/δ cells.[132,133] There is considerable functional overlap between these T cells with regard to their ability to support B cell differentiation, and even mice that lack T cells have considerable numbers of IgA-producing plasma cells.[77] Still, T cell signals are required for the response to TD antigens and GALT GC formation. Some studies indicate that GC formation may be neither required nor sufficient for TD SIgA responses. Hence, CD28-deficient mice respond to CT despite complete lack of GC; and even though GC form in mice without CD4$^+$ T cells they do not respond to oral immunization with CT.[56,99] Th17 cells were recently shown to be important for mucosal responses to CT, although it was not tested if this observation was a direct effect of perturbed T–B cell interaction, or whether it was an indirect effect due to that the whole gut microenvironment was changed in Th17-deficient mice.[96] Furthermore, recent data suggest that the origin for $T_{FH}$ cells in the GALT may be unique in that they can be derived from FoxP3-expressing $T_{reg}$ cells, rather than from Th1 or Th2 cells;[134,135] to induce this T cell transformation, interactions with B cells appear to be necessary. The converted $T_{reg}$ cells continue to express TGF-β and IL-10, which support IgA CSR, even after losing FoxP3 expression. Notably, interactions with microbial antigens can trigger the development of antigen-specific $T_{reg}$ cells in colon, and they may also play a role in supporting survival of SIgA-producing plasma cells in the LP.[134,136]

In GALT, interactions between DC and B cells appear to play an important role in the induction of IgA differentiation, especially during TI responses.[35] The composition of the DC compartment in the gut is complex, and there are also cells such as CX$_3$CR$^+$ and Tip DC that can be classified as either DC or macrophages.[137] Both the ILF and the LP contain large numbers of DC, and among these Tip and TLR5$^+$ DC especially have been found to support IgA B cell differentiation.[24,112] CX$_3$CR$^+$ DC can sample antigens by extending processes into the gut lumen.[138] As they are nonmigratory, they can then either activate B cells *in situ* or deliver antigen to migratory cells.[139] Alternatively, M cells in GALT FAE, but also in villous gut epithelium, can transfer antigen to migratory DC.[140,141] Tip DC, a rather poorly defined subset in the gut, have attracted attention because of experiments showing that iNOS-deficient mice have lowered levels of SIgA.[24,142] Gut-derived DC support IgA CSR *in vitro*, and in this function TGF-β, APRIL, BAFF, and RA are important factors.[26,35] DC are prominent producers of RA, a signal that induces expression of $\alpha_4\beta_7$ integrin and CCR9 on B and T lymphocytes to secure gut homing properties.[35] TNF-α from DC also induces expression of matrix metalloproteinase that cleaves and activates TGF-β.[126,143] DC may play a more important role outside of the PP than within them. In ILF, for example, DC and B cells make close contact.[60]

Nonhematopoietic cells also support IgA differentiation. MyD88-mediated bacterial stimulation, together with RA, induces expression of BAFF and TGF-β in FDC.[126] Thus, FDC may not only present tethered antigens to B cells in the mucosa but they may also promote IgA B cell differentiation. Other cell types that interact with B cells are stromal cells that produce chemokines and express LTβR and epithelial cells that secrete BAFF and APRIL.[13,60] The latter appear to be a consequence of TLR-mediated signals, although it is unclear how much bacterial material will actually reach the epithelium due to the mucus barrier.[13,144] The roles of these cell types have been difficult to asses *in vivo*, but a recent study demonstrated that overexpression of TLR4 (to increase TLR signals) in epithelial cells leads increased numbers of IgA plasma cells through production of APRIL.[145]

## The relative importance for IgA CSR inductive sites

The importance of different sites and pathways in overall gut IgA production is hard to adequately address. Numerous experimental models have pointed to a complex and, in several respects, redundant system for producing IgA critical for maintaining barrier function and securing homeostasis. This redundancy is, for example, evident in μMT mice, as even a small "leakage" of B cells in this strain could contribute significantly to levels of IgA.[146,147] Also, SIgA-producing plasma cells stimulated by TI antigens in mono-colonized, previously GF mice have very long gut survival time, whereas following additional colonization, the plasma cells are competed out from their gut LP niche by newly arriving plasma

cells.[59] Thus, IgA production in gene-deficient mice, relative to WT mice, does not always accurately reflect the importance of that particular IgA pathway during steady state conditions. Transfers of B cells into lymphopenic mice have a similar problem, as these types of experiment largely reflect the ability of the transferred cells to expand and invade niches rather than the importance of a certain pathway. The contribution of different pathways during steady state can therefore be accurately determined only in WT mice, or after careful transfer of cells into nonirradiated, nonlymphopenic mice. We have taken the strategy to investigate this matter in somewhat more detail by also comparing findings in laboratory mice with those obtained from wild-caught feral mice.[63] We believe the following observations can give important clues as to the importance of different IgA-inductive pathways for maintaining steady state and an intact gut mucosal barrier.

### Histology

In both laboratory and wild-caught mice few IgM-expressing cells are present in the LP (Figs 3 and 4). There are no signs of ongoing B cell proliferation outside of the GALT. In mice that lack functional PP, ILFs are larger and more activated than in normal WT mice.[49,51] A possible explanation for this finding is that the ILF expansion is driven by an overgrowth of the gut microbiota, as protective IgA is largely missing.[79,148] Interestingly, we find that wild-caught mice have enlarged PP and cP but small ILFs—in particular in the small intestine. Of note, even though the wild-caught mice should have a more diverse bacterial microbiota than laboratory mice and should have encountered more pathogens and more complex food antigens, ILF numbers were rather insignificant. Thus, it may be that ILFs primarily function more as a backup for IgA CSR, when other GALT inductive sites fail, rather than in response to the normal microbiota.

### V region sequences

In mice, 85% of the gut IgA plasma cells are mutated and have, on average, six mutations in their 300 bp long V regions.[114] The mutation rate of V regions in GC has been estimated to be at most $10^{-3}$ bp/cell division.[149] Gut IgA B cells must therefore have undergone many divisions before differentiating into IgA plasma cells. Furthermore, randomly cloned V regions from IgA B cells and plasma cells isolated from spatially separated sites, even from the small intestine and the colon, often have identical CDR3 regions.[114]

*Expression of IgA CSR-associated transcripts*
CTα switch transcripts have never convincingly been demonstrated in LP devoid of ILF. They have been reported by two studies, but neither of these have taken into account the possibility of confounding tissues from ILF.[14,145] In fact, all reports using LP from which ILF were specifically removed have failed to detect CTα in LP.[22,114,115] Moreover, in ILF, CTα transcripts are rare compared to PP, but previous studies have had no problem in detecting these transcripts, arguing that the sensitivity of the method would be adequate for detecting CTα transcripts also in the LP.[114] In PP, AID mRNA expression is high in GC and much lower in SED. Only few AID mRNA-expressing cells are found in ILF from WT mice, and in LP devoid of ILF no AID mRNA has been detected.[22,114,115] In addition, an AID-GFP gene reporter mouse had few GFP-expressing IgM+, but many GFP+ IgA+ B cells in the PP.[113] In the LP, a similar picture was found, but it is unclear if the isolated AID mRNA-expressing cells were plasma cells or plasmablasts, newly arriving to the LP or located to ILF and not present in the nonorganized LP at all.

Taken together, we would like to propose the following scheme of different IgA inductive pathways that contribute to the overall production of IgA in the gut during steady state. The majority of IgA-expressing plasma cells are generated from IgM+ B cells in PP. The cells enter GC after CSR, where they go through several rounds of proliferation with SHM before seeding the LP. The PP host both TD and TI IgA CSR, and possibly cells from both pathways enter into GC after CSR. Although cP can perform similar tasks as PP, they are usually less activated, possibly as a consequence of a thicker mucus layer.[62] TI IgA CSR can occur in ILF, but under normal conditions PP dominate over ILF as inductive sites for IgA CSR. Only if the PP fail to generate sufficient numbers of IgA-producing cells do ILFs mature into efficient IgA inductive sites to compensate, possibly as a consequence of changes to the gut microbiota. Although an attractive idea, the notion that IgA CSR occurs in the mouse gut LP under normal steady-state conditions finds very little support in the literature. Recent studies by Spencer and coworkers also argue against this phenomenon

in the human nonorganized LP.[150,151] Whether IgA CSR in the gut LP can occur under extreme conditions is an open question and cannot be excluded at the present time.

## Maintenance of IgA plasma and memory B cells

The ability of the gut immune system to protect the mucosa against pathogens by long-term production of antigen-specific IgA antibodies is pivotal to mucosal vaccine development. A recent elegant study by Macphearson and coworkers addressed the importance of mucosal memory after mono-colonization of GF mice with a commensal bacterial strain dependent on nutrients not present in the mammalian hosts.[59] Using this reversible colonization, the authors found that repeated immunizations gave rise to increasing, specific SIgA titers, but in an additive rather than a synergistic manner. Interestingly, in the absence of competing antigens, the half-life of the LP plasma cells was very long, whereas in the presence of other microbiota that stimulated the formation of new IgA plasma cells the life-span of the IgA plasma cells was dramatically reduced. Based on these observations, the authors concluded that memory B cells did not develop, and that, although LP plasma cells had the potential for longevity, they were normally short lived. These conclusions may be relevant for gut TI B cell responses driven by the microbiota, but they are definitely challenged by findings after oral immunizations with TD antigens, as discussed later.[77] It is likely that memory development at mucosal sites may be strikingly different when driven by TD and TI responses. Humans indeed maintain a sizable proportion of blood B cells that appear to be circulating IgA+ memory cells.[152–154]

Gut SIgA responses with long-lived plasma and memory B cells have, in fact, been described in mouse studies. We have performed extensive studies looking at memory development following oral immunization with CT. In human studies, ample documentation exists showing that cholera infection or oral cholera vaccination results in protection against disease for several years.[75] The response is dependent on the development of memory B cells, as production of specific antibodies vanishes within months, indicating that long-lived plasma cells prevail for only 6–12 months. A similar picture emerges from studies in mice, where oral CT immunizations stimulate anti-CT IgA antibodies in the gut and serum that vanishes within 6–12 months, while after this time still significant anti-CT IgA responses can be elicited from long-lived memory B cells by reexposure to CT.[155] Transfer studies have demonstrated that CT-specific memory B cells are present in spleen, MLN, and PP for more than a year following CT immunizations.[93,156–158] These memory B cells responded to either oral or intravenous challenge immunizations, indicating that mucosal and systemic memory B cells were generated by oral immunizations.[156] Memory B cells transferred from spleen gave stronger systemic responses after an oral challenge than did MLN memory cells. Thus, the route of challenge influenced the recall IgA memory response. Similar conclusions with regard to B cell memory have been reached using other models. For example, after a murine rotavirus infection, specific antibodies were produced long after the infection cleared, indicating the existence of long-lived plasma cells or ongoing recruitment of memory B cells into plasma cells.[159,160] When memory B cells from these mice were transferred into RAG-deficient mice chronically infected with rotavirus, the infection cleared.[161] Interestingly, splenic memory B cells with the ability to clear infection through SIgA production could be identified based on their expression of the $\alpha_4\beta_7$ integrin, whereas B cell lacking this integrin did not clear the infection, even though they produced specific IgG antibodies after transfer. Several interesting observations supporting differential maintenance of immunological memory between TI and TD gut responses were also recently made in mice lacking the chemokine receptor CCR10. These mice responded poorly to CT but had essentially normal steady-state levels of SIgA due to homeostatic TI pathways. In addition, they were deficient in maintenance of plasma cells and memory B cells after immunization, suggesting that these TI responses were not able to generate long-lived plasma and memory cells.[102]

Thus, mucosal responses against TD antigens are characterized by the development of a strong antigen-specific memory B cell population and long-lived plasma cells, whereas TI antigens, similar to systemic immune responses, do not appear to stimulate mucosal memory responses. Memory B cells formed after a mucosal immunization are, however, distinct from the ones formed after systemic immunization. They have undergone IgA

CSR, and may have distinct homing properties as determined by expression of distinct integrins. Expanding our knowledge about what regulates the development of long-lived IgA plasma cells and memory B cells after mucosal immunizations is critical for the development of better mucosal vaccines.

## IgA differentiation in humans

Although sharing many similarities, there are also disparities between the human and the mouse IgA system.[48] The most obvious difference between the two is the presence of two IgA classes in humans, IgA1 and IgA2, encoded by distinct C regions. Other differences include that ILF form before birth in humans, that human B cells do not express TLR4, and that IgM and IgG plasma cells are more prevalent in human than the mouse LP.[7,48] Furthermore, a distinct B1 population has not been identified in humans.[162,163] Specific gene-targeting or blockage of signaling pathways *in vivo* are rarely possible in humans, and the experimental systems available are, therefore, limited to immunizations with approved vaccines, analysis of histology of extracted tissues or isolated cells, or *in vitro* culture systems with human cells. Using these methods, however, very many similarities have been shown between mouse and human mucosal immune systems. In particular, the microanatomy of the mucosal immune system and especially the gut and GALT system appears to be very similar, although the distribution of IgA1 and IgA2 cells is unique in the human mucosal immune system.[117,164] Interestingly, the two classes appear to be skewed towards recognition of different types of antigen, with IgA1 recognizing protein antigens and IgA2 recognizing polysaccharides and LPS.[165] This difference may be related to that IgA1 posses an extended hinge region, potentially allowing for increased antigen binding but at the same time making it susceptible to microbial proteases.

The existence of a TI pathway in human IgA CSR is demonstrated by mucosal IgA production in patients lacking CD40 and in HIV-infected individuals lacking T cells.[13] It is also clear that APRIL and BAFF can induce human B cells to undergo IgA CSR *in vitro*.[13,26] Many cell types in LP, including DC, monocytes, macrophages, granulocytes, and epithelial cells, upregulate their expression of BAFF and APRIL following TLR stimulation.[116] Using immunofluorescent antibody staining or *in situ* hybridization, AID expressing cells in human colonic LP were identified and these cells appeared to be in contact with epithelial cells expressing APRIL. Hence, the presence of extrachromosomal switch circles in the LP were interpreted a sign of ongoing IgA CSR in the nonorganized LP.[13] Surprisingly, switch junctions indicative of IgA1 to IgA2 sequential switching were found, and sequential switching could be induced in IgA1-expressing cells *in vitro*. Based on these findings it was argued that a proportion of IgA2 in the human colon LP form as a consequence of APRIL-induced sequential switching from IgA1 to IgA2. A follow up study showed that TACI collaborated with TLR or CD40, and that TACI-induced activation of IgA CSR required MyD88 as an important signaling intermediate.[166] Whereas evidence for local LP proliferation has never been presented, one report found that the frequency of related V regions in gut biopsies may indicate local proliferation.[167] Other researchers, however, disagree with extensive LP IgA CSR in humans, as they have not been able to confirm AID expression outside of GALT using RT-PCR or immunohistochemistry.[168] Also, they have not found any direct evidence for local proliferation in LP, which is postulated to be required for IgA CSR.[168] In addition, sequencing of SIgA V regions showed that these had signs of extensive SHM, and that clonally related CDR3 regions were present simultaneously in LP and GALT.[150,151] These findings would argue for proliferation and IgA CSR taking place primarily in the GALT, rather than in LP, in the human gut mucosal immune system. Indeed, no research group has hitherto reported evidence for postswitch CTα gene transcripts in human.

## Summary

There are two distinct pathways for IgA CSR in the gut mucosal immune system. One is driven by TI antigens, while the other is responsive to TD antigens. These pathways differ with regard to the requirements and longevity for IgA responses. In both humans and mice, the vast majority of IgA producing plasma cells in the gut LP have mutated V regions, and related V regions are present in nonadjacent regions, indicating extensive proliferation and differentiation of the responding B cells prior to a synchronized distribution of IgA-switched plasmablasts (through blood) that differentiate to plasma cells at LP effector sites. Although AID mRNA expression has been observed in LP, B

cell or plasma cell proliferation has not. As CSR and SHM require proliferation, LP IgA CSR appears to play a minor (if any) role during steady-state conditions. Recent work in our laboratory has suggested a model in which IgA CSR occurs prior to cells entering GC-reactions, and is followed by extensive SHM in GC in PP before cells are distributed to the entire gut immune system, including both inductive and effector sites. The fact that GC are constantly present in PP and can be maintained independently of antigen specificity suggests that antigen-activated B cells may enter already preformed GC in multiple PP to undergo further expansion and affinity maturation. This provocative hypothesis is currently being tested in our laboratory. Better knowledge of the requirements for regulation of gut IgA responses is needed for the development of better, more efficacious mucosal vaccines. However, our recent studies have clearly demonstrated that multiple oral immunizations are required to drive a highly synchronized and oligoclonal, high affinity, IgA B cell response in the gut immune system.

## Acknowledgments

The authors are grateful to Prof. Jo Spencer and Joel Holmqvist for helpful comments on the manuscript, and Anneli Stenson for microscopy of mice tissues. This work was supported by grants from the Swedish Research Council, the Swedish Cancer Foundation, the Swedish Child Cancer foundation, Globvac/the Norwegian Research Council, the Wellcome Trust, the Sahlgrenska University Hospital Foundation LUA/ALF, and a Swedish Foundation for Strategic Research grant to the Mucosal Immunobiology and Vaccine Center (MIVAC).

## References

1. Russel, M.W. & M. Kilian. 2005. Biological activities of IgA. In *Mucosal Immunology*. J. Mestecky *et al.*, Eds.: 267–289. Elsevier Academic Press. Burlington, MA.

2. Holmgren, J. & C. Czerkinsky. 2005. Mucosal immunity and vaccines. *Nat. Med.* **11:** S45–S53.

3. Brandtzaeg, P. 2010. Update on mucosal immunoglobulin A in gastrointestinal disease. *Curr. Opin. Gastroenterol.* **26:** 554–563.

4. Macpherson, A.J. *et al.* 2008. The immune geography of IgA induction and function. *Mucosal Immunol.* **1:** 11–22.

5. Mestecky, J. *et al.* 2005. Mucosal immunoglobulins. In *Mucosal Immunology*. J. Mestecky *et al.*, Eds.: 153–181. Elsevier Academic Press. Burlington, MA.

6. Kaetzel, C.S. & M. K. 2005. Immunoglobulin transport and the polymeric Immunolglobulin receptor. In *Mucosal*

*Immunology*. J. Mestecky *et al.*, Eds.: 211–250. Elsevier Academic Press. Burlington, MA.

7. Brandtzaeg, P. 2010. Function of mucosa-associated lymphoid tissue in antibody formation. *Immunol. Invest.* **39:** 303–355.

8. Di Noia, J.M. & M.S. Neuberger. 2007. Molecular mechanisms of antibody somatic hypermutation. *Annu. Rev. Biochem.* **76:** 1–22.

9. Stavnezer, J., J.E.J. Guikema & C.E. Schrader. 2008. Mechanism and regulation of class switch recombination. *Annu. Rev. Immunol.* **26:** 261–292.

10. Nutt, S.L. & D.M. Tarlinton. 2011. Germinal center B and follicular helper T cells: siblings, cousins or just good friends? *Nat. Immunol.* **131:** 472–477.

11. Shen, H.M. *et al.* 2008. Expression of AID transgene is regulated in activated B cells but not in resting B cells and kidney. *Mol. Immunol.* **45:** 1883–1892.

12. Tangye, S.G. & P.D. Hodgkin. 2004. Divide and conquer: the importance of cell division in regulating B-cell responses. *Immunology* **112:** 509–520.

13. He, B. *et al.* 2007. Intestinal bacteria trigger T cell-independent immunoglobulin A(2) class switching by inducing epithelial-cell secretion of the cytokine APRIL. *Immunity* **26:** 812–826.

14. Fagarasan, S. *et al.* 2001. In situ class switching and differentiation to IgA-producing cells in the gut lamina propria. *Nature* **413:** 639–643.

15. Kinoshita, K. *et al.* 2001. A hallmark of active class switch recombination: transcripts directed by I promoters on looped-out circular DNAs. *Proc. Natl. Acad. Sci. USA* **98:** 12620–12623.

16. Harwood, N.E. & F.D. Batista. 2010. Early events in B cell activation. *Annu. Rev. Immunol.* **28:** 185–210.

17. Kurosaki, T., H. Shinohara & Y. Baba. 2010. B cell signaling and fate decision. *Annu. Rev. Immunol.* **28:** 21–55.

18. Dedeoglu, F. *et al.* 2004. Induction of activation-induced cytidine deaminase gene expression by IL-4 and CD40 ligation is dependent on STAT6 and NFkappaB. *Int. Immunol.* **16:** 395–404.

19. Vallabhapurapu, S. & M. Karin. 2009. Regulation and function of NF-kappaB transcription factors in the immune system. *Annu. Rev. Immunol.* **27:** 693–733.

20. Elgueta, R. *et al.* 2009. Molecular mechanism and function of CD40/CD40L engagement in the immune system. *Immunol. Rev.* **229:** 152–172.

21. Lanzavecchia, A. & F. Sallusto. 2007. Toll-like receptors and innate immunity in B-cell activation and antibody responses. *Curr. Opin. Immunol.* **19:** 268–274.

22. Bergqvist, P. *et al.* 2006. Gut IgA class switch recombination in the absence of CD40 does not occur in the lamina propria and is independent of germinal centers. *J. Immunol.* **177:** 7772–7783.

23. Pasare, C. & R. Medzhitov. 2005. Control of B-cell responses by Toll-like receptors. *Nature* **438:** 364–368.

24. Tezuka, H. *et al.* 2007. Regulation of IgA production by naturally occurring TNF/iNOS-producing dendritic cells. *Nature* **448:** 929–933.

25. Castigli, E. *et al.* 2005. TACI and BAFF-R mediate isotype switching in B cells. *J. Exp. Med.* **201:** 35–39.

26. Litinskiy, M.B. *et al.* 2002. DCs induce CD40-independent immunoglobulin class switching through BLyS and APRIL. *Nat. Immunol.* **3:** 822–829.

27. von Bülow, G.U., J.M. van Deursen & R.J. Bram. 2001. Regulation of the T-independent humoral response by TACI. *Immunity* **14:** 573–582.

28. Yan, M. *et al.* 2001. Activation and accumulation of B cells in TACI-deficient mice. *Nat. Immunol.* **2:** 638–643.

29. Varfolomeev, E. *et al.* 2004. APRIL-deficient mice have normal immune system development. *Mol. Cell. Biol.* **24:** 997–1006.

30. Castigli, E. *et al.* 2004. Impaired IgA class switching in APRIL-deficient mice. *Proc. Natl. Acad. Sci. USA* **101:** 3903–3908.

31. Stavnezer, J. & J. Kang. 2009. The surprising discovery that TGF beta specifically induces the IgA class switch. *J. Immunol.* **182:** 5–7.

32. Cazac, B.B. & J. Roes. 2000. TGF-beta receptor controls B cell responsiveness and induction of IgA in vivo. *Immunity* **13:** 443–451.

33. Borsutzky, S. *et al.* 2004. TGF-beta receptor signaling is critical for mucosal IgA responses. *J. Immunol.* **173:** 3305–3309.

34. Mora, J.R., M. Iwata & U.H. von Andrian. 2008. Vitamin effects on the immune system: vitamins A and D take centre stage. *Nat. Rev. Immunol.* **8:** 685–698.

35. Mora, J.R. *et al.* 2006. Generation of gut-homing IgA-secreting B cells by intestinal dendritic cells. *Science* **314:** 1157–1160.

36. Mora, J.R. & U.H. von Andrian. 2009. Role of retinoic acid in the imprinting of gut-homing IgA-secreting cells. *Semin. Immunol.* **21:** 28–35.

37. Park, M.-H. *et al.* 2011. Retinoic acid induces expression of Ig germ line α transcript, an IgA isotype switching indicative, through retinoic acid receptor. *Genes Genom.* **33:** 83–88.

38. Kaufman, D.R. *et al.* 2011. Vitamin A deficiency impairs vaccine-elicited gastrointestinal Immunity. *J. Immunol.* **187:** 1877–1883.

39. Fujieda, S. *et al.* 1996. Vasoactive intestinal peptide induces S(alpha)/S(mu) switch circular DNA in human B cells. *J. Clin. Invest.* **98:** 1527–1532.

40. Endsley, M.A. *et al.* 2009. Human IgA-inducing protein from dendritic cells induces IgA production by naive IgD+ B cells. *J. Immunol.* **182:** 1854–1859.

41. Strober, W., N. Lycke & S. Fagarasan. 2005. IgA B cell development. In *Mucosal Immunology*. J. Mestecky *et al.*, Eds.: 583–616. Elsevier Academic Press. Burlington, MA.

42. Avery, D.T. *et al.* 2008. IL-21-induced isotype switching to IgG and IgA by human naive B cells is differentially regulated by IL-4. *J. Immunol.* **181:** 1767–1779.

43. Dullaers, M. *et al.* 2009. A T cell-dependent mechanism for the induction of human mucosal homing immunoglobulin A-secreting plasmablasts. *Immunity* **30:** 120–129.

44. Seo, G.Y., J. Youn & P.H. Kim. 2009. IL-21 ensures TGF-1-induced IgA isotype expression in mouse Peye's patches. *J. Leukocyte Biol.* **85:** 744–750.

45. Tsuji, M. *et al.* 2008. Requirement for lymphoid tissue-inducer cells in isolated follicle formation and

T cell-independent immunoglobulin A generation in the gut. *Immunity* **29**: 261–271.

46. Yoshida, H. *et al.* 1999. IL-7 receptor alpha+ CD3(-) cells in the embryonic intestine induces the organizing center of Peyer's patches. *Int. Immunol.* **11**: 643–655.

47. Rennert, P.D. *et al.* 1996. Surface lymphotoxin alpha/beta complex is required for the development of peripheral lymphoid organs. *J. Exp. Med.* **184**: 1999–2006.

48. Gibbons, D.L. & J. Spencer. 2011. Mouse and human intestinal immunity: same ballpark, different players; different rules, same score. *Mucosal Immunol.* **4**: 148–157.

49. Hamada, H. *et al.* 2002. Identification of multiple isolated lymphoid follicles on the antimesenteric wall of the mouse small intestine. *J. Immunol.* **168**: 57–64.

50. Pabst, O. *et al.* 2005. Cryptopatches and isolated lymphoid follicles: dynamic lymphoid tissues dispensable for the generation of intraepithelial lymphocytes. *Eur. J. Immunol.* **35**: 98–107.

51. Lorenz, R.G. *et al.* 2003. Isolated lymphoid follicle formation is inducible and dependent upon lymphotoxin-sufficient B lymphocytes, lymphotoxin beta receptor, and TNF receptor I function. *J. Immunol.* **170**: 5475–5482.

52. Neutra, M.R. & J.P. Kraehenbuhl. 2005. Cellular and molecular basis for antigen transport across epithelial barriers. In *Mucosal Immunology*. J. Mestecky *et al.*, Eds.: 111–130. Elsevier Academic Press. Burlington, MA.

53. Kelsall, B.L. & W. Strober. 1996. Distinct populations of dendritic cells are present in the subepithelial dome and T cell regions of the murine Peyer's patch. *J. Exp. Med.* **183**: 237–247.

54. Kelsall, B.L. *et al.* 2005. Antigen handling and presentation by mucosal dendritic cells and macrophages. *In Mucosal Immunology*. J. Mestecky *et al.*, Eds.: 451–486. Elsevier Academic Press. Burlington, MA.

55. Bemark, M. *et al.* 2011. A unique role of the cholera toxin A1-DD adjuvant for long-term plasma and memory B cell development. *J. Immunol.* **186**: 1399–1410.

56. Hörnquist, C.E. *et al.* 1995. Paradoxical IgA immunity in CD4-deficient mice. Lack of cholera toxin-specific protective immunity despite normal gut mucosal IgA differentiation. *J. Immunol.* **155**: 2877–2887.

57. Bemark, M. *et al.* 2000. Somatic hypermutation in the absence of DNA-dependent protein kinase catalytic subunit (DNA-PK(cs)) or recombination-activating gene (RAG)1 activity. *J. Exp. Med.* **192**: 1509–1514.

58. Casola, S. *et al.* 2004. B cell receptor signal strength determines B cell fate. *Nat. Immunol.* **5**: 317–327.

59. Hapfelmeier, S. *et al.* 2010. Reversible microbial colonization of germ-free mice reveals the dynamics of IgA immune responses. *Science* **328**: 1705–1709.

60. Fagarasan, S. *et al.* 2010. Adaptive immune regulation in the gut: T cell-dependent and T cell-independent IgA synthesis. *Annu. Rev. Immunol.* **28**: 243–273.

61. Dohi, T. *et al.* 1999. Hapten-induced colitis is associated with colonic patch hypertrophy and T helper cell 2-type responses. *J. Exp. Med.* **189**: 1169–1180.

62. Johansson, M.E.V. *et al.* 2010. Bacteria penetrate the inner mucus layer before inflammation in the dextran sulfate colitis model. *PLoS ONE.* **5**: e12238.

63. Boysen, P., D.M. Eide & A.K. Storset. 2011. Natural killer cells in free-living Mus musculus have a primed phenotype. *Mol. Ecol.* **20**: 5103–5110.

64. Monteiro, R.C. & J.G.J. Van De Winkel. 2003. IgA Fc receptors. *Annu. Rev. Immunol.* **21**: 177–204.

65. Woof, J.M., M. van Egmond & M.A. Kerr. 2005. Fc receptors. In *Mucosal Immunology*. J. Mestecky, Eds.: 251–267. Elsevier Academic Press. Burlington, MA.

66. Harriman, G.R. *et al.* 1999. Targeted deletion of the IgA constant region in mice leads to IgA deficiency with alterations in expression of other Ig isotypes. *J. Immunol.* **162**: 2521–2529.

67. Brandtzaeg, P., I. Fjellanger & S.T. Gjeruldsen. 1968. Immunoglobulin M: local synthesis and selective secretion in patients with immunoglobulin A deficiency. *Science* **160**: 789–791.

68. Hendrickson, B.A. *et al.* 1995. Altered hepatic transport of immunoglobulin A in mice lacking the J chain. *J. Exp. Med.* **182**: 1905–1911.

69. Hendrickson, B.A. *et al.* 1996. Lack of association of secretory component with IgA in J chain-deficient mice. *J. Immunol.* **157**: 750–754.

70. Lycke, N. *et al.* 1999. Lack of J chain inhibits the transport of gut IgA and abrogates the development of intestinal antitoxic protection. *J. Immunol.* **163**: 913–919.

71. Johansen, F.-E. *et al.* 1999. Absence of epithelial immunoglobulin A transport, with increased mucosal leakiness, in polymeric immunoglobulin receptor/secretory component-deficient mice. *J. Exp. Med.* **190**: 915–922.

72. Shimada, S. *et al.* 1999. Generation of polymeric immunoglobulin receptor-deficient mouse with marked reduction of secretory IgA. *J. Immunol.* **163**: 5367–5373.

73. Lycke, N., L. Eriksen & J. Holmgren. 1987. Protection against cholera toxin after oral immunization is thymus-dependent and associated with intestinal production of neutralizing IgA antitoxin. *Scand. J. Immunol.* **25**: 413–419.

74. Lange, S. & J. Holmgren. 1978. Protective antitoxic cholera immunity in mice: influence of route and number of immunizations and mode of action of protective antibodies. *Acta Pathol. Microbiol. Scand.* **86C**: 145–152.

75. Holmgren, J. & C. Czerkinsky. 1992. Cholera as a model for research on mucosal immunity and development of oral vaccines. *Curr. Opin. Immunol.* **4**: 387–391.

76. Wei, M. *et al.* 2011. Mice carrying a knock-in mutation of Aicda resulting in a defect in somatic hypermutation have impaired gut homeostasis and compromised mucosal defense. *Nat. Immunol.* **12**: 264–270.

77. Macpherson, A.J. *et al.* 2000. A primitive T cell-independent mechanism of intestinal mucosal IgA responses to commensal bacteria. *Science* **288**: 2222–2226.

78. Macpherson, A.J. & T. Uhr. 2004. Induction of protective IgA by intestinal dendritic cells carrying commensal bacteria. *Science* **303**: 1662–1665.

79. Suzuki, K. *et al.* 2004. Aberrant expansion of segmented filamentous bacteria in IgA-deficient gut. *Proc. Natl. Acad. Sci. USA* **101**: 1981–1986.

80. Peterson, D.A. *et al.* 2007. IgA response to symbiotic bacteria as a mediator of gut homeostasis. *Cell Host Microbe.* **2**: 328–339.

81. Harris, N.L. *et al.* 2006. Mechanisms of neonatal mucosal antibody protection. *J. Immunol.* **177:** 6256–6262.

82. Kramer, D.R. & J.J. Cebra. 1995. Early appearance of "natural" mucosal IgA responses and germinal centers in suckling mice developing in the absence of maternal antibodies. *J. Immunol.* **154:** 2051–2062.

83. Allman, D. & S. Pillai. 2008. Peripheral B cell subsets. *Curr. Opin. Immunol.* **20:** 149–157.

84. Bos, N.A. *et al.* 1989. Serum immunoglobulin levels and naturally occurring antibodies against carbohydrate antigens in germ-free BALB/c mice fed chemically defined ultrafiltered diet. *Eur. J. Immunol.* **19:** 2335–2339.

85. Bos, N.A., H.Q. Jiang & J.J. Cebra. 2001. T cell control of the gut IgA response against commensal bacteria. *Gut.* **48:** 762–764.

86. Crabbe, P.A. *et al.* 1969. Antibodies of the IgA type in intestinal plasma cells of germfree mice after oral or parenteral immunization with ferritin. *J. Exp. Med.* **130:** 723–744.

87. Husband, A.J. & J.L. Gowans. 1978. The origin and antigen-dependent distribution of IgA-containing cells in the intestine. *J. Exp. Med.* **148:** 1146–1160.

88. Craig, S.W. & J.J. Cebra. 1971. Peyer's patches: an enriched source of precursors for IgA-producing immunocytes in the rabbit. *J. Exp. Med.* **134:** 188–200.

89. Yamamoto, M. *et al.* 2004. Role of gut-associated lymphoreticular tissues in antigen-specific intestinal IgA Immunity. *J. Immunol.* **173:** 762–769.

90. Fahlen-Yrlid, L. *et al.* 2009. CD11c(high)dendritic cells are essential for activation of CD4+ T cells and generation of specific antibodies following mucosal immunization. *J. Immunol.* **183:** 5032–5041.

91. Lycke, N. & W. Strober. 1989. Cholera toxin promotes B cell isotype differentiation. *J. Immunol.* **142:** 3781–3787.

92. Anosova, N.G. *et al.* 2008. Cholera toxin, E. coli heat-labile toxin, and non-toxic derivatives induce dendritic cell migration into the follicle-associated epithelium of Peyer's patches. *Mucosal Immunol.* **1:** 59–67.

93. Lycke, N. & M. Bemark. 2010. Mucosal adjuvants and long-term memory development with special focus on CTA1-DD and other ADP-ribosylating toxins. *Mucosal Immunol.* **3:** 556–566.

94. Vajdy, M. *et al.* 1995. Impaired mucosal immune responses in interleukin 4-targeted mice. *J. Exp. Med.* **181:** 41–53.

95. Bromander, A.K. *et al.* 1996. IL-6-deficient mice exhibit normal mucosal IgA responses to local immunizations and Helicobacter felis infection. *J. Immunol.* **156:** 4290–4297.

96. Datta, S.K. *et al.* 2010. Mucosal adjuvant activity of cholera toxin requires Th17 cells and protects against inhalation anthrax. *Proc. Natl. Acad. Sci. USA* **107:** 10638–10643.

97. Hörnquist, E. *et al.* 1996. CD8-deficient mice exhibit augmented mucosal immune responses and intact adjuvant effects to cholera toxin. *Immunology* **87:** 220–229.

98. Gärdby, E. & N.Y. Lycke. 2000. CD19-deficient mice exhibit poor responsiveness to oral immunization despite evidence of unaltered total IgA levels, germinal centers and IgA-isotype switching in Peyer's patches. *Eur. J. Immunol.* **30:** 1861–1871.

99. Gärdby, E. *et al.* 2003. Strong differential regulation of serum and mucosal IgA responses as revealed in CD28-deficient mice using cholera toxin adjuvant. *J. Immunol.* **170:** 55–63.

100. Gärdby, E., P. Lane & N.Y. Lycke. 1998. Requirements for B7-CD28 costimulation in mucosal IgA responses: paradoxes observed in CTLA4-H gamma 1 transgenic mice. *J. Immunol.* **161:** 49–59.

101. Kjerrulf, M. *et al.* 1997. Interferon-gamma receptor-deficient mice exhibit impaired gut mucosal immune responses but intact oral tolerance. *Immunology* **92:** 60–68.

102. Hu, S. *et al.* 2011. Critical roles of chemokine receptor CCR10 in regulating memory IgA responses in intestines. *Proc. Natl. Acad. Sci. USA* **108:** E1035–1044.

103. Morteau, O. *et al.* 2008. An indispensable role for the chemokine receptor CCR10 in IgA antibody-secreting cell accumulation. *J. Immunol.* **181:** 6309–6315.

104. Yamamoto, M. *et al.* 2000. Alternate mucosal immune system: organized Peyer's patches are not required for IgA responses in the gastrointestinal tract. *J. Immunol.* **164:** 5184–5191.

105. Uren, T.K. *et al.* 2003. Role of the polymeric Ig receptor in mucosal B cell homeostasis. *J. Immunol.* **170:** 2531–2539.

106. Deppong, C.M. *et al.* 2010. CTLA4-Ig inhibits allergic airway inflammation by a novel CD28-independent, nitric oxide synthase-dependent mechanism. *Eur. J. Immunol.*

107. Grohmann, U. *et al.* 2002. CTLA-4-Ig regulates tryptophan catabolism in vivo. *Nat. Immunol.* **3:** 1097–1101.

108. Pallotta, M.T. *et al.* 2011. Indoleamine 2,3-dioxygenase is a signaling protein in long-term tolerance by dendritic cells. *Nat. Immunol.* **12:** 870–878.

109. Guy-Grand, D., C. Griscelli & P. Vassalli. 1975. Peyer's patches, gut IgA plasma cells and thymic function: study in nude mice bearing thymic grafts. *J. Immunol.* **115:** 361–364.

110. Mombaerts, P. *et al.* 1994. Peripheral lymphoid development and function in TCR mutant mice. *Int. Immunol.* **6:** 1061–1070.

111. Franco, M.A. & H.B. Greenberg. 1997. Immunity to rotavirus in T cell deficient mice. *Virology* **238:** 169–179.

112. Uematsu, S. *et al.* 2008. Regulation of humoral and cellular gut immunity by lamina propria dendritic cells expressing Toll-like receptor 5. *Nat. Immunol.* **9:** 769–776.

113. Crouch, E.E. *et al.* 2007. Regulation of AID expression in the immune response. *J. Exp. Med.* **204:** 1145–1156.

114. Bergqvist, P. *et al.* 2010. T cell-independent IgA class switch recombination is restricted to the GALT and occurs prior to manifest germinal center formation. *J. Immunol.* **184:** 3545–3553.

115. Shikina, T. *et al.* 2004. IgA class switch occurs in the organized nasopharynx- and gut-associated lymphoid tissue, but not in the diffuse lamina propria of airways and gut. *J. Immunol.* **172:** 6259–6264.

116. Cerutti, A., K. Chen & A. Chorny. 2011. Immunoglobulin responses at the mucosal interface. *Annu. Rev. Immunol.* **29:** 273–293.

117. He, B., W. Xu & A. Cerutti. 2010. Comment on Gut-associated lymphoid tissue contains the molecular machinery to support T-cell-dependent and T-cell-independent class switch recombination. *Mucosal Immunol.* **3:** 92–94.

118. Schwickert, T.A. *et al.* 2009. Germinal center reutilization by newly activated B cells. *J. Exp. Med.* **206:** 2907–2914.

119. Schwickert, T.A. *et al.* 2011. A dynamic T cell-limited checkpoint regulates affinity-dependent B cell entry into the germinal center. *J. Exp. Med.* **208:** 1243–1252.

110. Talham, G.L. *et al.* 1999. Segmented filamentous bacteria are potent stimuli of a physiologically normal state of the murine gut mucosal immune system. *Infect. Immun.* **67:** 1992–2000.

111. Obata, T. *et al.* 2010. Indigenous opportunistic bacteria inhabit mammalian gut-associated lymphoid tissues and share a mucosal antibody-mediated symbiosis. *Proc. Natl. Acad. Sci. USA* **107:** 7419–7424.

112. Bouskra, D. *et al.* 2008. Lymphoid tissue genesis induced by commensals through NOD1 regulates intestinal homeostasis. *Nature* **456:** 507–510.

123. Fritz, J.H. *et al.* 2007. Nod1-mediated innate immune recognition of peptidoglycan contributes to the onset of adaptive Immunity. *Immunity* **26:** 445–459.

124. Ichinohe, T. *et al.* 2009. Inflammasome recognition of influenza virus is essential for adaptive immune responses. *J. Exp. Med.* **206:** 79–87.

125. Barr, T.A. *et al.* 2009. B cell intrinsic MyD88 signals drive IFN-gamma production from T cells and control switching to IgG2c. *J. Immunol.* **183:** 1005–1012.

126. Suzuki, K. *et al.* 2010. The sensing of environmental stimuli by follicular dendritic cells promotes immunoglobulin A generation in the gut. *Immunity* **33:** 71–83.

127. Suzuki, K. *et al.* 2010. Roles of B-1 and B-2 cells in innate and acquired IgA-mediated Immunity. *Immunol. Rev.* **237:** 180–190.

128. Thurnheer, M.C. *et al.* 2003. B1 cells contribute to serum IgM, but not to intestinal IgA, production in gnotobiotic Ig allotype chimeric mice. *J. Immunol.* **170:** 4564–4571.

129. Berberich, S., R. Förster & O. Pabst. 2007. The peritoneal micromilieu commits B cells to home to body cavities and the small intestine. *Blood* **109:** 4627–4634.

130. Ha, S.-A. *et al.* 2006. Regulation of B1 cell migration by signals through Toll-like receptors. *J. Exp. Med.* **203:** 2541–2550.

131. Rosado, M.M. *et al.* 2009. From the fetal liver to spleen and gut: the highway to natural antibody. *Mucosal Immunol.* **2:** 351–361.

132. Hayday, A. & D. Gibbons. 2008. Brokering the peace: the origin of intestinal T cells. *Mucosal Immunol.* **1:** 172–174.

133. Wan, Y.Y. 2010. Multi-tasking of helper T cells. *Immunology.* **130:** 166–171.

134. Cong, Y. *et al.* 2009. A dominant, coordinated T regulatory cell-IgA response to the intestinal microbiota. *Proc. Natl. Acad. Sci. USA* **106:** 19256–19261.

135. Tsuji, M. *et al.* 2009. Preferential generation of follicular B helper T cells from Foxp3+ T cells in gut Peyer's patches. *Science* **323:** 1488–1492.

136. Lathrop, S.K. *et al.* 2011. Peripheral education of the immune system by colonic commensal microbiota. *Nature* **478:** 250–254.

137. Pabst, O. & G. Bernhardt. 2010. The puzzle of intestinal lamina propria dendritic cells and macrophages. *Eur. J. Immunol.* **40:** 2107–2111.

138. Rescigno, M. 2011. The intestinal epithelial barrier in the control of homeostasis and immunity. *Trends Immunol.* **32:** 256–264.

139. Schulz, O. *et al.* 2009. Intestinal CD103+, but not CX3CR1+, antigen sampling cells migrate in lymph and serve classical dendritic cell functions. *J. Exp. Med.* **206:** 3101–3114.

140. Jang, M.H. *et al.* 2004. Intestinal villous M cells: an antigen entry site in the mucosal epithelium. *Proc. Natl. Acad. Sci. USA* **101:** 6110–6115.

141. Nochi, T. *et al.* 2007. A novel M cell-specific carbohydrate-targeted mucosal vaccine effectively induces antigen-specific immune responses. *J. Exp. Med.* **204:** 2789–2796.

142. Dominguez, P.M. & C. Ardavin. 2010. Differentiation and function of mouse monocyte-derived dendritic cells in steady state and inflammation. *Immunol. Rev.* **234:** 90–104.

143. Cerutti, A., I. Puga & M. Cols. 2011. Innate control of B cell responses. *Trends Immunol.* **32:** 202–211.

144. Johansson, M.E. & G.C. Hansson. 2011. Microbiology. Keeping bacteria at a distance. *Science* **334:** 182–183.

145. Shang, L. *et al.* 2008. Toll-like receptor signaling in small intestinal epithelium promotes B-cell recruitment and IgA production in lamina propria. *Gastroenterology* **135:** 529–538.

146. Hasan, M. *et al.* 2002. Incomplete block of B cell development and immunoglobulin production in mice carrying the muMT mutation on the BALB/c background. *Eur. J. Immunol.* **32:** 3463–3471.

147. Macpherson, A.J. *et al.* 2001. IgA production without mu or delta chain expression in developing B cells. *Nat. Immunol.* **2:** 625–631.

148. Fagarasan, S. *et al.* 2002. Critical roles of activation-induced cytidine deaminase in the homeostasis of gut flora. *Science* **298:** 1424–1427.

149. Berek, C. & C. Milstein. 1987. Mutation drift and repertoire shift in the maturation of the immune response. *Immunol. Rev.* **96:** 23–41.

150. Barone, F. *et al.* 2011. IgA-producing plasma cells originate from germinal centers that are induced by B-cell receptor engagement in humans. *Gastroenterology* **140:** 947–956.

151. Boursier, L. *et al.* 2005. Human intestinal IgA response is generated in the organized gut-associated lymphoid tissue but not in the lamina propria. *Gastroenterology* **128:** 1879–1889.

152. Klein, U., K. Rajewsky & R. Kuppers. 1998. Human immunoglobulin (Ig)M+IgD+ peripheral blood B cells expressing the CD27 cell surface antigen carry somatically mutated variable region genes: CD27 as a general marker for somatically mutated (memory) B cells. *J. Exp. Med.* **188:** 1679–1689.

153. Tengvall, S. *et al.* 2010. BAFF, stimulatory DNA and IL-15 stimulates IgA(+) memory B cells and provides a novel approach for analysis of memory responses to mucosal vaccines. *Vaccine* **28:** 5445–5450.

154. Harris, A.M. *et al.* 2009. Antigen-specific memory B-cell responses to Vibrio cholerae O1 infection in Bangladesh. *Infect. Immun.* **77:** 3850–3856.

155. Lycke, N. & J. Holmgren. 1987. Long-term cholera antitoxin memory in the gut can be triggered to antibody formation

associated with protection within hours of an oral challenge immunization. *Scand. J. Immunol.* **25:** 407–412.

156. Lycke, N. & J. Holmgren. 1989. Adoptive transfer of gut mucosal antitoxin memory by isolated B cells 1 year after oral immunization with cholera toxin. *Infect. Immun.* **57:** 1137–1141.

157. Vajdy, M. & N. Lycke. 1993. Stimulation of antigen-specific T- and B-cell memory in local as well as systemic lymphoid tissues following oral immunization with cholera toxin adjuvant. *Immunology* **80:** 197–203.

158. Vajdy, M. & N. Lycke. 1995. Mucosal memory B cells retain the ability to produce IgM antibodies 2 years after oral immunization. *Immunology* **86:** 336–342.

159. Burns, J.W. *et al.* 1995. Analyses of homologous rotavirus infection in the mouse model. *Virology* **207:** 143–153.

160. McNeal, M.M. & R.L. Ward. 1995. Long-term production of rotavirus antibody and protection against reinfection following a single infection of neonatal mice with murine rotavirus. *Virology* **211:** 474–480.

161. Williams, M.B. *et al.* 1998. The memory B cell subset responsible for the secretory IgA response and protective humoral immunity to rotavirus expresses the intestinal homing receptor, alpha4beta7. *J. Immunol.* **161:** 4227–4235.

162. Boursier, L. *et al.* 2002. IgVH gene analysis suggests that peritoneal B cells do not contribute to the gut immune system in man. *Eur. J. Immunol.* **32:** 2427–2436.

163. Bemark, M. *et al.* 2012. Reconstitution after haematopoietic stem cell transplantation: revelation of B cell developmental pahtways and lineage phenotypes. *Clin. Exp. Immunol.* **167:** 15–25. doi:10.1111/j.1365-2249.2011.04469.x.

164. Spencer, J. & F. Barone. 2010. Reply to "Gut-associated lymphoid tissue contains the molecular machinery to support T-cell- dependent and T-cell-independent class switch recombination". *Mucosal Immunol.* **3:** 94–95.

165. Woof, J.M. & J. Mestecky. 2005. Mucosal immunoglobulins. *Immunol. Rev.* **206:** 64–82.

166. He, B. *et al.* 2010. The transmembrane activator TACI triggers immunoglobulin class switching by activating B cells through the adaptor MyD88. *Nat. Immunol.* **11:** 836–845.

167. Yuvaraj, S. *et al.* 2009. Evidence for local expansion of IgA plasma cell precursors in human ileum. *J. Immunol.* **183:** 4871–4878.

168. Barone, F. *et al.* 2009. Gut-associated lymphoid tissue contains the molecular machinery to support T-cell-dependent and T-cell-independent class switch recombination. *Mucosal Immunol.* **2:** 495–503.

Ann. N.Y. Acad. Sci. ISSN 0077-8923

ANNALS OF THE NEW YORK ACADEMY OF SCIENCES
Issue: *The Year in Immunology*

# New and emerging disease modifying therapies for multiple sclerosis

Shiv Saidha,[1,*] Christopher Eckstein,[2,*] and Peter A. Calabresi[1]

[1]Department of Neurology, Johns Hopkins University School of Medicine, Baltimore, Maryland. [2]Department of Neurology, University of South Alabama College of Medicine, Mobile, Alabama

Address for correspondence: Peter A. Calabresi, M.D., 600 N. Wolfe Street, Pathology 627, Baltimore, MD 21287. calabresi@jhmi.edu

Several disease-modifying drugs (DMDs) are currently approved for the treatment of multiple sclerosis (MS). Recently, there has been increased identification and development of potential new treatments that may modulate the MS disease process, including oral therapies. Many of the newly approved MS therapies, as well as those in ongoing clinical trials, have the advantage of improved efficacy and/or being oral and more convenient, as compared to conventional injectable first-line MS therapies. However, many of these new and emerging MS treatments are known to be associated with serious adverse events, some of which may be potentially life threatening. Of additional concern, there is limited experience and long-term safety data for many of these drugs, and thus the true potential for complications associated with these agents remains ambiguous. With an anticipated explosion in the artillery of available MS therapies in the near future, neurologists will need to carefully weigh drug efficacy, convenience, safety, and tolerability when making therapeutic decisions. In this review, we describe the known mechanisms of action, efficacy, and side-effect profiles of new and emerging MS DMDs.

Keywords: multiple sclerosis; fingolimod; cladribine; laquinimod; teriflunomide; BG12; alemtuzumab; daclizumab; anti-CD20; monoclonal antibodies

## Introduction and brief overview of existing disease-modifying therapies

Multiple sclerosis (MS), a complex immune-mediated disorder of the central nervous system (CNS), is the most common nontraumatic cause of neurologic disability in early to middle adulthood.[1] Although the precise etiology of MS remains incompletely elucidated, pathologic hallmarks of MS lesions include inflammation, demyelination, gliosis, axonal degeneration, and neuronal loss.[2–5] Axonal and neuronal degeneration, the principal pathological substrates of permanent disability in MS,[6–12] are primarily regarded as sequelae of the inflammatory demyelination that occurs central to MS.[13–16] Although a detailed overview of the immunopathophysiology of MS is beyond the scope of this review, it is worth briefly summarizing current hypotheses regarding the complex cellular and humoral mechanisms underlying MS. MS is primarily considered an inflammatory demyelinating CNS disorder characterized by lymphocyte and macrophage infiltrates, and glial cell activation.[17] Changes in several lymphocyte subsets have been found in MS, most notably increased expression of Th1 $CD4^+$ cells, which secrete proinflammatory cytokines such as interferon-$\gamma$ and tumor necrosis factor $\alpha$.[18] Decreased activity of Th2 $CD4^+$ cells, which principally secrete cytokines such as interleukin-4, interleukin-5, and interleukin-13, may contribute to impaired regulation in MS. Th17 $CD4^+$ cells, which secrete the proinflammatory cytokine interleukin-17, have also been implicated in the immunopathogenesis of MS. In addition to $CD4^+$ T cells, changes in cytotoxic and regulatory $CD8^+$ T cells have been described in MS. Clonal and oligoclonal expansions of $CD8^+$ T cells are often found in MS plaques,

---

*Co-first authors/contributed equally to this work.

doi: 10.1111/j.1749-6632.2011.06272.x

and in some studies CD8$^+$ T cells have been found to outnumber CD4$^+$ T cells, raising the possibility that in some instances inflammation in MS may be driven more by CD8$^+$ than CD4$^+$ T cells.[19] A subset of CD4$^+$ T cells, called T regulatory cells (CD4$^+$CD25$^+$T$_{reg}$ cells), that express CD25, the $\alpha$ chain of the interleukin-2 receptor, have been shown to have a critical role in the regulation of inflammation. Reduced suppressive properties of this cell type may have an important role in the immunopathophysiology of MS.[20,21]

In addition to T cell dysfunction, humoral immunity is also thought to play an important role in MS, as evidenced by antigen-driven B cell clonal expansion and oligoclonal immunoglobulin synthesis in the cerebrospinal fluid (CSF) of MS patients. In addition, it is now known that lymphoid follicles containing expanded antigen-experienced B cell clones are also found in both the meninges and brain parenchyma of MS patients.[22] Moreover, B cells have a number of antibody-independent proinflammatory functions, which are discussed later in this review. Given the critical role of inflammation in MS, a key goal of MS therapy continues to be reduction or abolishment of related CNS inflammatory activity, with different therapies attempting to target different aspects of the aberrant immune responses recognized to occur in MS, as outlined above. In addition to the known efficacy of anti-inflammatory therapies, the potential benefits of alternative strategies that may accomplish neuroprotection and/or remyelination in MS are recognized.[23–29] We will first review notable updates to the existing approved MS disease-modifying drugs (DMDs) and then focus on those drugs in late-stage development, which could be available in the next few years. Both oral and infrequently injected monoclonal antibodies (mAbs) will be considered. Early phase trials of other drugs, some with remyelinating potential, are beyond the scope of this review.

Several DMDs are currently approved for the management of relapsing-remitting MS (RRMS) in the United States and internationally. Interferon-$\beta$ (IFN-$\beta$) and glatiramer acetate (GA), the longest approved MS DMDs, are relatively safe and commonly used first-line agents.[30–34] IFN-$\beta$ has been available for the treatment of MS for over two decades and GA was licensed for the treatment of MS in the United States in 1996.[31,33–35] Signif-

icant global experience with these therapies has enabled detailed characterization of their side-effect profiles.[36,37] Depending on the formulation, IFN-$\beta$ is administered either subcutaneously (SC) or intramuscularly (IM), and either on alternate days, three times per week, or once weekly. It is worth noting, however, that a longer acting formulation of IFN-$\beta$ requiring less frequent injection (PEGylated IFN-$\beta$1a) is currently under evaluation in a phase 3 placebo-controlled trial. Adverse events (AEs) of IFN-$\beta$ include injection-site reactions, flu-like symptoms, leukopenia, deranged liver enzymes, and depression. Common AEs of GA (a once-daily SC injection) include local injection-site reactions, postinjection systemic reactions, and lipodystrophy (with long-term therapy). Since MS commonly afflicts females of childbearing age, determination and consideration of the potential effects of therapies on pregnancy are important. Both IFN-$\beta$ and GA are not regarded as teratogenic, although IFN-$\beta$ may possess abortofacient properties.[38–40]

Since inflammatory activity may be most intense,[16,41] and the long-term benefits of DMDs might be greatest during early MS,[42–44] early recognition, diagnosis, and implementation of appropriate therapy are important goals in MS. IFN-$\beta$ and GA have relatively comparable efficacy, reducing relapse rate (RR) by approximately 30–40% in MS.[45,46] As the pathophysiological processes underpinning MS continue to be unraveled, strategies to modulate or suppress the immune system have also evolved, often with improved efficacy. A monoclonal antibody, Natalizumab, blocks the interaction between $\alpha$4-integrin on mononuclear leucocytes and vascular cell adhesion molecule-1 on endothelial cells and, possibly, other ligands within the CNS such as fibronectin and osteopontin, preventing the migration of leucocytes across the blood–brain barrier (BBB) into the brain parenchyma, or their interaction with resident CNS cells.[47–49] Natalizumab (administered IV every four weeks) was shown to reduce RR by 68%, and sustained progression of disability at two years by 42% in RRMS in the placebo-controlled phase 3 AFFIRM trial.[50] Natalizumab was initially approved for the treatment of MS in the United States in 2004.[51] In the SENTINEL trial, patients received the combination of once-weekly IM IFN-$\beta$, with once-monthly IV natalizumab, or once-monthly IV placebo.[52] During this study, it became apparent that natalizumab therapy may be associated with progressive multiofocal leucoencephalopathy (PML), a potentially life-threatening complication. Consequently, natalizumab was withdrawn in 2005, before being relicensed in 2006 under revised prescription guidelines and with the implementation of a surveillance program for monitoring the safety of natalizumab-treated MS patients.[51] PML, an opportunistic brain infection, principally of oligodendrocytes, results in CNS demyelination and may be associated with severe morbidity and mortality.[53,54] PML is thought to be caused by reactivation of the polyoma JC virus, primarily in the setting of immunosuppression.[55] It was initially suspected that PML may only represent a potential complication of natalizumab during concomitant IFN therapy, and the risk of PML with natalizumab may be approximately 1/1000.[56] With experience, it has become evident that PML is a complication of natalizumab monotherapy, and that the risk of PML with natalizumab may be increased by longer duration of treatment (particularly beyond 24 months), especially in those with concomitant or prior exposure to immunosuppressants.[57,58] Because natalizumab is a highly effective MS therapy, methods to stratify patients according to risk of developing PML are being actively investigated. One promising method is the detection of serum anti-JC virus antibodies, for which approximately 50–60% of MS patients may be positive. In one study, all MS patients who developed PML during natalizumab therapy, from whom sera were available prenatalizumab, had a positive JC virus antibody status months-to-years before developing PML.[59] In natalizumab-treated patients diagnosed with PML, plasma exchange has been shown to reduce natalizumab saturation of α4-integrin receptors on immune cells, thereby allowing reconstitution of their migratory function. While this has dramatically reduced the mortality of PML from nearly 100% to less than 30%, many patients are left with severe disability related to PML itself, or the exuberant immune response—immune reconstitution inflammatory syndrome (IRIS)—that occurs following the release of previously trapped immune cells.[60–62] Other AEs of natalizumab include infusion-related hypersensitivity reactions, lymphocytosis, and hepatotoxicity. The effects of natalizumab during pregnancy are unclear, and patients should be advised to ensure strict contraception.[63]

Long-term self-administration of injections or receipt of IV drugs may be burdensome for some patients. As such, two new efficacious oral agents have been approved for the treatment of MS: fingolimod in the United States and Europe, and cladribine in Australia and Russia (although this drug was declined approval for the treatment of MS in both the United States and Europe).[64] However, these and many other potential DMDs under investigation in MS may be associated with serious AEs, some of which may be potentially life threatening. As new therapies continue to emerge, recent experience with natalizumab emphasizes the need to exert caution and a careful assessment of the risks versus potential benefits of these therapies. Indeed, cladribine was not approved by U.S. and European regulatory agencies. Moving forward, neurologists will need to carefully consider not only drug efficacy and convenience, but also drug safety, realizing that it can take time for the true risks of therapies to become clear. The purpose of this review is to describe the mechanisms of action, efficacy, and safety of newly approved and emerging DMDs for MS (summarized in Table 1).

## Oral therapies

### Fingolimod

Oral fingolimod was approved for the treatment of MS by the Food and Drug Administration (FDA) and the European Medicines Agency (EMA) in 2010. Fingolimod is licensed for use as a first-line agent in the United States, but only as a second-line agent for active MS in Europe. Fingolimod is FTY720, a structural analog of intracellular sphingosine that is phosphorylated by sphingosine kinase 2 *in vivo*, and exerts its effects by mimicking sphingosine 1-phosphate (S1P) and binding to four of five S1P receptors on lymphocytes (agents selective for different S1P receptor subtypes are also in development). Fingolimod binding to S1P receptors results in internalization of activated S1P receptors, and prolonged downregulation of these receptors. Without signals from S1P receptors, $CD4^+$ and $CD8^+$ T cells and B cells are unable to egress from secondary lymphoid tissue,[65–67] resulting in a marked decrease of these cells in the periphery and their reduced recruitment to sites of inflammation, although the impact on $CD4^+$ T cells and B cells in the CSF compartment may be less pronounced than in the periphery.[68] Fingolimod may not be a general

**Table 1.** Summary of mechanism of action, efficacy, AEs, and ongoing studies of new and emerging MS therapies

| Drug | Mechanism of action | Efficacy | Adverse events | Ongoing trials |
|---|---|---|---|---|
| Fingolimod (oral) | Sphingosine-1-phosphate (S1P) receptor modulator; prevents egress of $CD4^+$ & $CD8^+$ T cells, and B cells from secondary lymphoid tissue; possible contribution to CNS neuroprotection and/or remyelination | Phase 3 FREEDOMS: 54–60% ARR reduction; reduced risk of disability progression; fewer new/enlarging T2 lesions, $Gd^+$ lesions, and brain volume loss (compared to placebo) Phase 3 TRANSFORMS: 38–52% ARR reduction (compared to once-weekly IM IFN-β) | Herpes virus infections; bradycardia & atrioventricular conduction block during initiation; hypertension; elevated liver enzymes; macular edema; lower respiratory tract infections; lymphopenia; possibly malignancies (e.g., skin cancer) | INFORMS (phase 3 trial in PPMS) |
| Cladribine (oral) | Antilymphocytic; adenosine deaminase resistant analog of purine nucleoside adenosine; incorporates into DNA of dividing cells, disrupting DNA synthesis and repair, leading to dose-dependent, sustained, and progressive ablation of $CD4^+$ and $CD8^+$ T cells | Phase 3 CLARITY: 55–58% ARR reduction; reduced risk of disability progression; 86–88% reduction in $Gd^+$ lesions (compared to placebo) | Lymphopenia, neutropenia, thrombocytopenia, pancytopenia, dermatomal herpes zoster reactivation, possible malignancy | ONWARD (phase 3 add-on trial to IFN-β) ORACLE (phase 3 trial in CIS) |
| Teriflunomide (oral) | Active ring malononitrile metabolite A771726 of pro-drug leflunomide; mitochondrial dihydroorate dehydrogenase inhibitor; prevents *de novo* pyrimidine synthesis, proliferation, and effector functions of activated T and B cells | Phase 2: Suppression of worsening disability; 61% reduction in $Gd^+$ lesions (compared to placebo) Phase 3 TEMSO results announced: 31% ARR reduction; reduction in sustained disease progression (compared to placebo) | Diarrhea, nausea, dyspepsia, increased liver enzymes, alopecia, skin rashes, infections, neutropenia, paresthesia, hypertension | TOWER (phase 3 trial comparing to placebo) TOPIC (phase 3 trial in CIS) |

*Continued*

**Table 1.** *Continued*

| Drug | Mechanism of action | Efficacy | Adverse events | Ongoing trials |
|------|---------------------|----------|----------------|----------------|
| BG12 (oral) | Dimethyl fumarate; second-generation fumaric acid; directly targets Nrf2; antioxidative and immunomodulatory; may be neuroprotective by attenuating oxidative-stress mediated damage | Phase 2b: 32% ARR reduction; 69% reduction in Gd$^+$ lesions, 48% reduction new T2 lesions (compared to placebo) Phase 3 DEFINE results announced: 53% ARR reduction, 85% reduction new/enlarging T2 lesions, 90% reduction new Gd$^+$ lesions, and 38% reduction in disability progression (compared to placebo) | Flushing, headaches, gastrointestinal symptoms (abdominal pain, nausea, vomiting, diarrhea), dose-related elevations in liver enzymes | CONFIRM (phase 3 trial comparing to glatiramer acetate and placebo) |
| Laquinimod (oral) | Second-generation quinolone-3-carboxamide; related to linomide; promotes shift from pro-inflammatory Th1 to anti-inflammatory Th2 profile; may provide neuroprotection by promoting production of neuroprotective factors | Phase 2b: 40% reduction in Gd$^+$ lesions; significant reduction new T2 and T1 lesions (compared to placebo) Phase 3 ALLEGRO results announced: 23% ARR reduction; 36% reduction in disability progression; 33% reduction in progression of brain atrophy (compared to placebo) Phase 3 BRAVO results announced: 21% ARR reduction, 33% reduction in disability progression; 27% reduction in progression of brain atrophy (compared to placebo) | Dose-dependent increases in liver enzymes, arthralgia, local herpes virus reactivation | No phase 3 trials currently in progress |
| Alemtuzumab (intra-venous) | Humanized mAb directed against CD52; complement and cell-mediated lysis of CD4$^+$ & CD8$^+$ T cells, B cells, NK cells, and monocytes; duration of B cell depletion less than T cell depletion | Phase 2 CAMMS223: 74% ARR reduction; 71% reduction in risk of sustained disability; net gain of 0.77 points in EDSS; significant reduction in brain volume loss (compared to SC IFN-β three times per week) Phase 3 CARE-MS 1 results recently announced: 55% RR reduction, no improvement in time to six-month sustained disability accumulation (compared to SC IFN-β three times per week) | Thyroid autoimmunity, immune thrombocytopenic purpura, autoimmune neutropenia, autoimmune hemolytic anemia, Goodpasture's syndrome; infusion reactions, respiratory tract infections, recurrent oral herpes, possibly meningitis, possibly malignancies | CARE-MS II (phase 3 trial comparing to IFN-β) |

*Continued*

**Table 1.** *Continued*

| Drug | Mechanism of action | Efficacy | Adverse events | Ongoing trials |
|---|---|---|---|---|
| Daclizumab (intra-venous) | Humanized mAb directed against CD25 (alpha subunit of human high-affinity IL-2 receptor) expressed on activated T cells; expansion in CD56^bright NK cells; inhibition of activated T cell proliferation | Phase 2 CHOICE: Reduced number of new or enlarged Gd$^+$ lesions with high-dose daclizumab (compared to IFN-β) | Rashes, infections, lymphadenopathy, elevated liver enzymes, fever, fatigue | SELECT (phase 3 trial comparing to IFN-β) DECIDE (phase 3 trial comparing to placebo) |
| Rituximab (intra-venous) | CD20 chimeric IgG1 mAb; depletes B cells and attenuates antibody independent pro-inflammatory B cell functions | Phase 2: 91% reduction in Gd$^+$ lesions; reduced proportions of patients with relapses (compared to placebo) Phase 2/3 PPMS trial: reduced time to confirmed progression in those < 51 years of age and/or Gd$^+$ lesions at baseline (compared to placebo) | Infusion reactions, urinary tract infections, sinusitis, PML | No phase 3 trials currently in progress |
| Ocrelizumab (intra-venous) | CD20 humanized mAb; depletes B cells and attenuates antibody independent pro-inflammatory B cell functions | Phase 2: 73–80% ARR reduction; 89–96% reduction in Gd$^+$ lesions (compared to placebo) | Infusion reactions (mainly with first infusion), opportunistic infections (in RA and SLE patients with prior methotrexate exposure) | Phase 3 trials in RRMS and PPMS |
| Ofatumumab (intra-venous) | CD20 humanized mAb; depletes B cells and attenuates antibody independent pro-inflammatory B cell functions | Phase 1/2: 99.8% reduction in new Gd$^+$ lesions; similar reductions in new/enlarging T2 lesions (compared to placebo) | Insufficient data | No phase 3 trials currently in progress |

immunosuppressant since it has not been shown to affect the egress of memory T lymphocytes from lymph nodes and has no effect on effector function such as release of inflammatory cytokines. Fingolimod is also highly lipophilic, easily crosses the BBB and is thought to exert effects directly on resident CNS cells, which also express S1P receptors, thereby possibly contributing to neuroprotection and/or remyelination.[69] For these reasons, fingolimod is currently being investigated in primary progressive MS (PPMS) (INFORMS study).

The clinical efficacy of fingolimod in RRMS was initially demonstrated in a six-month, placebo-controlled, phase 2 trial of 281 RRMS patients, in which fingolimod 1.25 and 5 mg/day significantly reduced the number of magnetic resonance imaging (MRI) gadolinium enhancing (Gd+) lesions.[70] The 24-month dose-blinded extension of this study revealed those patients originally in the placebo group that were switched to fingolimod, as well as those continuing fingolimod from the study onset, experienced significant reductions in annualized relapse rate (ARR), Gd+ lesions, and new T2 lesions.[71] The three-year open-label extension results of this study demonstrated that 88–89% and 70–78% of patients were free from Gd+ lesions and new T2 lesions, respectively, at three years, and that 68–73% remained relapse free at three years.[72]

Two pivotal phase 3 trials have been performed with fingolimod. The two-year placebo-controlled FREEDOMS study of over 1000 RRMS patients investigated fingolimod 0.5 and 1.25 mg/day.[73] The ARR was lower with both fingolimod doses compared to placebo (0.5 mg/day: 0.18; 1.25 mg/day: 0.16; placebo: 0.40), with an aggregate reduction in ARR by 54–60%. It is worth noting the ARR in the placebo arm of FREEDOMS appears to be considerably lower than ARRs in the placebo arms of the pivotal IFN-β1a (0.90) and IFN-β1b (1.27) studies from the 1990s,[31,33] similar to other recent MS trials. The discrepancy in ARR between placebo arms of recent and earlier trials may be a reflection of earlier diagnosis and/or intervention in MS practice nowadays and makes it difficult to interpret current relative to historic findings. Risk of disability progression was also reduced with fingolimod in the FREEDOMS study (cumulative probability of disease progression confirmed after three months was 16.6–17.7% with fingolimod and 24.1% with placebo). The number of new or enlarging T2 lesions, Gd+ lesions, and brain volume loss were also improved with both fingolimod doses.

In the one-year, double-dummy designed phase 3 TRANSFORMS study of 1292 RRMS patients, fingolimod 0.5 and 1.25 mg/day were compared to once-weekly IM IFN-β1a (30 μg).[74] ARR was significantly lower with fingolimod compared to IFN-β (0.5 mg/day: 0.16, 1.25 mg/day: 0.20, IFN-β: 0.33; representing 38–52% reductions in ARR with fingolimod compared to IFN-β). Reduc-tions in ARR did not differ significantly between both fingolimod doses. More patients in the fingolimod group were relapse free at one year, compared to the IFN-β group (80–83% vs. 69%). Although MRI outcomes supported the primary study results, disability progression was not significantly different between study groups in this short study.

Similar proportions of patients in the fingolimod (86–91%) and IFN-β (92%) arms of the TRANSFORMS study experienced AEs, although they lead to greater discontinuation of therapy in the fingolimod groups (6–10% vs. 4%). Headache, nasopharyngitis, and fatigue were the most common AEs reported with fingolimod. Two fatal herpes virus infections occurred in the 1.25 mg fingolimod group. One patient, without chickenpox history and with negative baseline varicella zoster virus (VZV) antibodies, developed disseminated primary VZV infection following exposure to a child with chicken pox, while receiving corticosteroids for an MS relapse. The other patient developed herpes simplex encephalitis, during which a course of IV methylprednisolone was administered for suspected MS relapse, and acyclovir therapy was delayed due to initial misdiagnosis. Additional AEs associated with drug treatment in the TRANSFORMS study included transient reductions in heart rate during fingolimod initiation (8–12 beats/min), increased blood pressure (2–3 mmHg), elevated liver enzymes (in 7–8%), localized skin cancers (in 8 patients), and macular edema (in 8 patients). Similar AEs were likewise observed in the longer FREEDOMS study. Although the overall incidence of infection was similar between the fingolimod and placebo groups in this study, lower respiratory tract infections were more common with fingolimod (9.6–11.4% vs. 6%). While the incidence of herpes virus infections did not differ between the fingolimod and placebo groups, both serious herpes infections were observed in the fingolimod groups (one at each dosage). Bradycardia and atrioventricular conduction block were again noted during fingolimod initiation. Consistent with fingolimod's mechanism of action, lymphopenia was frequently observed with fingolimod. In the FREEDOMS study, average reduction in peripheral blood lymphocyte counts of 73% were observed with 0.5 mg/day of fingolimod. In healthy individuals peripheral blood lymphocyte counts in general increase within two to three days of discontinuing fingolimod and recover by 74% within four weeks, although the recovery of peripheral blood lymphocyte counts has been documented to be slow in some individuals.[75] In addition to skin cancer, breast cancer and malignant lymphoma have also occurred in fingolimod treated patients, although causality remains unclear. Severe vasospasm, posterior reversible encephalopathy syndrome, and hemorrhaging focal encephalitis have also been described in association with fingolimod.[76,77] Given the potential AEs that may be associated with fingolimod, as described above, safety assessment plans have been recommended in the United States and Europe. Within six months of starting treatment, peripheral white cell counts, liver transaminases, and bilirubin should be assessed. An electrocardiogram should be obtained within six months of starting fingolimod in those at risk, or with history of bradycardia or atrioventricular conduction block. In the United States, an ophthalmological assessment should be performed prior to commencing therapy, while in Europe, this is only recommended for patients at risk for macular edema. VZV serology should be considered in those without chicken pox history or without VZV vaccination. If VZV serology is negative, VZV vaccination should be considered (not recommended to commence fingolimod until one month after vaccination). Live-attenuated vaccines should, however, be avoided. At the time of first-dose administration, baseline pulse and blood pressure should be checked beforehand, and monitored for six hours afterwards. Liver enzymes should be monitored at regular intervals. In Europe, it is recommended to monitor white blood cell counts at regular intervals and to interrupt treatment if lymphocyte counts fall below $0.2 \times 10^9$/L. All women of childbearing age should be counseled regarding the importance of contraception during fingolimod therapy.

## Oral cladribine

Cladribine, an antilymphocytic drug, is an analog of the purine nucleoside adenosine.[78,79] In its parenteral form, cladribine is indicated for the treatment of hairy cell leukemia, other leukemias, and lymphoma.[80] Similar to other antineoplastic drugs, cladribine is considered a teratogen. Oral cladribine is licensed for the treatment of MS in Russia and Australia. However, cladribine received a negative European recommendation by the Committee for Medicinal Products for Human Use in September 2010. In March 2011, the FDA likewise rejected licensure for cladribine for the treatment of MS in the United States. The FDA concluded in their complete response letter that substantial evidence for the effectiveness of cladribine was provided, but that a better understanding of the drug's safety risks and overall benefit–risk profile were needed. Cladribine is a prodrug that preferentially accumulates in lymphocytes. Lymphocytes have high amounts of the enzyme deoxycytidine kinase that activate cladribine through phosphorylation and low amounts of the enzyme deoxynucleotidase (unlike the vast majority of other cell types) that degrade cladribine. Furthermore, cladribine is resistant to adenosine deaminase, a deactivating enzyme found in lymphocytes. Activated cladribine incorporates itself into the DNA of dividing cells, disrupting DNA synthesis and repair, leading to a dose-dependent, sustained, and progressive depletion of $CD4^+$ and $CD8^+$ T lymphocytes.[78]

In the pivotal 96-week, double-blind, randomized, placebo-controlled phase 3 CLARITY study of 1326 RRMS patients, 3.5 and 5.25 mg/kg of oral cladribine were compared to placebo.[81] Cladribine is taken in two short courses during the first year, one month apart, and again in two short courses during the following year. ARR was significantly lower with both cladribine doses than placebo (3.5 mg/kg: 0.14; 5.25 mg/kg: 0.15; placebo: 0.33; representing reductions in ARR of 55–58% with cladribine compared to placebo). There was also a relative reduction in the risk of three-month sustained progression of disability with both cladribine doses (3.5 mg/kg: 33%; 5.25 mg/kg: 31%) and an 86–88% reduction in $Gd^+$ lesions, compared with placebo.

Consistent with cladribine's mechanism of action, the most common AE reported in the CLARITY trial was lymphopenia. Neutropenia, thrombocytopenia, and pancytopenia were also observed. More patients receiving cladribine than placebo discontinued treatment because of AEs (3.5–7.9% vs. 2.1%) and experienced more serious AEs (8.7–9% vs. 6.4%). Although the frequency of infections were comparable between the cladribine and placebo groups, more patients administered cladribine developed restricted dermatomal herpes zoster reactivations ($n = 20$) (mild herpes zoster was also associated with SC cladribine).[79] In addition, three patients receiving cladribine developed self-limiting primary VZV infections. One patient receiving cladribine died from reactivation of latent tuberculosis. Uterine fibroids were reported more frequently in cladribine patients ($n = 5$). In addition, five malignancies were observed in the cladribine group (ovarian, cervical, and pancreatic cancers; a malignant melanoma; and a choriocarcinoma, nine months after study completion). No malignancies occurred in the placebo arm of CLARITY. In a prior study of IV cladribine and cyclophosphamide in chronic lymphocytic leukemia (CLL) ($n = 29$), one patient developed PML.[82] While the doses of oral cladribine investigated in MS may not be sufficient to elicit the profound bone marrow suppression or intense immunosuppression observed with higher doses of parenteral cladribine investigated in oncology, it should be remembered that oral cladribine is a chemotherapeutic agent. There is a lack of long-term safety data available from cladribine's usage in oncological disorders, since many of these conditions are rare and associated with short survival times. The implications for long-lasting lymphocytotoxicity with cladribine are unclear, particularly with respect to risk of future infections and malignancies. Sustained lymphocyte depletion may also restrict future treatment options in MS. Two ongoing phase 3 trials are investigating the safety and effectiveness of oral cladribine. In one study, cladribine is being investigated as an add-on therapy to IFN-β (ONWARD), and in another cladribine is being investigated in clinically isolated syndromes (CIS) (ORACLE).

## Teriflunomide

Teriflunomide is the active ring malononitrile metabolite A771726 of the prodrug lenflunomide.[83] Leflunomide has been FDA approved since 1998 for the treatment of mild–moderate rheumatoid arthritis (RA) and tested in other autoimmune disorders. Other than teratogenicity (in animal models) leflunomide has a relatively favorable safety profile.[84,85] Female patients receiving teriflunomide are likely to require efficient measures of contraception, based on preclinical data of the teratogenic effects of leflunomide in animal models. In addition, male patients receiving teriflunomide are advised to discontinue treatment if they wish to father a child, although it is unclear if there is an increased risk of male-mediated fetal toxicity associated with

teriflunomide (or leflunomide). Teriflunomide inhibits mitochondrial dihydroorate dehydrogenase, the rate limiting enzyme in *de novo* pyrimidine synthesis, an action that can be overcome with the administration of exogenous uridine.[86] Because activated lymphocytes depend on *de novo* pyrimidine synthesis and resting and homeostatically expanding lymphocytes rely on the salvage pathway, teriflunomide suppresses proliferation and effector functions of activated T and B lymphocytes.[83,87] Teriflunomide may also have immunomodulatory mechanisms of action—independent of pyrimidine depletion—that are not overcome by administration of exogenous uridine including, reduced T cell production of IFN-γ and interleukin-10, disrupted interaction between T cells and APCs, and disrupted integrin signaling during T cell activation.[88] High doses of teriflunomide may also inhibit tyrosine kinases and cyclooxygenase 2 *in vitro*.[89,90] It is also worth noting that teriflunomide may have a long half-life via the enterohepatic circulation, and that without washing out teriflunomide from the enterohepatic circulation with an agent such as cholestyramine, it may continue to exert potential teratogenic effects for many months after discontinuation of the drug. Physicians should be particularly vigilant in educating male and female patients regarding this concern.

In the randomized, double-blind, placebo-controlled phase 2 study of 157 RRMS patients and 29 secondary progressive MS patients with relapses, 7 and 14 mg/day of teriflunomide were investigated.[91] Compared to placebo, both doses reduced the number of Gd+ lesions by 61%. There was also a reduction in the total number of T1 and T2 lesions, over the 36-week treatment period. The higher dose of teriflunomide was associated with suppression of worsening disability, as estimated by expanded disability status scale (EDSS) scores. ARR was not significantly reduced with teriflunomide in this phase 2 study. Results of the two-year randomized, double-blind, placebo-controlled, phase 3 TEMSO trial of 1088 relapsing MS patients, in which 7 and 14 mg/day of teriflunomide were compared to placebo, were recently announced.[92,93] In this study, both teriflunomide doses reduced the ARR by 31%, compared to placebo (ARR teriflunomide group: 0.37; ARR placebo group: 0.539). Sustained disease progression was only significantly reduced with the higher dose of teriflunomide. MRI outcomes were reached for both doses of teriflunomide. Currently, three phase 3 trials investigating teriflunomide are ongoing in MS. In TOWER, 7 and 14 mg/day of teriflunomide are being compared to placebo, in TENERE, these same doses are being compared to SC IFN-β1a, and in TOPIC, teriflunomide is being investigated in CIS. Interestingly, the primary outcome in TOPIC is time to conversion to clinically definite MS, according to POSER criteria, rather than commonly used McDonald criteria.[94,95]

In phase 2, and TEMSO trials of teriflunomide in MS, similar numbers of AEs and serious AEs occurred in the teriflunomide and placebo groups. Common AEs observed with teriflunomide included diarrhea, nausea, dyspepsia, increased liver enzymes, alopecia, skin rashes, weight loss, infections, neutropenia, paresthesia, and hypertension.[96] The increase in liver enzymes observed with teriflunomide may be in keeping with known AEs of leflunomide, which is known to be associated with liver toxicity, and in rare cases, severe hepatic injury leading to death.[85] In addition, leflunomide has been shown to increase the risk of interstitial lung disease in RA patients with pre-existing pulmonary conditions or those previously treated with methotrexate.[97] It is unclear if teriflunomide may also be associated with this risk. There is also a single case of PML reported in a systemic lupus erythematosus (SLE) patient that received leflunomide for five months, but had also received several other immunomodulatory therapies including azathioprine, cyclosporine, and methotrexate.[98]

### BG12

BG12 is an oral formulation of dimethyl fumarate, a second-generation fumaric acid. Fumaric acid has been used in psoriasis since the 1950s and has been shown to have a favorable safety profile.[99,100] Although the precise mode of action of BG12 is unclear, it is thought fumaric acid esters have dual mechanisms of action, modulating the immune system and activating antioxidative pathways.[101,102] BG12 reduces inflammatory gene expression, including that of proinflammatory cytokines and chemokines, and increases anti-inflammatory expression,[103–105] effects likely to contribute to its antipsoriasis efficacy. BG12 can suppress NF-κB (nuclear factor κB)-dependent transcription,[103,106] thus accounting for some of its anti-inflammatory effects. BG12 can also activate the Nrf2 (nuclear factor-erythroid 2 p45 subunit-related factor 2) pathway. By cleaving the cytoplasmic complex between Nrf2 and Keap1 (kelch-like erythroid cell-derived protein with cap"n"collar homology-associated protein 1), Nrf2 is free to cross the nuclear membrane. Entry and accumulation of Nrf2 into nuclei result in activation and expression of a multitude of cytoprotective and detoxification genes, critical for attenuating oxidative stress.[101] By attenuating oxidative stress-mediated CNS damage, BG12 may provide neuroprotection.[107,108] In addition, Nrf2 attenuates proinflammatory stimuli by modulating cytokine signaling and through its role in glutathione homeostasis.[101,102]

In the randomized, double-blind, placebo-controlled phase 2b study of 257 RRMS, BG12 120 mg once daily, three times daily, or 240 mg three times daily were investigated.[109] Compared to placebo, the mean total number of Gd$^+$ lesions was reduced by 69% with the highest dose of BG12 tested. Although reductions in the mean total number of Gd$^+$ lesions were also observed with the lower doses of BG12 tested, these results were not statistically significant. In addition, the highest dose of BG12 significantly reduced the mean total number of new T2 lesions by 48% and new T1 hypo-intensities by 53%, compared to placebo. Furthermore, BG12 reduced the evolution of Gd$^+$ enhancing lesions into T1 hypo-intensities by 32%, compared to placebo.[110] Although the study was not powered to demonstrate significant differences in clinical outcomes, the highest dose of BG12 tested lowered the ARR by 32%, compared to placebo. Results of the randomized, placebo-controlled, phase 3 DEFINE trial, of more than 1200 MS patients, were recently announced[a] but are not yet published. In this study, BG12 240 mg twice daily, or three times daily, was evaluated. Both doses met the primary study endpoint, demonstrating significant reductions in the proportions of RRMS patients who relapsed at two years, compared with placebo (49% reduction with the 240 mg twice daily dose). Both doses also met all of the secondary study endpoints, providing significant reductions in ARRs (53% reduction with the 240 mg twice daily dose),

---

[a]www.biogenidec.com/press_release_details.aspx?ID= 5981&ReqId=1548648, www.nature.com/nrd/journal/ v10/n6/full/nrd3465

number of new or enlarging T2 lesions (85% reduction), number of new Gd$^+$ lesions (90% reduction), and disability progression at two years (38% reduction with the 240 mg twice daily dose), compared with placebo. More detailed results from the DEFINE trial are still awaited. Another phase 3 trial of BG12 (CONFIRM) is currently ongoing. This study is evaluating BG12, and an active reference comparator, GA, against placebo.

The long-term safety profile of fumaric acid esters appears to be good, with over 50,000 patient-years recorded from its use in psoriasis. In a retrospective study of psoriasis patients treated for up to 14 years, the most frequently reported AEs with fumaric acid esters were flushing, diarrhea, and nausea.[111] Other relevant AEs reported with fumaric acid esters include lymphopenia and eosinophilia.[112] The second-generation fumaric acid BG12 was, in part, developed to reduce gastrointestinal complications. During the phase 2b trial of BG 12 common AEs were flushing, headaches and gastrointestinal symptoms (30–41% with BG12 vs. 25% with placebo), including abdominal pain, nausea, vomiting, and diarrhea, which decreased over time. In general, flushing with BG12 began within 30 minutes of administration and subsided within 90 minutes. Dose-related elevations in liver enzymes were also observed with BG12. Rates of infections between the BG12 groups, or BG12 and placebo groups, did not differ. During the first 24 weeks of the phase 2b study, the frequency of AEs leading to drug discontinuation increased slightly with increasing doses of BG12 (8% of patients receiving BG12 120 mg once daily, 11% of patients receiving BG12 120 mg three times daily, and 13% of patients receiving BG12 240 mg three times daily). Drug discontinuation during the second part of the study was less in those patients receiving BG12 for the entire study duration, than for those transitioned from placebo to BG12 240 mg three times daily (4% vs. 15%). The most common reasons for BG12 discontinuation were AEs (2%) or voluntary discontinuation (2%) in patients receiving BG12 for the entire study duration, and poor tolerance in those changed from placebo to BG12 240 mg three times daily (7%). The safety profile of BG12 in the phase 3 DEFINE trial was announced to be consistent with that observed in the phase 2b study.

### Laquinimod

Laquinimod, a second-generation quinolone-3-carboxamide, is structurally related to linomide, a compound previously found to be effective in reducing MRI lesions in RRMS.[113,114] However, a phase 3 trial of linomide was prematurely terminated one month after complete enrollment because of serious cardiopulmonary toxicity, including myocardial infarction, pericarditis, pluritis, and death.[115] Fortunately, similar cardiopulmonary toxicity has not been observed with laquinimod in clinical trials, as laquinimod is thought to be chemically and pharmacologically distinct from linomide.[116] Laquinimod has been shown to be 20 times more potent than linomide in experimental autoimmune encephalomyelitis.[117] Although the precise mechanism of action of laquinimod in MS remains incompletely elucidated, preclinical studies suggest that laquinimod induces a shift from the proinflammatory Th1 profile to the anti-inflammatory Th2 profile, decreasing CNS leukocyte infiltration.[118] Additionally, laquinimod may provide neuroprotection by increasing production of brain-derived neurotrophic factor, as well as by exerting other potential neuroprotective effects.[119]

Two phase 2 clinical trials investigated laquinimod in RRMS. In the first randomized, double-blind, placebo-controlled phase 2 trial of 209 RRMS patients, laquinimod 0.3 mg/day was investigated.[116] Although laquinimod reduced the cumulative number of Gd$^+$ lesions over 24 weeks by 44% compared to placebo ($P = 0.05$), this reduction was less pronounced and not statistically significant in an intent-to-treat analysis. The subsequent randomized, double-blind, parallel-group, placebo-controlled 36-week phase 2b trial of 306 RRMS patients investigated laquinimod 0.3 and 0.6 mg/day.[120] Only the higher dose of laquinimod in this study reduced the cumulative number of Gd$^+$ lesions (40% reduction compared to placebo). This dose also significantly reduced the cumulative number of new T2 hyperintensities and T1 hypointensities. The 36-week, double-blind, active extension of this study found those switched from placebo to laquinimod, and those who continued laquinimod, had significant reductions in the mean number of Gd$^+$ lesions.[121] It is unclear why conflicting results were obtained with the 0.3 mg/day dose of laquinimod between both phase 2 studies, although differences in gadolinium dosing, MRI, and/or study populations may have contributed. Results of the two-year, randomized, double-blind, placebo-controlled phase 3 ALLEGRO trial of 1106 MS patients, in which laquinimod 0.6 mg/day was investigated, were recently announced[b], but are not yet published. Laquinimod significantly reduced the ARR by 23%, and disability progression by 36%, compared to placebo. Laquinimod therapy was also associated with a 33% reduction in progression of brain atrophy. More detailed results from the AL-LEGRO trial are awaited. Results of the two-year, randomized, double-blind, parallel-group, placebo-controlled BRAVO study of 1331 MS patients were also recently announced[c] but are not yet published. This study was designed to compare the safety, efficacy, and tolerability of laquinimod 0.6 mg/day to placebo, and to provide a descriptive comparison of the risk-benefit profiles of laquinimod and once-weekly IM IFN-β1a. The primary outcome was the efficacy of daily laquinimod, as measured by the ARR, as compared to placebo. Secondary outcome measures included the effect of laquinimod on disability and brain atrophy progression. Although the primary endpoint of reduction in ARR was not met with laquinimod compared to placebo ($P = 0.075$), and randomization in BRAVO was adequately performed, there was dissimilarity in two of the baseline characteristics on MRI between the groups. According to a standard and prespecified sensitivity analysis included within the original statistical analysis plan, when this imbalance was corrected, laquinimod demonstrated a significant reduction in the ARR ($21.3\%$, $P = 0.026$), in the risk of disability progression as measured by EDSS ($33.5\%$, $P = 0.044$), and in brain volume loss ($27.5\%$, $P < 0.0001$), as compared to placebo. More detailed results from the BRAVO trial are awaited.

In phase 2 trials, laquinimod was generally well tolerated, although some patients experienced dose-dependent increases in liver enzymes. Other possible laquinimod-related AEs included arthralgia, and reactivation of herpes simplex and herpes zoster, which were local and self-limited. In addition, two

serious AEs were reported as being possibly laquinimod related. One patient who was found to suffer from hypercoagubility secondary to Factor V Leiden mutation developed a Budd–Chiari syndrome (thrombotic venous outflow obstruction of the liver), and another patient developed marked elevation of liver enzymes without clinical signs.

## Monoclonal antibodies

### Alemtuzumab
Alemtuzumab is a humanized mAb directed against CD52. CD52 is expressed on the surface of lymphocytes, eosinophils, and thymocytes, but not plasma cells or hematological precursor cells.[122,123] While the physiological role of CD52 remains unclear, binding of alemtuzumab to CD52 results in complement and cell-mediated lysis of expressing cells, resulting in rapid and sustained depletion of CD4[+] and CD8[+] T cells, B cells, natural killer (NK) cells, and monocytes.[124] Consequently, alemtuzumab has been used in the treatment of various leukemias. Within one hour of alemtuzumab therapy, lymphocytes are depleted from the blood. Although alemtuzumab only has a half-life of approximately six days, and alemtuzumab does not affect precursor cells, CD4[+] and CD8[+] T cells do not return to baseline levels until a median of 61 months and 30 months, respectively. In contrast, B cells are only depleted for approximately three months and thereafter may rise to higher than pretreatment levels.[124,125] Differences in the repletion of repertoires of B cells and T cells following alemtuzumab may contribute to the described propensity for developing autoimmune complications following alemtuzumab.[126–130]

In the randomized, blinded, phase 2 CAMMS223 trial of 334 previously untreated early RRMS patients, two doses of annual IV cycles of alemtuzumab were compared with SC IFN-β1a (44 μg three times per week).[131] Although alemtuzumab was planned to be administered by IV infusion on five consecutive days during the first month, and three consecutive days at months 12 and 24, alemtuzumab therapy was suspended early after immune thrombocytopenic purpura (ITP) developed in three patients, one of whom died from a cerebral hemorrhage. At the time of dose suspension, only two patients (1%) had not received the second cycle of alemtuzumab at month 12, whereas 75% of patients were precluded from receiving the third cycle of

---

[b]www.tevapharm.com/pr/2011/pr_1004.asp
[c]www.tevapharm.com/en-US/Media/News/Pages/Bravo.aspx

alemtuzumab at month 24. There were no significant differences between the lower (12 mg) and higher doses of alemtuzumab (24 mg), in terms of outcome measures or AEs. Compared to IFN-β, alemtuzumab reduced the risk of sustained disability by 71%. The number of patients needed to treat with alemtuzumab instead of IFN-β to avoid one sustained disability event over 36 months was 5.8. There was a risk reduction of 64% in sustained disability at 3 months with alemtuzumab. Mean EDSS score at 36 months improved in the alemtuzumab groups by 0.39 points, while mean disability scores deteriorated by 0.38 points in the IFN-β group, equating to a net advantage of 0.77 points in those treated with alemtuzumab ($P < 0.001$). Alemtuzumab reduced RR by 74% compared to IFN-β (ARR in alemtuzumab group: 0.10; ARR in IFN-β group: 0.36, at 36 months). Proportions of patients who remained relapse free at 36 months were 80% for alemtuzumab, and 52% for IFN-β. The number of patients needed to treat with alemtuzumab instead of IFN-β to prevent one patient from having a relapse at 36 months was 3.5. While there were no significant differences in safety or treatment effect on disability between alemtuzumab patients who received two cycles of therapy, instead of three, there was evidence of waning of treatment efficacy on RR. T2-weighted lesion volumes were significantly reduced from baseline, at 12 months, and 24 months with alemtuzumab. The reduction in brain volume between baseline and month 36 was significantly less among patients receiving alemtuzumab than IFN-β. Results of the two-year, randomized, rater-blinded phase 3 CARE-MS 1 clinical trial to determine the efficacy and safety of alemtuzumab in early, active, treatment-naive RRMS, in which 581 patients were included, were recently announced[d] but are not yet published. In this study, two annual cycles of alemtuzumab therapy resulted in a 55% reduction in RR over the two-year study period, as compared to SC IFN-β1a (44 μg three times per week) ($P < 0.0001$), meeting the first primary endpoint of the study. Statistical significance was not however met for the second primary endpoint of the study (time to six month sustained accumulation of disability, as compared to IFN-β1a). At two

years, 8% of alemtuzumab-treated patients had a sustained increase in their EDSS score, while 11% of IFN-β1a-treated patients had a sustained increase in their EDSS score at the same time point (hazard ratio = 0.70, $P = 0.22$). Further results from the CARE-MS 1 study are awaited.

Almost all study participants in the CAMMS223 trial reported at least one AE, and although the numbers of patients with serious AEs were similar between the three study groups, more patients discontinued IFN-β than alemtuzumab, possibly because of difficulty in concealing blinding, such that 59% of patients in the IFN group completed the study, compared with 83% of alemtuzumab patients. On account of the initial three cases of ITP, a program was implemented as part of the study to ensure prompt identification and appropriate management of ITP, including monthly blood counts. Three further cases of ITP were identified following alemtuzumab suspension. Chronic asymptomatic ITP also developed in one patient receiving IFN-β. Four of the ITP cases occurred in patients treated with the higher dose of alemtuzumab, and the two cases of ITP that occurred with the lower dose, occurred following three cycles of therapy. ITP required therapy with corticosteroids, IV immunoglobulin, or rituximab in four patients, but was reversible with no recurrences. AEs affecting the thyroid (transient hyperthyroidism, sustained hyperthyroidism, sustained hypothyroidism, hypothyroidism followed by hyperthyroidism) were more frequent in the alemtuzumab group (22.7% of patients), than the IFN-β group (2.8% of patients), were associated with thyroid autoantibodies in 96% of cases, and occurred up to 30 months after the last dose of administration. Serious infusion reactions occurred in three patients (1.4%) in the alemtuzumab group. Mild-to-moderate infections (particularly of the respiratory tract) were more common in the alemtuzumab groups. Recurrent oral herpes simplex virus type 1 was observed in three patients immediately following each alemtuzumab cycle. One case of viral meningitis and one case of listeria meningitis occurred in the alemtuzumab arm of the study. In addition, three cases of malignancy occurred in alemtuzumab-treated patients: non-EBV associated Burkitt lymphoma, breast cancer, and cervical carcinoma *in situ*. Other AEs described following alemtuzumab include Goodpasture's syndrome with acute renal

---

[d]www.businesswire.com/news/genzyme/201107100-05114/en

failure,[132] autoimmune neutropenia, and autoimmune hemolytic anemia.[125] In the recently announced results of the phase 3 CARE-MS I clinical trial, the most common AE observed with alemtuzumab was infusion reactions, characterized commonly by headache, rash, fever, nausea, flushing, hives, and chills. An increased incidence of infections was also noted with alemtuzumab therapy, with the most common infections including upper respiratory, urinary tract, and oral herpetic infections. Another phase 3 clinical trial (CARE-MS II) comparing alemtuzumab to IFN-β1a in RRMS patients who have relapsed while on other DMDs is currently ongoing.

### Daclizumab

Daclizumab, a humanized IgG1 mAb directed against CD25, has been approved by the FDA for the treatment of renal allograft rejections since 1997.[133] CD25, the alpha subunit of the human high-affinity interleukin-2 receptor, is expressed on the surface of activated and regulatory T cells, activated B cells, myeloid precursor cells, and thymocytes.[134] Although the rationale for testing daclizumab in autoimmune disorders was based on its potential to inhibit activated T cell proliferation, lymphocyte subpopulation analyses in daclizumab-treated patients reveal normal numbers of circulating T and B cells, but marked expansion of CD56[bright] NK cells.[135] In addition, daclizumab appears to affect the capacity of dendritic cells to present antigen to T cells.[136]

In the randomized, double-blind, placebo-controlled, phase 2 CHOICE trial, 230 active RRMS patients on IFN-β were randomly assigned add-on SC daclizumab 2 mg/kg two-weekly (high-dose daclizumab group), daclizumab 1 mg/kg four-weekly (low-dose daclizumab group), or placebo (IFN-β alone group), for 24 weeks.[135] The adjusted mean number of new or enlarged Gd[+] lesions was 1.32 in the high-dose daclizumab group, 3.58 in the low-dose daclizumab group, and 4.75 in the IFN-β alone group. Pharmacodynamic analyses comparing daclizumab and IFN-β alone treated patients did not demonstrate significant changes in absolute numbers of T cells, B cells, NK cells, or T cell proliferative responses, but rather seven- to eightfold increases in numbers of CD56[bright] NK cells, which normalized within two to three months of discontinuing daclizumab. Common AEs were equally distributed across all groups in the study. AEs reported with daclizumab in prior trials include rashes, infections, lymphadenopathy, elevated liver enzymes, fever, and fatigue.[137,138] Currently, there are two ongoing phase 3 trials, SELECT and DECIDE, comparing daclizumab 150 or 300 mg four times weekly to IM IFN-β or placebo.

### CD20 monoclonal antibodies

CD20 is expressed on B cell lineage from the pre-B cell stage to the memory B cell stage, but not on plasma cells.[139] CD20 mAbs result in B cell depletion.[140,141] Rituximab, the first chimeric CD20 IgG1 mAb found to target and efficiently deplete circulating CD20[+] B cells in humans,[142] was approved for the treatment of non-Hodgkins lymphoma in 1997 and RA in 2006. Pharmacokinetic and pharmacodynamic analyses conducted during phase 1 and 2 RRMS trials confirmed almost complete depletion of circulating CD19[+] B cells within two weeks of administration.[143,144] While it was anticipated benefit of CD20 mAbs in MS would result from depletion of pathogenic autoantibodies, it now appears that their effectiveness instead relates to attenuation of antibody-independent proinflammatory B cell functions. Several studies demonstrate that CD20 mAbs in MS have little to no impact on serum or CSF IgG levels or oligoclonal IgG banding patterns.[143–146] Antibody-independent functions of B cells include antigen presentation, T cell activation, production of effector cytokines, innate-adaptive interfacing, and the formation and maintenance of new lymphoid foci, including in the CNS.[147] CD20 mAb therapies result in the reduction of both B cells and T cells in the CSF.[146] This may reflect either reduced CNS recruitment of T cells by B cells, or reduced activation of CNS or peripheral T cells by B cells.[144]

The 48-week, double-blind, placebo-controlled, phase 2 clinical trial of rituximab included 104 RRMS patients. In this study, patients received IV rituximab 1,000 mg (on days 1 and 15), or placebo.[148] Compared to placebo, there was a relative reduction of Gd[+] lesions with rituximab of approximately 91%. In addition, proportions of patients with relapses in the rituximab group were significantly lower than in the placebo group (20% vs. 40%). In the double-blind, placebo-controlled phase 2/3 study of 439 PPMS patients, rituximab (two 1000 mg infusions two weeks apart) or placebo were administered every 24 weeks until week 96.[149] Although the primary endpoint (time to confirmed disease progression) was not significantly different between rituximab and placebo, increases in T2 lesion volumes were significantly lower with rituximab. Subgroup analyses did however reveal rituximab significantly reduced time to confirmed progression in patients under 51 years of age, in patients with Gd$^+$ lesions at baseline, and most noticeably in patients fulfilling both of these criteria.

In the phase 2 study of rituximab, antichimeric antibodies developed in approximately 24% of patients, but did not affect AEs or treatment efficacy. Infusion-associated AEs (mostly mild–moderate in severity) were encountered more with rituximab than placebo in both studies. Overall, no differences were observed in the incidence of serious AEs or infections between groups in these studies, although urinary tract infections and sinusitis were reported more commonly with rituximab. While fatal infusion reactions have been reported in lymphoma patients treated with rituximab, these patients tended to have high tumor mass and concurrent cardiovascular or pulmonary disease.[150] Several cases of PML have been reported with rituximab in RA and lymphoma.[151] While most of these patients received prior or concomitant treatment with other immunosupressants, there is at least one known case of PML reported in a RA patient not previously treated with any other immunosuppressive therapies.[152]

Ocrelizumab, a humanized CD20 mAb, binds to a different but overlapping epitope of CD20 as rituximab, and unlike rituximab, primarily depletes B cells through antibody-dependent cellular cytotoxicity, rather than complement-dependent cytotoxicity (CDC). This different mechanism of action may potentially improve efficacy, and reduce infusion reactions.[153,154] In the phase 2 randomized, placebo-controlled study of ocrelizumab, 220 RRMS patients received either ocrelizumab 600 or 2000 mg over two-infusions (on days 1 and 15), once-weekly intramuscular IFN-β1a, or placebo.[155] Ocrelizumab 600 and 2000 mg reduced Gd$^+$ lesions by 89% and 96%, respectively, compared to placebo. Both doses were also superior to weekly IFN-β1a at reducing Gd$^+$ lesions. The 600 and 2000 mg doses of ocrelizumab also significantly reduced RR by 80% and 73%, respectively, compared to placebo.

More serious AEs occurred with high-dose ocrelizumab than low-dose ocrelizumab. Although infusion-related AEs were more common with ocrelizumab than placebo during the first infusion (34.5–43.6% vs. 9.3%), rates with the second infusion were comparable to placebo. One patient who received high-dose ocrelizumab died from acute-onset microangiopathy. Although there was no difference in frequencies of serious infections among groups, ocrelizumab is no longer being pursued in RA or SLE, due to the development of lethal opportunistic infections in high-dose ocrelizumab-treated patients, with prior methotrexate exposure. Currently, phase 3 trials of ocrelizumab are in progress in RRMS and PPMS.

Ofatumumab, a fully human CD20 mAb, binds to a distinct CD20 epitope, dissociates more slowly from CD20, and exhibits predominantly CDC activity.[156–159] Ofatumumab was approved by the FDA for the treatment of refractory CLL in 2009. Ofatumumab has also been tested in RA, where it appears to demonstrate efficacy, without increased risk of opportunistic infections.[160] Ofatumumab has been studied in RRMS in a small phase 1/2 randomized, placebo-controlled trial. In this study, three IV doses of ofatumumab (100, 200, and 700 mg) given in two courses, six months apart, were compared to placebo.[161] The mean cumulative number of new Gd$^+$ lesions was 0.04 in the combined ofatumumab group and 9.69 in the placebo group (estimated relative reduction: 99.8%). Similar reductions were also found for new and enlarging T2 lesions.

## Conclusions

As the availability of MS DMDs continues to grow, so too may the complexity of individual patient care. Many of the new and emerging MS therapies differ with respect to their route of administration, mechanism of action, efficacy, and safety. As these drugs become available, their roles in the treatment algorithm of MS will need to be defined. Although oral therapies may be convenient, and potentially improve adherence, particularly in needle-phobic patients or patients intolerant of injectable first-line agents, they should not be considered synonymous with safe. Some oral therapies may require risk-mitigation plans, as is the case with fingolimod. Although potentially inconvenient, currently approved injectable first-line agents are overall relatively safe and have well-characterized safety profiles. Neurologists should be cautious selecting therapies based purely on efficacy. Treatment safety and tolerability also need to be carefully considered. It warrants emphasis that many of the new and emerging MS therapies lack long-term safety data; it is unclear what their long-term complications may be, or if their use may restrict future therapeutic options. Establishing safety profiles for these drugs will be critical for effective and balanced therapeutic decision making.

Further comparative trials, as well as trials assessing combinations of new and emerging MS therapies with other DMDs may be indicated. Studies comparing these therapies in treatment-naive MS patients, previously treated MS patients, as well as MS patients of varying severity may be illuminating. Moving forward, identification of safer, yet efficacious therapies, including neuroprotective and remyelinating agents are major goals in MS.

## Conflicts of interest

Dr. Shiv Saidha has received consulting fees from MedicalLogix for the development of continuing medical education programs in neurology and has received educational grant support from Teva Neurosciences. Dr. Christopher Eckstein has no disclosures. Dr. Peter Calabresi has provided consultation services to Novartis, EMD-Serono, Teva, Biogen-IDEC, Vertex, Vaccinex, Genzyme, Genentech and has received grant support from EMD-Serono, Teva, Biogen-IDEC, Genentech, Bayer, Abbott, and Vertex.

## References

1. Anderson, D.W., J.H. Ellenberg, C.M. Leventhal, *et al.* 1992. Revised estimate of the prevalence of multiple sclerosis in the United States. *Ann. Neurol.* **31:** 333–336.
2. Marburg, O. 1906. Die sogennate akute multiple Sklerose. *Jahrb. Psychiatrie* **27:** 211–312.
3. Putnam, T. 1936. Studies in multiple sclerosis. *Arch. Neurol. Psych.* **35:** 1289–1308.
4. Prineas, J. 2001. Pathology of multiple sclerosis. In *Handbook of Multiple Sclerosis*. *In Anonymous*. S. Cook, Ed.: 289–324. Marcel Dekker. New York.
5. Frohman, E.M., M.K. Racke & C.S. Raine. 2006. Multiple sclerosis—the plaque and its pathogenesis. *N. Engl. J. Med.* **354:** 942–955.
6. van Waesberghe, J.H., W. Kamphorst, C.J. De Groot, *et al.* 1999. Axonal loss in multiple sclerosis lesions: magnetic resonance imaging insights into substrates of disability. *Ann. Neurol.* **46:** 747–754.
7. De Stefano N., S. Narayanan, G.S. Francis, *et al.* 2001. Evidence of axonal damage in the early stages of multiple sclerosis and its relevance to disability. *Arch. Neurol.* **58:** 65–70.
8. Compston, A. & A. Coles. 2002. Multiple sclerosis. *Lancet* **359:** 1221–1231.
9. Miller, D.H. 2004. Biomarkers and surrogate outcomes in neurodegenerative disease: lessons from multiple sclerosis. *NeuroRx* **1:** 284–294.
10. Minneboo A., B.M. Uitdehaag, P. Jongen, *et al.* 2009. Association between MRI parameters and the MS severity scale: a 12 year follow-up study. *Mult. Scler.* **15:** 632–637.
11. Calabrese M., M. Atzori, V. Bernardi, *et al.* 2007. Cortical atrophy is relevant in multiple sclerosis at clinical onset. *J. Neurol.* **254:** 1212–1220.
12. Calabrese M., F. Agosta, F. Rinaldi, *et al.* 2009. Cortical lesions and atrophy associated with cognitive impairment in relapsing-remitting multiple sclerosis. *Arch. Neurol.* **66:** 1144–1150.
13. Rawes, J.A., V.P. Calabrese, O.A. Khan, *et al.* 1997. Antibodies to the axolemma-enriched fraction in the cerebrospinal fluid and serum of patients with multiple sclerosis and other neurological diseases. *Mult. Scler.* **3:** 363–369.
14. Madigan, M.C., N.S. Rao, W.N. Tenhula, *et al.* 1996. Preliminary morphometric study of tumor necrosis factor-alpha (TNF alpha)-induced rabbit optic neuropathy. *Neurol. Res.* **18:** 233–236.
15. Shindler, K.S., E. Ventura, M. Dutt, *et al.* 2008. Inflammatory demyelination induces axonal injury and retinal ganglion cell apoptosis in experimental optic neuritis. *Exp. Eye Res.* **87:** 208–213.
16. Frischer, J.M., S. Bramow, A. Dal-Bianco, *et al.* 2009. The relation between inflammation and neurodegeneration in multiple sclerosis brains. *Brain* **132:** 1175–1189.
17. Delgado, S. & W.A. Sheremata. 2006. The role of CD4+ T-cells in the development of MS. *Neurol. Res.* **28:** 245–249.
18. Mosmann, T.R., H. Cherwinski, M.W. Bond, *et al.* 1986. Two types of murine helper T cell clone: I. Definition according to profiles of lymphokine activities and secreted proteins. *J. Immunol.* **136:** 2348–2357.
19. Crawford, M.P., S.X. Yan, S.B. Ortega, *et al.* 2004. High prevalence of autoreactive, neuroantigen-specific CD8+ T cells in multiple sclerosis revealed by novel flow cytometric assay. *Blood* **103:** 4222–4231.
20. Haas, J., A. Hug, A. Viehover, *et al.* 2005. Reduced suppressive effect of CD4+CD25 high regulatory T cells on the T cell immune response against myelin oligodendrocyte glycoprotein in patients with multiple sclerosis. *Eur. J. Immunol.* **35:** 3343–3352.
21. Kumar M., N. Putzki, V. Limmroth, *et al.* 2006. CD4+CD25+FoxP3+ T lymphocytes fail to suppress myelin basic protein-induced proliferation in patients with multiple sclerosis. *J. Neuroimmunol.* **180:** 178–184.
22. Lovato L., S.N. Willis, S.J. Rodig, *et al.* 2011. Related B cell clones populate the meninges and parenchyma of patients with multiple sclerosis. *Brain* **134:** 534–541.
23. Lo, A.C., J.A. Black & S.G. Waxman. 2002. Neuroprotection of axons with phenytoin in experimental allergic encephalomyelitis. *Neuroreport* **13:** 1909–1912.

24. Lo, A.C., C.Y. Saab, J.A. Black, *et al.* 2003. Phenytoin protects spinal cord axons and preserves axonal conduction and neurological function in a model of neuroinflammation in vivo. *J. Neurophysiol.* **90:** 3566–3571.

25. Kapoor, R. 2010. Lamotrigine for neuroprotection in secondary progressive multiple sclerosis: a randomised, double-blind, placebo-controlled, parallel-group trial. *Lancet Neurol.* **9:** 681–688.

26. Mi S., B. Hu, K. Hahm, *et al.* 2007. LINGO-1 antagonist promotes spinal cord remyelination and axonal integrity in MOG-induced experimental autoimmune encephalomyelitis. *Nat. Med.* **13:** 1228–1233.

27. Calza L., M. Fernandez & L. Giardino. 2010. Cellular approaches to central nervous system remyelination stimulation: thyroid hormone to promote myelin repair via endogenous stem and precursor cells. *J. Mol. Endocrinol.* **44:** 13–23.

28. Frohman, E.M., J.G. Fujimoto, T.C. Frohman, *et al.* 2008. Optical coherence tomography: a window into the mechanisms of multiple sclerosis. *Nat. Clin. Pract. Neurol.* **4:** 664–675.

29. Saidha S., C. Eckstein & J.N. Ratchford. 2010. Optical coherence tomography as a marker of axonal damage in multiple sclerosis. *CML—Multiple Sclerosis* **2:** 33–43.

30. Paty, D.W. & D.K. Li.UBC MS/MRI Study Group and the IFNB Multiple Sclerosis Study Group. 1993. Interferon beta-1b is effective in relapsing-remitting multiple sclerosis: II. MRI analysis results of a multicenter, randomized, double-blind, placebo-controlled trial. *Neurology* **43:** 662–667.

31. The IFNB Multiple Sclerosis Study Group. 1993. Interferon beta-1b is effective in relapsing-remitting multiple sclerosis: I. Clinical results of a multicenter, randomized, double-blind, placebo-controlled trial. *Neurology* **43:** 655–661.

32. PRISMS (Prevention of Relapses and Disability by Interferon beta-1a Subcutaneously in Multiple Sclerosis) Study Group. 1998. Randomised double-blind placebo-controlled study of interferon beta-1a in relapsing/remitting multiple sclerosis. *Lancet* **352:** 1498–1504.

33. Jacobs, L.D., D.L. Cookfair, R.A. Rudick, *et al.* The Multiple Sclerosis Collaborative Research Group (MSCRG). 1996. Intramuscular interferon beta-1a for disease progression in relapsing multiple sclerosis. *Ann. Neurol.* **39:** 285–294.

34. Johnson, K.P., B.R. Brooks, J.A. Cohen, *et al.*The Copolymer 1 Multiple Sclerosis Study Group. 1995. Copolymer 1 reduces relapse rate and improves disability in relapsing-remitting multiple sclerosis: results of a phase III multicenter, double-blind placebo-controlled trial. *Neurology* **45:** 1268–1276.

35. Racke, M.K. & A.E. Lovett-Racke. 2011. Glatiramer acetate treatment of multiple sclerosis: an immunological perspective. *J. Immunol.* **186:** 1887–1890.

36. Reder, A.T., G.C. Ebers, A. Traboulsee, *et al.* 2010. Cross-sectional study assessing long-term safety of interferon-beta-1b for relapsing-remitting MS. *Neurology* **74:** 1877–1885.

37. Ford C., A.D. Goodman, K. Johnson, *et al.* 2010. Continuous long-term immunomodulatory therapy in relapsing multiple sclerosis: results from the 15-year analysis of the US prospective open-label study of glatiramer acetate. *Mult. Scler.* **16:** 342–350.

38. Sandberg-Wollheim M., D. Frank, T.M. Goodwin, *et al.* 2005. Pregnancy outcomes during treatment with interferon beta-1a in patients with multiple sclerosis. *Neurology* **65:** 802–806.

39. Weber-Schoendorfer, C. & C. Schaefer. 2009. Multiple sclerosis, immunomodulators, and pregnancy outcome: a prospective observational study. *Mult. Scler.* **15:** 1037–1042.

40. Salminen, H.J., H. Leggett & M. Boggild. 2010. Glatiramer acetate exposure in pregnancy: preliminary safety and birth outcomes. *J. Neurol.* **257:** 2020–2023.

41. Kuhlmann T., G. Lingfeld, A. Bitsch, *et al.* 2002. Acute axonal damage in multiple sclerosis is most extensive in early disease stages and decreases over time. *Brain* **125:** 2202–2212.

42. Kappos L., M.S. Freedman, C.H. Polman, *et al.* 2007. Effect of early versus delayed interferon beta-1b treatment on disability after a first clinical event suggestive of multiple sclerosis: a 3-year follow-up analysis of the BENEFIT study. *Lancet* **370:** 389–397.

43. Jacobs, L.D., R.W. Beck, J.H. Simon, *et al.*CHAMPS Study Group. 2000. Intramuscular interferon beta-1a therapy initiated during a first demyelinating event in multiple sclerosis. *N. Engl. J. Med.* **343:** 898–904.

44. Comi, G. 2009. Shifting the paradigm toward earlier treatment of multiple sclerosis with interferon beta. *Clin. Ther.* **31:** 1142–1157.

45. Mikol, D.D., F. Barkhof, P. Chang, *et al.* 2008. Comparison of subcutaneous interferon beta-1a with glatiramer acetate in patients with relapsing multiple sclerosis (the REbif vs Glatiramer Acetate in Relapsing MS Disease [REGARD] study): a multicentre, randomised, parallel, open-label trial. *Lancet Neurol.* **7:** 903–914.

46. O'Connor P., M. Filippi, B. Arnason, *et al.* 2009. 250 microg or 500 microg interferon beta-1b versus 20 mg glatiramer acetate in relapsing-remitting multiple sclerosis: a prospective, randomised, multicentre study. *Lancet Neurol.* **8:** 889–897.

47. Yednock, T.A., C. Cannon, L.C. Fritz, *et al.* 1992. Prevention of experimental autoimmune encephalomyelitis by antibodies against alpha 4 beta 1 integrin. *Nature* **356:** 63–66.

48. Osborn L., C. Hession, R. Tizard, *et al.* 1989. Direct expression cloning of vascular cell adhesion molecule 1, a cytokine-induced endothelial protein that binds to lymphocytes. *Cell* **59:** 1203–1211.

49. Elices, M.J., L. Osborn, Y. Takada, *et al.* 1990. VCAM-1 on activated endothelium interacts with the leukocyte integrin VLA-4 at a site distinct from the VLA-4/fibronectin binding site. *Cell* **60:** 577–584.

50. Polman, C.H., P.W. O'Connor, E. Havrdova, *et al.* 2006. A randomized, placebo-controlled trial of natalizumab for relapsing multiple sclerosis. *N. Engl. J. Med.* **354:** 899–910.

51. Naismith, R.T. & D. Bourdette. 2011. Interruption of natalizumab therapy for multiple sclerosis: What are the risks? *Neurology* **76:** 1854–1855.

52. Rudick, R.A., W.H. Stuart, P.A. Calabresi, *et al.* 2006. Natalizumab plus interferon beta-1a for relapsing multiple sclerosis. *N. Engl. J. Med.* **354:** 911–923.

53. Major, E.O. 2010. Progressive multifocal leukoencephalopathy in patients on immunomodulatory therapies. *Annu. Rev. Med.* **61:** 35–47.

54. Ransohoff, R.M. 2010. PML risk and natalizumab: more questions than answers. *Lancet Neurol.* **9:** 231–233.

55. Koralnik, I.J. 2006. Progressive multifocal leukoencephalopathy revisited: Has the disease outgrown its name? *Ann. Neurol.* **60:** 162–173.

56. Hutchinson, M. 2007. Natalizumab: a new treatment for relapsing remitting multiple sclerosis. *Ther. Clin. Risk Manag.* **3:** 259–268.

57. Sandrock A., C. Hotermans, S. Richman, *et al.* 2011. Risk stratification for progressive mulitfocal leukoencephalopathy (PML) in MS patients: role of prior immunosuppressant use, natalizumab treatment duration, and anti-JCV antibody status [abstract]. *Neurology* **76**(Suppl. 4): A248.

58. Clifford, D.B., A. De Luca, D.M. Simpson, *et al.* 2010. Natalizumab-associated progressive multifocal leukoencephalopathy in patients with multiple sclerosis: lessons from 28 cases. *Lancet Neurol.* **9:** 438–446.

59. Gorelik L., M. Lerner, S. Bixler, *et al.* 2010. Anti-JC virus antibodies: implications for PML risk stratification. *Ann. Neurol.* **68:** 295–303.

60. Khatri, B.O., S. Man, G. Giovannoni, *et al.* 2009. Effect of plasma exchange in accelerating natalizumab clearance and restoring leukocyte function. *Neurology* **72:** 402–409.

61. Vermersch P., L. Kappos, R. Gold, *et al.* 2011. Clinical outcomes of natalizumab-associated progressive multifocal leukoencephalopathy. *Neurology* **76:** 1697–1704.

62. Tan K., R. Roda, L. Ostrow, *et al.* 2009. PML-IRIS in patients with HIV infection: clinical manifestations and treatment with steroids. *Neurology* **72:** 1458–1464.

63. Hellwig K., A. Haghikia & R. Gold. 2011. Pregnancy and natalizumab: results of an observational study in 35 accidental pregnancies during natalizumab treatment. *Mult. Scler.*

64. Gold, R. 2011. Oral therapies for multiple sclerosis: a review of agents in phase III development or recently approved. *CNS Drugs* **25:** 37–52.

65. Brinkmann, V. 2004. FTY720: mechanism of action and potential benefit in organ transplantation. *Yonsei Med. J.* **45:** 991–997.

66. Brinkmann V., A. Billich, T. Baumruker, *et al.* 2010. Fingolimod (FTY720): discovery and development of an oral drug to treat multiple sclerosis. *Nat. Rev. Drug Discov.* **9:** 883–897.

67. Matloubian M., C.G. Lo, G. Cinamon, *et al.* 2004. Lymphocyte egress from thymus and peripheral lymphoid organs is dependent on S1P receptor 1. *Nature* **427:** 355–360.

68. Kowarik, M.C., H.L. Pellkofer, S. Cepok, *et al.* 2011. Differential effects of fingolimod (FTY720) on immune cells in the CSF and blood of patients with MS. *Neurology* **76:** 1214–1221.

69. Miron, V.E., A. Schubart & J.P. Antel. 2008. Central nervous system-directed effects of FTY720 (fingolimod). *J. Neurol. Sci.* **274:** 13–17.

70. Kappos L., J. Antel, G. Comi, *et al.* 2006. Oral fingolimod (FTY720) for relapsing multiple sclerosis. *N. Engl. J. Med.* **355:** 1124–1140.

71. O'Connor P., G. Comi, X. Montalban, *et al.* 2009. Oral fingolimod (FTY720) in multiple sclerosis: two-year results of a phase II extension study. *Neurology* **72:** 73–79.

72. Comi G., P. O'Connor, X. Montalban, *et al.* 2010. Phase II study of oral fingolimod (FTY720) in multiple sclerosis: 3-year results. *Mult. Scler.* **16:** 197–207.

73. Kappos L., E.W. Radue, P. O'Connor, *et al.* 2010. A placebo-controlled trial of oral fingolimod in relapsing multiple sclerosis. *N. Engl. J. Med.* **362:** 387–401.

74. Cohen, J.A., F. Barkhof, G. Comi, *et al.* 2010. Oral fingolimod or intramuscular interferon for relapsing multiple sclerosis. *N. Engl. J. Med.* **362:** 402–415.

75. Schmouder R., S. Aradhye, P. O'Connor, *et al.* 2006. Pharmacodynamic effects of oral fingolimod (FTY720) [abstract]. *Mult. Scler.* **12:** S101–S102.

76. Schwarz A., M. Korporal, W. Hosch, *et al.* 2010. Critical vasospasm during fingolimod (FTY720) treatment in a patient with multiple sclerosis. *Neurology* **74:** 2022–2024.

77. Leypoldt F., A. Munchau, F. Moeller, *et al.* 2009. Hemorrhaging focal encephalitis under fingolimod (FTY720) treatment: a case report. *Neurology* **72:** 1022–1024.

78. Beutler, E. 1992. Cladribine (2-chlorodeoxyadenosine). *Lancet* **340:** 952–956.

79. Sipe, J.C. 2005. Cladribine for multiple sclerosis: review and current status. *Expert Rev. Neurother.* **5:** 721–727.

80. Beutler, E. 1994. New chemotherapeutic agent: 2-chlorodeoxyadenosine. *Semin. Hematol.* **31:** 40–45.

81. Giovannoni G., G. Comi, S. Cook, *et al.* 2010. A placebo-controlled trial of oral cladribine for relapsing multiple sclerosis. *N. Engl. J. Med.* **362:** 416–426.

82. Montillo M., A. Tedeschi, S. O'Brien, *et al.* 2003. Phase II study of cladribine and cyclophosphamide in patients with chronic lymphocytic leukemia and prolymphocytic leukemia. *Cancer* **97:** 114–120.

83. Bruneau, J.M., C.M. Yea, S. Spinella-Jaegle, *et al.* 1998. Purification of human dihydro-orotate dehydrogenase and its inhibition by A77 1726, the active metabolite of leflunomide. *Biochem. J.* **336**(Pt 2): 299–303.

84. Bartlett, R.R., M. Dimitrijevic, T. Mattar, *et al.* 1991. Leflunomide (HWA 486), a novel immunomodulating compound for the treatment of autoimmune disorders and reactions leading to transplantation rejection. *Agents Actions.* **32:** 10–21.

85. Alcorn N., S. Saunders & R. Madhok. 2009. Benefit-risk assessment of leflunomide: an appraisal of leflunomide in rheumatoid arthritis 10 years after licensing. *Drug Saf.* **32:** 1123–1134.

86. Williamson, R.A., C.M. Yea, P.A. Robson, *et al.* 1995. Dihydroorotate dehydrogenase is a high affinity binding protein for A77 1726 and mediator of a range of biological effects of the immunomodulatory compound. *J. Biol. Chem.* **270:** 22467–22472.

87. Cherwinski, H.M., R.G. Cohn, P. Cheung, *et al.* 1995. The immunosuppressant leflunomide inhibits lymphocyte proliferation by inhibiting pyrimidine biosynthesis. *J. Pharmacol. Exp. Ther.* **275:** 1043–1049.

88. Zeyda M., M. Poglitsch, R. Geyeregger, *et al.* 2005. Disruption of the interaction of T cells with antigen-presenting cells by the active leflunomide metabolite teriflunomide:

involvement of impaired integrin activation and immuno-logic synapse formation. *Arthritis Rheum.* **52:** 2730–2739.

89. Elder, R.T., X. Xu, J.W. Williams, *et al.* 1997. The im-munosuppressive metabolite of leflunomide, A77 1726, af-fects murine T cells through two biochemical mechanisms. *J. Immunol.* **159:** 22–27.

90. Hamilton, L.C., I. Vojnovic & T.D. Warner. 1999. A771726, the active metabolite of leflunomide, directly inhibits the activity of cyclo-oxygenase-2 in vitro and in vivo in a substrate-sensitive manner. *Br. J. Pharmacol.* **127:** 1589–1596.

91. O'Connor, P.W., D. Li, M.S. Freedman, *et al.* 2006. A phase II study of the safety and efficacy of teriflunomide in mul-tiple sclerosis with relapses. *Neurology* **66:** 894–900.

92. O'Connor P., J. Wolinsky, C. Confavreux, *et al.* 2010. A placebo-controlled phase III trial (TEMSO) of oral teri-flunomide in relapsing multiple sclerosis: clinical efficacy and safety outcomes [abstract]. *Mult. Scler.* **16**(Suppl. 10): S23.

93. Wolinsky J., P. O'Connor, C. Confavreux, *et al.* 2010. A placebo-controlled phase III trial (TEMSO) of oral teri-flunomide in relapsing multiple sclerosis: magnetic reso-nance imaging (MRI) outcomes [abstract]. *Mult. Scler.* **16:** S347–S348.

94. Polman, C.H., S.C. Reingold, G. Edan, *et al.* 2005. Diag-nostic criteria for multiple sclerosis: 2005 revisions to the "McDonald Criteria". *Ann. Neurol.* **58:** 840–846.

95. Polman, C.H., S.C. Reingold, B. Banwell, *et al.* 2011. Diag-nostic criteria for multiple sclerosis: 2010 revisions to the McDonald criteria. *Ann. Neurol.* **69:** 292–302.

96. Claussen, M.C. & T. Korn. 2011. Immune mech-anisms of new therapeutic strategies in MS–Teriflunomide. *Clin. Immunol.* Epub ahead of print. doi:10.1016/j.clim.2011.02.011.

97. Suissa S., M. Hudson & P. Ernst. 2006. Leflunomide use and the risk of interstitial lung disease in rheumatoid arthritis. *Arthritis Rheum.* **54:** 1435–1439.

98. Warnatz K., H.H. Peter, M. Schumacher, *et al.* 2003. In-fectious CNS disease as a differential diagnosis in systemic rheumatic diseases: three case reports and a review of the literature. *Ann. Rheum. Dis.* **62:** 50–57.

99. Reich K., D. Thaci, U. Mrowietz, *et al.* 2009. Efficacy and safety of fumaric acid esters in the long-term treatment of psoriasis–a retrospective study (FUTURE). *J. Dtsch. Der-matol. Ges.* **7:** 603–611.

100. Moharregh-Khiabani D., R.A. Linker, R. Gold, *et al.* 2009. Fumaric acid and its esters: an emerging treatment for mul-tiple sclerosis. *Curr. Neuropharmacol.* **7:** 60–64.

101. Osburn, W.O. & T.W. Kensler. 2008. Nrf2 signaling: an adaptive response pathway for protection against environ-mental toxic insults. *Mutat. Res.* **659:** 31–39.

102. Harvey, C.J., R.K. Thimmulappa, A. Singh, *et al.* 2009. Nrf2-regulated glutathione recycling independent of biosynthesis is critical for cell survival during oxidative stress. *Free Radic. Biol. Med.* **46:** 443–453.

103. Stoof, T.J., J. Flier, S. Sampat, *et al.* 2001. The antipsori-atic drug dimethylfumarate strongly suppresses chemokine production in human keratinocytes and peripheral blood mononuclear cells. *Br. J. Dermatol.* **144:** 1114–1120.

104. Loewe R., W. Holnthoner, M. Groger, *et al.* 2002. Dimethyl-fumarate inhibits TNF-induced nuclear entry of NF-kappa B/p65 in human endothelial cells. *J. Immunol.* **168:** 4781–4787.

105. Seidel P., I. Merfort, J.M. Hughes, *et al.* 2009. Dimethyl-fumarate inhibits NF-{kappa}B function at multiple levels to limit airway smooth muscle cell cytokine secretion. *Am. J. Physiol. Lung Cell. Mol. Physiol.* **297:** L326–39.

106. Gerdes S., K. Shakery & U. Mrowietz. 2007. Dimethyl-fumarate inhibits nuclear binding of nuclear factor kap-paB but not of nuclear factor of activated T cells and CCAAT/enhancer binding protein beta in activated human T cells. *Br. J. Dermatol.* **156:** 838–842.

107. Shih, A.Y., S. Imbeault, V. Barakauskas, *et al.* 2005. Induc-tion of the Nrf2-driven antioxidant response confers neu-roprotection during mitochondrial stress in vivo. *J. Biol. Chem.* **280:** 22925–22936.

108. Johnson, J.A., D.A. Johnson, A.D. Kraft, *et al.* 2008. The Nrf2-ARE pathway: an indicator and modulator of oxida-tive stress in neurodegeneration. *Ann. N. Y. Acad. Sci.* **1147:** 61–69.

109. Kappos L., R. Gold, D.H. Miller, *et al.* 2008. Efficacy and safety of oral fumarate in patients with relapsing-remitting multiple sclerosis: a multicentre, randomised, double-blind, placebo-controlled phase IIb study. *Lancet* **372:** 1463–1472.

110. MacManus, D.G., D. Miller, L. Kappos, *et al.* 2008. The effect of BG00012 on conversion of gadolinium-enhancing lesions to T1-hypointense lesions [abstract]. *Mult.Scler.* **14:** S163.

111. Hoefnagel, J.J., H.B. Thio, R. Willemze, *et al.* 2003. Long-term safety aspects of systemic therapy with fumaric acid esters in severe psoriasis. *Br. J. Dermatol.* **149:** 363–369.

112. Nast A., I. Kopp, M. Augustin, *et al.* 2007. German evidence-based guidelines for the treatment of Psoriasis vulgaris (short version). *Arch. Dermatol. Res.* **299:** 111–138.

113. Andersen O., J. Lycke, P.O. Tollesson, *et al.* 1996. Linomide reduces the rate of active lesions in relapsing-remitting mul-tiple sclerosis. *Neurology* **47:** 895–900.

114. Karussis, D.M., Z. Meiner, D. Lehmann, *et al.* 1996. Treat-ment of secondary progressive multiple sclerosis with the immunomodulator linomide: a double-blind, placebo-controlled pilot study with monthly magnetic resonance imaging evaluation. *Neurology* **47:** 341–346.

115. Noseworthy, J.H., J.S. Wolinsky, F.D. Lublin, *et al.,* North American Linomide Investigators. 2000. Linomide in re-lapsing and secondary progressive MS: part I. Trial design and clinical results. *Neurology* **54:** 1726–1733.

116. Polman C., F. Barkhof, M. Sandberg-Wollheim, *et al.* 2005. Treatment with laquinimod reduces development of active MRI lesions in relapsing MS. *Neurology* **64:** 987–991.

117. Brunmark C., A. Runstrom, L. Ohlsson, *et al.* 2002. The new orally active immunoregulator laquinimod (ABR-215062) effectively inhibits development and relapses of experimen-tal autoimmune encephalomyelitis. *J. Neuroimmunol.* **130:** 163–172.

118. Yang, J.S., L.Y. Xu, B.G. Xiao, *et al.* 2004. Laquinimod (ABR-215062) suppresses the development of experimental

autoimmune encephalomyelitis, modulates the Th1/Th2 balance and induces the Th3 cytokine TGF-beta in Lewis rats. *J. Neuroimmunol.* **156:** 3–9.

119. Tselis, A. 2010. Laquinimod, a new oral autoimmune modulator for the treatment of relapsing-remitting multiple sclerosis. *Curr. Opin. Investig Drugs* **11:** 577–585.

120. Comi G., A. Pulizzi, M. Rovaris, *et al.* 2008. Effect of laquinimod on MRI-monitored disease activity in patients with relapsing-remitting multiple sclerosis: a multicentre, randomised, double-blind, placebo-controlled phase IIb study. *Lancet* **371:** 2085–2092.

121. Comi G., O. Abramsky, T. Arbizu, *et al.* 2010. Oral laquinimod in patients with relapsing-remitting multiple sclerosis: 36-week double-blind active extension of the multicentre, randomized, double-blind, parallel-group placebo-controlled study. *Mult. Scler.* **16:** 1360–1366.

122. Gilleece, M.H. & T.M. Dexter. 1993. Effect of Campath-1H antibody on human hematopoietic progenitors in vitro. *Blood* **82:** 807–812.

123. Jones, J.L. & A.J. Coles. 2008. Campath-1H treatment of multiple sclerosis. *Neurodegener Dis.* **5:** 27–31.

124. Coles, A.J., A. Cox, E. Le Page, *et al.* 2006. The window of therapeutic opportunity in multiple sclerosis: evidence from monoclonal antibody therapy. *J. Neurol.* **253:** 98–108.

125. Jones, J.L., C.L. Phuah, A.L. Cox, *et al.* 2009. IL-21 drives secondary autoimmunity in patients with multiple sclerosis, following therapeutic lymphocyte depletion with alemtuzumab (Campath-1H). *J. Clin. Invest.* **119:** 2052–2061.

126. Thompson, S.A., J.L. Jones, A.L. Cox, *et al.* 2010. B cell reconstitution and BAFF after alemtuzumab (Campath-1H) treatment of multiple sclerosis. *J. Clin. Immunol.* **30:** 99–105.

127. Coles, A.J., M. Wing, S. Smith, *et al.* 1999. Pulsed monoclonal antibody treatment and autoimmune thyroid disease in multiple sclerosis. *Lancet* **354:** 1691–1695.

128. Otton, S.H., D.L. Turner, R. Frewin, *et al.* 1999. Autoimmune thrombocytopenia after treatment with Campath 1H in a patient with chronic lymphocytic leukaemia. *Br. J. Haematol.* **106:** 261–262.

129. Haider, I. & M. Cahill. 2004. Fatal thrombocytopaenia temporally related to the administration of alemtuzumab (MabCampath) for refractory CLL despite early discontinuation of therapy. *Hematology* **9:** 409–411.

130. Loh Y., Y. Oyama, L. Statkute, *et al.* 2007. Development of a secondary autoimmune disorder after hematopoietic stem cell transplantation for autoimmune diseases: role of conditioning regimen used. *Blood* **109:** 2643–2548.

131. CAMMS223 Trial Investigators, A.J. Coles, D.A. Compston, *et al.* 2008. Alemtuzumab vs. interferon beta-1a in early multiple sclerosis. *N. Engl. J. Med.* **359:** 1786–1801.

132. Clatworthy, M.R., E.F. Wallin & D.R. Jayne. 2008. Anti-glomerular basement membrane disease after alemtuzumab. *N. Engl. J. Med.* **359:** 768–769.

133. Schippling, D.S. & R. Martin. 2008. Spotlight on anti-CD25: daclizumab in MS. *Int. MS J.* **15:** 94–98.

134. Waldmann, T.A. 2007. Anti-Tac (daclizumab, Zenapax) in the treatment of leukemia, autoimmune diseases, and in the prevention of allograft rejection: a 25-year personal odyssey. *J. Clin. Immunol.* **27:** 1–18.

135. Wynn D., M. Kaufman, X. Montalban, *et al.* 2010. Daclizumab in active relapsing multiple sclerosis (CHOICE study): a phase 2, randomised, double-blind, placebo-controlled, add-on trial with interferon beta. *Lancet Neurol.* **9:** 381–390.

136. Wuest, S.C., J.H. Edwan, J.F. Martin, *et al.* 2011. A role for interleukin-2 trans-presentation in dendritic cell-mediated T cell activation in humans, as revealed by daclizumab therapy. *Nat. Med.* **17:** 604–609.

137. Bielekova B., N. Richert, T. Howard, *et al.* 2004. Humanized anti-CD25 (daclizumab) inhibits disease activity in multiple sclerosis patients failing to respond to interferon beta. *Proc. Natl. Acad. Sci. U.S.A.* **101:** 8705–8708.

138. Rojas, M.A., N.G. Carlson, T.L. Miller, *et al.* 2009. Long-term daclizumab therapy in relapsing-remitting multiple sclerosis. *Ther. Adv. Neurol. Disord.* **2:** 291–297.

139. Stashenko P., L.M. Nadler, R. Hardy, *et al.* 1980. Characterization of a human B lymphocyte-specific antigen. *J. Immunol.* **125:** 1678–1685.

140. Reff, M.E., K. Carner, K.S. Chambers, *et al.* 1994. Depletion of B cells in vivo by a chimeric mouse human monoclonal antibody to CD20. *Blood* **83:** 435–445.

141. Deans, J.P., H. Li & M.J. Polyak. 2002. CD20-mediated apoptosis: signalling through lipid rafts. *Immunology* **107:** 176–182.

142. Maloney, D.G., T.M. Liles, D.K. Czerwinski, *et al.* 1994. Phase I clinical trial using escalating single-dose infusion of chimeric anti-CD20 monoclonal antibody (IDEC-C2B8) in patients with recurrent B cell lymphoma. *Blood* **84:** 2457–2466.

143. Bar-Or A., P.A. Calabresi, D. Arnold, *et al.* 2008. Rituximab in relapsing-remitting multiple sclerosis: a 72-week, open-label, phase I trial. *Ann. Neurol.* **63:** 395–400.

144. Bar-Or A., L. Fawaz, B. Fan, *et al.* 2010. Abnormal B cell cytokine responses a trigger of T cell-mediated disease in MS? *Ann. Neurol.* **67:** 452–461.

145. Monson, N.L., P.D. Cravens, E.M. Frohman, *et al.* 2005. Effect of rituximab on the peripheral blood and cerebrospinal fluid B cells in patients with primary progressive multiple sclerosis. *Arch. Neurol.* **62:** 258–264.

146. Cross, A.H., J.L. Stark, J. Lauber, *et al.* 2006. Rituximab reduces B cells and T cells in cerebrospinal fluid of multiple sclerosis patients. *J. Neuroimmunol.* **180:** 63–70.

147. Barun, B. & A. Bar-Or. 2011. Treatment of multiple sclerosis with anti-CD20 antibodies. *Clin. Immunol.*

148. Hauser, S.L., E. Waubant, D.L. Arnold, *et al.* 2008. B cell depletion with rituximab in relapsing-remitting multiple sclerosis. *N. Engl. J. Med.* **358:** 676–688.

149. Hawker K., P. O'Connor, M.S. Freedman, *et al.* 2009. Rituximab in patients with primary progressive multiple sclerosis: results of a randomized double-blind placebo-controlled multicenter trial. *Ann. Neurol.* **66:** 460–471.

150. Waubant, E. 2008. Spotlight on anti-CD20. *Int. MS J.* **15:** 19–25.

151. Carson, K.R., A.M. Evens, E.A. Richey, *et al.* 2009. Progressive multifocal leukoencephalopathy after rituximab therapy in HIV-negative patients: a report of 57 cases from the Research on Adverse Drug Events and Reports project. *Blood* **113:** 4834–4840.

152. Allison, M. 2010. PML problems loom for Rituxan. *Nat. Biotechnol.* **28:** 105–106.

153. Kausar F., K. Mustafa, G. Sweis, *et al.* 2009. Ocrelizumab: a step forward in the evolution of B cell therapy. *Expert Opin. Biol. Ther.* **9:** 889–895.

154. Genovese, M.C., J.L. Kaine, M.B. Lowenstein, *et al.* 2008. Ocrelizumab, a humanized anti-CD20 monoclonal antibody, in the treatment of patients with rheumatoid arthritis: a phase I/II randomized, blinded, placebo-controlled, dose-ranging study. *Arthritis Rheum.* **58:** 2652–2661.

155. Kappos L., P. Calabresi, P. O'Connor, *et al.* 2010. Efficacy and safety of ocrelizumab in patients with relapsing–remitting multiple sclerosis: results of a phase II randomised placebo-controlled multicentre trial. *Mult. Scler.* **16**(Suppl. 10): S33–S34.

156. Zhang, B. 2009. Ofatumumab. *MAbs* **1:** 326–331.

157. Teeling, J.L., R.R. French, M.S. Cragg, *et al.* 2004. Characterization of new human CD20 monoclonal antibodies with potent cytolytic activity against non-Hodgkin lymphomas. *Blood* **104:** 1793–1800.

158. Teeling, J.L., W.J. Mackus, L.J. Wiegman, *et al.* 2006. The biological activity of human CD20 monoclonal antibodies is linked to unique epitopes on CD20. *J. Immunol.* **177:** 362–371.

159. Pawluczkowycz, A.W., F.J. Beurskens, P.V. Beum, *et al.* 2009. Binding of submaximal C1q promotes complement-dependent cytotoxicity (CDC) of B cells opsonized with anti-CD20 mAbs ofatumumab (OFA) or rituximab (RTX): considerably higher levels of CDC are induced by OFA than by RTX. *J. Immunol.* **183:** 749–758.

160. Ostergaard M., B. Baslund, W. Rigby, *et al.* 2010. Ofatumumab, a human anti-CD20 monoclonal antibody, for treatment of rheumatoid arthritis with an inadequate response to one or more disease-modifying antirheumatic drugs: results of a randomized, double-blind, placebo-controlled, phase I/II study. *Arthritis Rheum.* **62:** 2227–2238.

161. Sorensen, P.S., J. Drulovic, E. Havrdova, *et al.* 2010. Magnetic resonance imaging (MRI) efficacy of ofatumumab in relapsing-remitting multiple sclerosis (RRMS)—24-week results of a phase II study [abstract]. *Mult. Scler.* **16**(Suppl 10): S37–S38.

Ann. N.Y. Acad. Sci. ISSN 0077-8923

ANNALS OF THE NEW YORK ACADEMY OF SCIENCES
Issue: *The Year in Immunology*

# Treatment of systemic lupus erythematosus: new advances in targeted therapy

Mindy S. Lo[1,2] and George C. Tsokos[2,3]

[1]Division of Immunology, Children's Hospital Boston, Boston, Massachusetts. [2]Harvard Medical School, Boston, Massachusetts. [3]Division of Rheumatology, Beth Israel Deaconess Medical Center, Boston, Massachusetts

Address for correspondence: George Tsokos, M.D., Beth Israel Deaconess Medical Center, 330 Brookline Ave, CLS 937, Boston, MA 02115. gtsokos@bidmc.harvard.edu

Treatment for systemic lupus erythematosus (SLE) has traditionally been restricted to broad-based immunosuppression, with glucocorticoids being central to care. Recent insights into lupus pathogenesis promise new, selective therapies with more favorable side effect profiles. The best example of this is belimumab, which targets the B cell cytokine BLyS and has now received Food and Drug Administration (FDA) approval for its use in SLE. Strategies targeting other cytokines, such as interleukin 6 (IL-6) and interferon (IFN)-$\alpha$, are also on the horizon. Blockade of costimulatory interactions between immune cells offers another opportunity for therapeutic intervention, as do small molecule inhibitors that interfere with cell signaling pathways. We review here the current strategies for SLE treatment, with particular focus on therapies now in active pharmaceutical development. We will also discuss new understandings in lupus pathogenesis that may lead to future advances in therapy.

Keywords: systemic lupus erythematosus; belimumab; tolerance; Syk; biologic

## Introduction

This year (2011) has brought a new advance in the treatment of systemic lupus erythematosus (SLE), a complex and heterogeneous disease. For many years, SLE has been treated with broad-spectrum immunosuppressive agents, with varying degrees of success. In March of 2011 the FDA granted approval for a new targeted therapy for the treatment of SLE:[1] belimumab, the first medication to receive such a designation in over 50 years. The development of belimumab and was based on new understanding about SLE pathophysiology. In clinical trials, the number of patients that achieved clinical responses after receiving belimumab appeared to be only modestly increased when compared to that of patients receiving standard of care. Nevertheless, this successful example of taking benchside innovation to the patient bedside promises much for the future of SLE therapy.

In this review, we will discuss some of the current approaches for SLE treatment and new therapies currently being investigated in clinical and preclin-ical trials. We will also consider new insights being made at the basic science level and their potential for future therapeutic development.

## Current immunosuppressive therapy

### Corticosteroids

Glucocorticoids have broad immunosuppressive effects, with the ability to downregulate both innate and adaptive inflammatory immune responses. Prostaglandin and cytokine production are reduced.[2] Glucocorticoids can also directly inhibit cell proliferation and promote apoptosis of T and B cells and macrophages.[3] The effects of glucocorticoids on immune cells are mediated through many diverse mechanisms that have been well studied but remain incompletely understood. One example is glucocorticoid repression of gene upregulation by NF-$\kappa$B, a primary mediator of inflammation.[4]

In SLE, glucocorticoids remain the most important and most effective short-term therapy. Multiple studies have shown improvement in survival with glucocorticoid use.[5] Despite the necessity of glucocorticoids in the treatment of SLE, long-term

doi: 10.1111/j.1749-6632.2011.06263.x

Ann. N.Y. Acad. Sci. 1247 (2012) 138–152 © 2012 New York Academy of Sciences.

toxicities limit their use. These dose-dependent effects include decreased bone mineral density, weight gain, Cushingoid features, hypertension, diabetes mellitus, glaucoma, and cataract formation.[6] In addition, the degree of immunocompromise achieved with high-dose glucocorticoids and the risk for opportunistic infections should not be underestimated.

### Antimalarials

Like corticosteroids, antimalarial medications have long been used for the treatment of SLE despite limited understanding of their mechanism of action. Chloroquine and hydroxychloroquine are the most common antimalarials used for SLE. They are thought to affect leukocyte phagocytosis and migration, in part via inhibition of lysosome acidification. This latter property may also explain hydroxychloroquine's inhibition of antigen processing and presentation[7] and negative effect on Toll-like receptor (TLR) activation in response to antigen.[8]

Antimalarial medications are most useful for limiting disease flares[9] and delaying accrual of further autoimmune disease in patients with early SLE.[10] Several studies have shown that hydroxychloroquine may reduce the frequency of thrombotic events.[11] More recent data suggest that hydroxychloroquine use in pregnancy may lower the risk for congenital heart block associated with neonatal lupus.[12] Although hydroxychloroquine is not used as primary treatment for major organ involvement in lupus, it has a relatively benign side effect profile and is inexpensive. Toxicity is unusual and for the most part limited to occasional conduction defects and cardiomyopathy, and even more rarely, retinal toxicity.[13]

### Cyclophosphamide

Cyclophosphamide is an alkylating agent that causes cell death and is therefore highly immunosuppressive. Its use is reserved for severe manifestations of autoimmune disease and for certain malignancies. Cyclophosphamide has until recently been the standard of care for proliferative lupus nephritis. Commonly used regimens are based on protocols employing monthly or biweekly IV cyclophosphamide infusions in conjunction with steroids.[14,15]

The use of cyclophosphamide is unfortunately limited by significant toxicity. In the short term, cyclophosphamide confers risk for opportunistic infections including *Pneumocystis jiroveci* and fungal disease. Cyclophosphamide is also associated with renal and bladder toxicity. Long term, cyclophosphamide is associated with premature ovarian failure, infertility, and increased risk for malignancies.[16,17] Reproductive side effects are proportional to cumulative cyclophosphamide dose, and the age of the patient at onset of treatment.[18,19]

### Mycophenolate mofetil

Due to the concerning toxicities associated with cyclophosphamide it is usually not the preferred maintenance therapy for SLE. Mycophenolate mofetil (MMF), an inhibitor of DNA synthesis first used as an antirejection agent for renal transplantation, has been increasingly used for moderate and severe SLE. Its effects are mediated by inhibition of T and B lymphocyte proliferation. An initial open label randomized controlled trial suggested possible superiority of MMF over cyclophosphamide when used as induction therapy for lupus nephritis.[20] Another study evaluating the use of MMF, azathioprine, and cyclophosphamide as maintenance agents following cyclophosphamide induction showed better relapse-free survival rates and fewer adverse events with MMF or azathioprine over cyclophosphamide.[21] However, a larger international study of induction therapy showed no significant differences between MMF and cyclophosphamide in terms of efficacy or adverse events.[22,23] Subgroup analyses suggest that MMF may have particular benefit in patients of African American and Hispanic ethnicities.[24]

MMF is generally well tolerated, with nausea, abdominal cramping, and diarrhea being the most common side effects. Leukopenia has also been described. Opportunistic infections also remain a concern; in transplant patients on combined immunosuppressive agents, the use of MMF may increase the risk for cytomegalovirus (CMV) infection as compared with other regimens.[25]

### Azathioprine

Azathioprine, a purine analog, is converted in the body to its active metabolite, 6-mercaptopurine (6-MP). Azathioprine and 6-MP inhibit DNA synthesis and lymphocyte proliferation; both are commonly used in the treatment of inflammatory bowel disease. In hematopoietic cells, 6-MP is cleared predominantly by thiopurine methyltransferase (TPMT). Polymorphisms in TPMT affecting enzyme activity are common and can lead to increased toxicity, including myelosuppression and hepatotoxicity.[26]

Azathioprine is inferior to cyclophosphamide and MMF as induction therapy for proliferative lupus nephritis.[27] Still, azathioprine can be useful as an alternative maintenance regimen to MMF or cyclophosphamide.[21,28]

## Methotrexate

Methotrexate is a folic acid analog that inhibits purine synthesis and adenosine deaminase activity. It is used primarily in the treatment of arthritis and cutaneous manifestations of SLE. Methotrexate may also be useful in the treatment of Sjogren's syndrome or Sjogren's features in SLE patients.[29] The overall effect of methotrexate on SLE disease activity appears to be modest[30] and it is not used for major organ system involvement. Toxicity of low-dose methotrexate includes hepatotoxicity (including fibrosis), pulmonary damage, myelosuppression, and, rarely, a photosensitive rash.[31] Organ disease related to methotrexate toxicity, therefore, has the potential to be confused with SLE disease activity.

## Hematopoietic stem cell transplantation

Intense immunosuppression with chemotherapy followed by autologous or allogeneic hematopoietic stem cell transplantation (HSCT) rescue has been tried with anecdotal success for patients with severe lupus and other autoimmune diseases. It is hypothesized that this induces a "resetting" of the immune system; studies have reported normalization of the T cell repertoire, a shift from memory to naive B cell predominance, and improvement in other serologic markers of disease. However, the risk for transplant-related mortality remains a serious concern.[32,33]

## B cell targeted strategies

SLE is a disease characterized by the production of autoantibodies. Retrospective studies have shown that the development of autoantibodies precedes the development of clinical manifestations, in many cases by several years.[34,35] However, only some of these autoantibodies have been shown to play a direct contributory role to pathogenesis. Loss of tolerance on multiple levels contributes to the overactive B cell response. Improper clearance of apoptotic debris and immune complexes may lead to excessive antigen stimulation. This may be further worsened by increased costimulatory signals provided by T cells. A number of strategies have been attempted to dampen such overactive B cell responses.

## B cell depletion

Rituximab is a chimeric monoclonal antibody directed against CD20, a surface marker of mature B cells. Treatment with rituximab induces depletion of circulating B cells; penetration of this effect into secondary lymphoid organs is less quantifiable and likely difficult to achieve. Rituximab was initially developed for the treatment of nonHodgkin's lymphoma and remains an important part of the treatment regimens for several different types of lymphoma and chronic lymphocytic leukemia.[36] In 2006, FDA approval was granted for the use of rituximab to treat rheumatoid arthritis; approval was also granted in 2011 for treatment of ANCA-associated vasculitis. Rituximab has gained acceptance in the treatment of many other autoimmune diseases, including idiopathic/immune-mediated thrombocytopenic purpura (ITP), autoimmune hemolytic anemia, multiple sclerosis, pemphigus vulgaris, and Sjogren's syndrome.

Importantly, CD20 is not expressed on plasma cells, and because plasma cells are not directly depleted by rituximab therapy, the effect on circulating pathogenic autoantibody levels is variable. The rapid efficacy of rituximab in certain clinical scenarios (often far earlier than a measurable change in antibody levels) suggests alternative mechanisms of action. One hypothesis is that clearance of rituximab-opsonized B cells diverts complement, macrophages, and neutrophils from the kidney and other target organs; rapid B cell depletion would also affect T cell activation and inflammatory cytokine production.[37]

Pilot studies of rituximab in SLE were promising.[38,39] A review of off-label use also suggested significant response rates and improvement in serologic markers.[40] Unfortunately, two large randomized, double-blinded phase II/III trials showed no superiority of rituximab over standard therapy and did not reach primary or secondary endpoints.[41,42] *Post hoc* analysis did suggest that there may be a reduction in severe flares in patients treated with rituximab.[43] Despite these overall discouraging results, both studies were noted to have significant design shortcomings that limit their applicability.[44] Furthermore, strategies combining rituximab with cyclophosphamide administration, especially in patients with moderate to severe lupus, may still have merit.[45] Although usually well tolerated, adverse events related to rituximab include severe infusion reactions, including those associated with human antichimeric antibodies (HACA). Rituximab, like other immunosuppressive therapies, is associated with reports of progressive multifocal leukoencephalopathy, a rare but fatal viral encephalitis.[46]

Evaluation of another anti-CD20 antibody, ocrelizumab, was stopped prematurely due to an increase in serious infections. Other B cell-depleting strategies include antibodies directed against CD22 (expressed on mature B cells), CD19 (expressed throughout B cell development from pro-B precursors to mature B cells), and plasma cell-depleting therapy.

Epratuzumab, a humanized anti-CD22 monoclonal antibody, also has inhibitory effects on B cell signaling and is now undergoing phase III study for SLE treatment.[47]

### B cell cytokine activation

B cell activation and function has also been successfully targeted in the treatment of SLE. The cytokine B lymphocyte stimulator (BLyS), also known as B cell activating factor of the TNF family (BAFF), is produced by myeloid cells and provides necessary signaling for B cell maturation, survival, and immunoglobulin production. The BLyS/BAFF receptor (BAFFR) is found on most types of B cells and effector T cells. A second receptor, TACI (transmembrane activator and CAML interactor), is expressed on activated B cells and mediates signaling to induce class switch recombination. APRIL (a proliferation inducing ligand), a cytokine similar to BLyS/BAFF, also binds to TACI to mediate overlapping effects (Fig. 1).[48] Both BLyS/BAFF and APRIL can bind to a third receptor B cell maturation antigen (BCMA), although the affinity of BLyS/BAFF for BCMA is relatively weak. TACI mutations have been associated with common variable immunodeficiency (CVID) and CVID-related autoimmunity.[49,50] Several conditions have been associated with increased circulating levels of BLyS/BAFF, including autoimmune diseases such as SLE, allergic diseases, and certain infections.[51]

Belimumab, a fully humanized monoclonal antibody against BAFF, was approved for the treat-

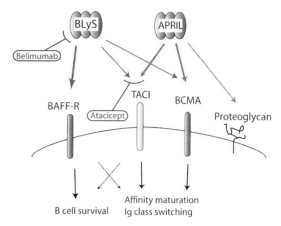

**Figure 1.** BLyS/BAFF and APRIL signaling. BLyS and APRIL are heterotrimers that bind to receptors with distinct but overlapping functions. BLyS signals most strongly through the BAFF receptor (BAFFR) to promote B cell survival and maturation. TACI is highly expressed on memory B cell subsets and also promotes class switching and B cell proliferation. BCMA, B cell maturation protein.

ment of SLE based on two large randomized controlled trials, BLISS 52 and BLISS 76. In BLISS 52, more patients receiving belimumab met the threshold for clinical response compared to those receiving placebo, and there were fewer flares in the belimumab-treated group.[52] BLISS 76 showed a similar benefit at 52 weeks, although the difference from placebo was not as great.[53] This benefit was lost by 76 weeks. Notably, patients with severe active lupus nephritis or CNS lupus were excluded from both trials. Another concern has been that all patients, including the placebo comparison group, received aggressive background immune suppression and, therefore, the high response rates seen overall may have masked some of the drug's effects. Belimumab was well tolerated in both trials.

BLyS/BAFF signaling has also been targeted through the use of a soluble TACI receptor. Atacicept is a fusion protein combining the extracellular domain of TACI with the Fc portion of human IgG. As APRIL also signals through TACI, atacicept could provide additional benefit over belimumab. Initial exploratory studies of atacicept in SLE patients have shown proof of principle, with decrease in B cell and immunoglobulin (Ig) levels.[54,55] Phase II/III trials are ongoing.

Briobacept is another recombinant fusion protein with two BAFF receptors attached to the Fc portion of IgG. Studies of briobacept in humans have not yet been published.

## B cell tolerogens

Another innovative strategy has been to target pathogenic autoantibodies themselves. Edratide is a synthetic peptide that binds the complementarity determining region of anti-DNA antibodies.[56] In mouse models, this peptide could be used to induce tolerance in mice challenged with anti-DNA antibodies.[57] A small study of nine SLE patients showed improvement in serologic markers and disease activity after treatment with edratide.[58] However, a phase II study did not meet its primary endpoint over a 26-week treatment period.

Abetimus (previously LJP-394) is another synthetic drug comprising four double-stranded oligonucleotides that bind to anti-double strand DNA (dsDNA) antibodies. This compound can also cross-link the B cell receptor on cells making antibodies to dsDNA, inducing death or anergy of these pathogenic cells.[59] For this reason, it was hoped that abetimus would act as a B cell "tolerogen." Initial studies in humans showed that abetimus reduced anti-dsDNA antibody titers in SLE patients.[60–62] A phase III randomized controlled trial showed fewer disease flares and improved disease activity scores in the group receiving abetimus; unfortunately, the primary endpoint (time to renal flare) was not met.[63] A larger follow-up study was halted due to apparent lack of efficacy.

## Fcγ receptor modulation

There are several different receptors for the Fc region of IgG. Most have activating functions, but FcγRIIB signals through an immunoreceptor tyrosine-based inhibitory motif (ITIM) and therefore has inhibitory effect when bound to immune-complexed IgG. FcγRIIB is expressed on B cells, macrophages, granulocytes, and dendritic cells. Polymorphisms in FcγRIIB are associated with SLE in some populations.[64,65] The anti-inflammatory effects of intravenous immunoglobulin (Iv1g[b], used to treat a variety of autoimmune conditions, may be mediated in part by binding to FcγRIIB.[66] Targeting FcγRIIB directly through monoclonal antibodies, receptor cross-linking, and other techniques has been proposed for the treatment of B cell malignancies; similar approaches might also be useful for the treatment of autoimmunity.[67]

## Cytokine directed therapy

### Interleukin 6

Interleukin 6 (IL-6) is a proinflammatory cytokine secreted by activated T cells, monocytes, endothelial cells, and fibroblasts. IL-6 plays a variety of roles in both the adaptive and innate immune systems but is particularly notable for its activating and differentiating effect on B and T cells. Levels of IL-6 are increased in the serum of patients with SLE and correlate with disease activity.[68] IL-6 polymorphisms have also been described in some patients with SLE.[69,70] Tocilizumab is a humanized monoclonal antibody directed against the IL-6 receptor that received FDA approval for the treatment of rheumatoid arthritis in 2010. A phase I trial of tocilizumab in 16 SLE patients showed significant improvement in disease activity for most patients, although neutropenia was a frequent side effect.[71]

### Tumor necrosis factor

Infliximab is a monoclonal antibody directed against tumor necrosis factor (TNF-α), another proinflammatory cytokine. The development of infliximab and other anti-TNF agents has had a significant impact on the treatment of rheumatoid arthritis. As some SLE patients have been reported to have elevated TNF-α levels, this strategy has also been tried in patients with lupus with anecdotal success.[72] However, a phase II/III trial was terminated prematurely. Drug-induced lupus triggered by infliximab is also a well-recognized phenomenon, further limiting the enthusiasm for this approach.[73,74]

### Interleukin 10

IL-10 is an inhibitory cytokine produced by lymphocytes and monocytes. The role of IL-10 in SLE is as yet incompletely defined: despite its ability to downregulate T cell activation and cytokine production, IL-10 also promotes Ig class switching and antibody secretion. IL-10 levels have been found to be increased in patients with SLE and an anti-IL-10 monoclonal antibody showed beneficial effects in a small study of six patients.[75]

### Interleukins 17 and 23

T cells secreting IL-17 have been described to play a pathogenic role in a number of autoimmune conditions, including SLE, multiple sclerosis, and psoriasis. Th17 cells, a subset of the helper T cell population, are the predominant producers of IL-17, although CD8[+] and other T cells have also been reported to secrete IL-17. Production of IL-17 in peripheral tissue serves as a local inflammatory signal, inducing recruitment and activation of other immune effector cells. As an example, cells secreting IL-17 can be found infiltrating the kidneys of patients with lupus nephritis.[76] Serum levels of IL-17 are also increased in SLE patients.[77] The pathogenic role of IL-17 in SLE has been further supported by mouse models of lupus.[78,79] Although anti-IL-17 therapies have not yet been studied in patients with SLE, an anti-IL-17 monoclonal antibody is now in clinical trials for the treatment of psoriasis, arthritis, and uveitis.[80]

IL-23, a cytokine critical for the differentiation and proliferation of Th17 cells, has been targeted for the treatment of psoriasis. Ustekinumab, a monoclonal antibody against IL-23, showed superiority over a TNF inhibitor in a brief trial of patients with psoriasis.[81] Whether these results can be extrapolated for the treatment of SLE remains to be seen.

### Interferon-α

Several reports have demonstrated increased type-I interferon (IFN) signaling in patients with SLE based on gene expression arrays showing upregulation of IFN-inducible genes.[82] This has been termed the "interferon signature." IFN-α levels are also higher in patients with SLE.[83,84] Excessive IFN-α production is primarily due to TLR stimulation of plasmacytoid dendritic cells; consequences of this excess include increased lymphocyte activation and upregulation of costimulatory molecules and other cytokines. Neutrophils in SLE patients show increased rates of "NETosis," a different form of cell death, releasing nuclear material that stimulates plasmacytoid dendritic cells to produce IFN-α.[85] A phase Ia trial showed that the IFN signature in lupus patients could be modified by an anti-IFN-α monoclonal antibody.[86] A phase II study is currently underway.

## Costimulation

Overproduction of autoantibodies in SLE is multifactorial. In addition to cytokine stimulation, B cell activation requires multiple costimulatory interactions with T cells. Both CD4[+] and CD8[+] T cells from SLE patients express higher levels of CD40L; B cells from these patients may also be more sensitive to CD40:CD40L stimulation.[87,88] An initial study of an anti-CD40L monoclonal antibody in five SLE pa-

tients showed reduction in total IgG and anti-DNA antibody levels shortly after treatment.[89] Disruption of CD40:CD40L interaction was also promising in early studies of patients with ITP,[90] and in 28 patients with proliferative lupus nephritis.[91] However, the latter study was stopped prematurely due to an increase in thromboembolic events. The reason for this unexpected side effect is unclear but may be related to platelet activation by anti-CD40L-containing immune complexes.[92] Another phase II study of a different anti-CD40L antibody did not show any beneficial effect and did not meet its primary endpoint.[93]

Costimulatory interaction via CD28 on T cells with B7 expressed on B cells is another important activation pathway (Fig. 2). Cytotoxic T lymphocyte antigen-4 (CTLA-4), expressed on regulatory T cells and other activated T cells, is a homolog of CD28 that has higher affinity to B7 than CD28 itself. Abatacept, a fusion protein of the CTLA-4 extracellular domain with the Fc portion of Ig, takes advantage of this affinity by disrupting the CD28:B7 interaction, thus inhibiting both B and T cell activation. Abatacept is FDA-approved for the treatment of rheumatoid arthritis. A recent phase IIb study of abatacept in patients with non-life-threatening SLE showed a mild reduction in serious flares, more pronounced in patients with arthritis.[94] However, the primary and secondary endpoints (total flares and time to flare) were not met. Belatacept is a similar CTLA-4 fusion protein with even higher affinity for B7; it is now approved for prevention of renal transplant rejection.[95] Conversely, CTLA-4 transmits an inhibitory signal on T cells that has been targeted for another therapeutic purpose: monoclonal antibodies blocking CTLA-4 are used to augment T cell antitumor responses for the treatment of melanoma. A side effect of this blockade, however, is potentiation of autoimmune phenomena.[96]

Inducible T-cell costimulator (ICOS) is another member of the CD28 family of costimulatory molecules, expressed on activated T cells as well as NK cells. The interaction between ICOS and its ligand B7 related peptide 1 (B7RP1) plays an important role in the development of Th17 and follicular helper T cells. T cells from patients with SLE express higher levels of ICOS compared to normal controls.[97] Preliminary reports from animal studies suggest that blocking ICOS:B7RP1 interaction may be useful for the treatment of autoimmune disease.[98,99]

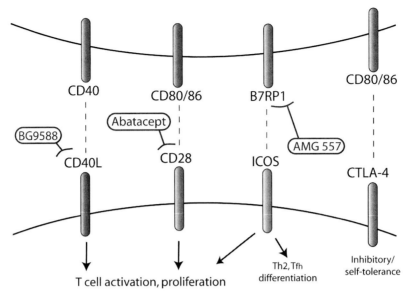

**Figure 2.** T cell costimulatory interactions. CD40:CD40L interactions lead to activating and pro-differentiating signals for both B and T cells, respectively. Ligation of CD28, expressed constitutively on T cells, provides necessary costimulation for naive cells. Signaling through ICOS, which is induced on activated T cells, promotes Th2 differentiation and is important for follicular helper cell development. CTLA-4 is highly homologous to CD28, but has much stronger affinity for CD80/86. CTLA-4 activation provides an inhibitory signal that promotes self-tolerance.

A humanized monoclonal antibody against B7RP1 is currently being investigated in a phase I study.

## T cells and cell signaling targets

Intrinsic T cell abnormalities also play an important role in SLE pathogenesis. T cell dysfunction in SLE has been characterized on multiple levels, from its costimulatory interaction with B cells to excessive IL-17 secretion. SLE patient-derived T cells ("SLE T cells") T cells also express lower levels of IL-2 when compared to normal controls.[100] Although the reason for this decreased IL-2 expression is not completely understood, IL-2 is necessary for the survival and function of regulatory T cells, reported to be deficient in SLE patients.[101] A defect in IL-2 may, therefore, contribute to loss of tolerance in lupus patients.

Many intracellular signaling pathways, perhaps best characterized in T cells, have been reported to be abnormal in SLE. Strategies described thus far targeting cytokines, receptors, and specific cell types have required the use of biologic proteins. In contrast, intracellular signaling is more readily amenable to modulation by small molecule inhibitors. These inhibitors are typically easier to dose

and administer, and may have more favorable side effect profiles.

### Syk

Spleen tyrosine kinase (Syk) is a critical component for signal transduction through the B cell receptor. Syk is also found in a number of other cell types, including macrophages, neutrophils, mast cells, and platelets. Overactive signaling through Syk may play a role in lupus pathogenesis. Normal T cells express CD3ζ as part of the T cell receptor (TCR) signaling complex. CD3ζ in turn signals through the tyrosine kinase zeta-associated protein 70 (ZAP70). In contrast, SLE T cells express lower levels of CD3ζ, substituting an alternative receptor, FcRγ, in the TCR complex.[102] FcRγ signals through Syk rather than ZAP70, and T cells in SLE show higher levels of Syk expression.[103] Calcium flux induced by signaling through FcRγ and Syk is both stronger and faster than that of normal T cells, and may contribute to the overactive T cell phenotype seen in SLE. Fostamatinib, a Syk inhibitor, corrected this aberrant signaling *in vitro. In vivo*, fostamatinib attenuated both cutaneous findings and renal disease in lupus-prone mice.[104] Although there are no trials of Syk inhibitors in SLE, the use of fostamatinib to

**Table 1.** New therapies in development for SLE. RA, rheumatoid arthritis. ITP, idiopathic thrombocytopenic purpura. ROS, reactive oxygen species.

| Target | Drug | Study phase | Status | Reference and/or Clinical trial number |
|---|---|---|---|---|
| B cell | | | | |
| CD20 | Rituximab | Phase II/III, EXPLORER and LUNAR | Did not meet primary endpoint | 41–43 |
| | Ocrelizumab | Phase III | Halted due to infections | NCT00539838, NCT00626197 |
| | Ofatumumab | Trials in lymphoma and leukemia | No studies in SLE | – |
| | Veltuzumab | Phase I/II studies in RA, ITP, and lymphoma | No studies in SLE | – |
| CD22 | Epratuzumab | Phase III | In progress | NCT01261793 |
| BLyS/BAFF | Belimumab | Phase III, BLISS52/BLISS76 | FDA approved | 52,53 |
| | Atacicept | Phase II/III | Initially halted for infections; new study in progress | NCT00573157, NCT01369628 |
| | Briobacept | Preclinical development | – | |
| B cell tolerogen | Edratide | Phase II | Did not meet primary endpoint | NCT00203151 |
| | Abetimus | Phase III | Second phase III study halted for lack of efficacy | 62,63 |
| Cytokines | | | | |
| IL-6 | Tocilizumab | Phase I | Larger study planned | 71 |
| TNF-α | Infliximab | Phase II/III | Terminated | NCT00368264 |
| IL-17 | AIN457 | Phase I/II studies for psoriasis, uveitis, RA | No studies in SLE | – |
| IL-23 | Ustekinumab | Phase III studies for psoriasis, Crohn's | No studies in SLE | – |
| IFN-α | Rontalizumab | Phase II | In progress | NCT00962832 |
| IFN-γ | AMG 811 | Phase I | In progress | NCT00818948 |
| Costimulation | | | | |
| CD40:CD40L | BG9588 | Phase II | Halted due to thromboembolic complications | 91, NCT00001789 |
| | IDEC-131 | Phase II | Did not meet primary endpoint | 93 |

*Continued*

**Table 1.** *Continued*

| Target | Drug | Study phase | Status | Reference and/or Clinical trial number |
|---|---|---|---|---|
| CD28:B7 | Abatacept | Phase IIb | In progress | 94, NCT00774852 |
|  | Belatacept | Phase I/II in RA and renal transplant | No studies in SLE | – |
| ICOS:B7RP1 | AMG 557 | Phase I | In progress | NCT00774943 |
| Cell signaling |  |  |  |  |
| Syk | Fostamatinib | Phase II studies for RA | No studies in SLE | – |
| Jak | Tofacitinib | Phase III studies for RA | No studies in SLE | – |
|  | LY3009104 | Phase II studies for RA | No studies in SLE | – |
| Other |  |  |  |  |
| ROS | N-acetylcysteine | Phase I/II | In progress | NCT00775476 |
| Metabolism | Sirolimus | Phase II | In progress | NCT00779194 |
| Complement C5 | Eculizumab | Phase I/II | Terminated | 131 |
| ROCK | Fasudil | Phase I for Raynaud's | In progress | NCT0049865 |
| TLR7, TLR9 | DV1179 | Phase I | Planned to begin 2011 | – |

treat other diseases, including ITP and lymphoma, is currently being investigated. Fostamatinib was also both safe and effective in a phase II trial of patients with rheumatoid arthritis.[105] Although the side effect profile seen with fostamatinib thus far has been relatively benign, the ubiquitous expression of Syk in such a wide variety of cell types warrants careful examination of the effects of Syk inhibition before widespread use in humans.

## Jak

The Janus kinases (Jak) are tyrosine kinases that bridge signaling between cytokine receptors and the signal transducer and activator of transcription (STAT) proteins. Different combinations of Jak and STAT protein activation lead to upregulation of different patterns of gene expression. Type I IFN, for example, signals through the Jak kinases Jak1 and Tyk2 to activate STAT1 and STAT2. In contrast, IL-6 signals primarily through Jak1 and Jak2 to activate STAT3 and STAT1. Tofacitinib, a Jak inhibitor that shows preference for Jak1 and Jak3 (and to a lesser extent Jak2), inhibits both Th1 and Th17 differentiation *in vitro*.[106] A phase III trial of tofacitinib in rheumatoid arthritis patients met all primary endpoints for efficacy, although the results have yet to be published.[107] An earlier phase IIa trial of 264 patients randomized to receive varying doses of tofacitinib for six weeks showed that

the drug was well tolerated, with no serious adverse events.[108]

One concern raised with nonselective Jak inhibition has been the shared use of these kinases in multiple signaling pathways. As Jak3 is critical for IL-2 signaling and Jak3 deficiency results in severe immunodeficiency, a more selective inhibitor may have less risk for immunocompromise. A phase IIb trial of LY3009104, a selective inhibitor of Jak1 and Jak2, for the treatment of rheumatoid arthritis is currently in progress. The relatively low IL-2 levels in SLE may contribute to decreased numbers of regulatory T cells.[109] It may, therefore, be especially useful to avoid Jak3 inhibition in the treatment of lupus.

## Calmodulin kinase

The calcium-activated calmodulin kinases (CaMKs) are serine-threonine kinases known to be involved in regulation of Jak/STAT activation. In human macrophages, a CaMK inhibitor decreased STAT1α activation responses to IFN-α.[77] CaMKs have also been implicated in regulation of IL-2 production. The defect in IL-2 production in SLE T cells is due in part to increased expression of the cyclic AMP response element modulator (CREM). CREM binds to the IL-2 gene promoter, acting as a repressor of transcription. This increased CREM expression is in turn secondary to increased CaMKIV activity in SLE T cells.[110] A CaMK inhibitor has been tested in lupus-prone mice; KN-93 significantly alleviated both nephritis and cutaneous disease in these mice.[111]

### Calcineurin

As described earlier, T cells from SLE patients show an increased calcium flux response to activation, leading to hyperactive calcineurin/NF-AT signaling. Calcineurin inhibitors, such as cyclosporine and tacrolimus, are sometimes used as second-line agents in SLE therapy. Despite a number of trials showing good efficacy for both induction and maintenance therapy, the use of cyclosporine and tacrolimus is limited by their renal toxicity in patients with nephritis, as well as a number of other side effects.[112] Recently, dipyridamole, an inhibitor of platelet aggregation used in stroke prevention, was also found to affect calcineurin signaling. SLE T cells treated with dipyridamole showed a decrease in IL-17 production and CD40L upregulation. Dipyridamole also delayed and attenuated disease manifestations in lupus-prone mice.[113]

### Rho kinase

Tissue inflammation requires cell homing, migration, and adhesion. T cells from patients with lupus express variant isoforms of the CD44 membrane adhesion molecule. In particular, CD44v3 and CD44v6 isoforms predominate in SLE T cells.[114] CD44 signals through its intracellular partners ezrin, radixin, and moesin (collectively known as ERM), which are also dependent on phosphorylation by the rho kinase (ROCK). ERM phosphorylation is increased in SLE T cells and correlates with enhanced adhesion and migration.[115] A ROCK-specific inhibitor reduced both polar cap formation and adhesion of SLE T cells. Recently, ROCK2 was found to regulate IL-17 production and Th17 differentiation through phosphorylation of interferon regulatory factor-4 (IRF-4). Treatment of lupus-prone mice with fasudil, a ROCK inhibitor, resulted in decreased IL-17 and IL-21 production as well as less proteinuria.[116] Fasudil also has vasodilatory properties, and is currently under phase I investigation for the treatment of Raynaud's phenomenon.

## Other immunomodulatory strategies

### Oxidative stress

Free radical-mediated damage has been proposed to contribute to lupus pathogenesis. Reactive oxygen species generated as byproducts of metabolism can damage DNA and other cellular components, triggering abnormal apoptosis and necrosis. In a recent study of 72 SLE patients and 36 matched healthy controls, the SLE patients demonstrated significantly higher serum levels of oxidative stress markers, and these levels correlated with disease activity.[117] Oxidant damage in SLE is likely multifactorial in etiology, with contributory influences from diet, environmental exposures, and genetic polymorphisms in metabolic pathways.[118] N-acetylcysteine (NAC) is a strong antioxidant that has improved survival in a mouse model of lupus, and there are case reports of its use in patients with SLE.[119,120] A phase I trial of NAC for the treatment of SLE is currently underway.

T cell dysfunction in lupus is also influenced by abnormal mitochondrial oxidative metabolism. Lymphocytes from SLE patients showed higher production of reactive oxygen intermediates, lower ATP content, and increased rates of necrosis.[121] Mitochondrial transmembrane potential is controlled by the mammalian target of rapamycin (mTOR). Treatment of SLE patients with rapamycin, an mTOR inhibitor (also known as sirolimus), led to normalization of CD3ζ expression and calcium flux in T cells.[122] Lupus-prone mice treated with sirolimus showed reduced proteinuria, nephritis, and anti-dsDNA antibodies.[123] In a preliminary report, seven of nine SLE patients refractory to conventional immunosuppression showed an improvement in disease activity scores after treatment with sirolimus.[124] Phase II trials of sirolimus in SLE and lupus nephritis are in progress.

### Epigenetic modification

Single gene defects account for a small fraction of SLE patients. Increasingly, epigenetic regulation of gene expression patterns has been shown to influence lupus pathogenesis. In SLE lymphocytes, genes show an overall hypomethylated state as compared to normal controls. Hypomethylation correlates with increased expression of a number of genes previously implicated in SLE pathogenesis, including IL-10, CD154/CD40L, and the protein phosphatase 2A.[125–127] Gene expression is also regulated by modifications to the nucleosome, including histone acetylation, ubiquitination, and phosphorylation, among others. Histone acetylation in particular has been investigated in the development of autoimmune disease. As an example, CREM repression of IL-2 transcription in SLE T cells is mediated by recruitment of histone deacetylase 1 (HDAC1) to the IL-2 gene promoter.[128] Administration of an HDAC inhibitor attenuated disease in two different mouse models of lupus.[129] However, application of these results to human disease requires further investigation.

## Complement regulation

Complement abnormalities are a seminal feature of SLE, particularly lupus nephritis. Complement proteins play a variety of both protective and pro-inflammatory roles in lupus. Excessive immune complex deposition contributes to renal damage. Eculizumab, a monoclonal antibody that binds C5, preventing its cleavage to C5 and C5b, has been tested in ischemia-reperfusion injury, paroxysmal nocturnal hemoglobinuria, and idiopathic membranous nephropathy. This approach significantly improved nephritis in lupus mouse models,[130] and a phase I study of eculizumab in SLE patients was also encouraging. However, a phase II trial was ultimately halted.[131]

## Toll-like receptors

Chloroquine and hydroxychloroquine, as mentioned above, derive part of their activity in lupus via inhibition of TLR signaling. Notably, TLR9 activation by double-stranded CpG DNA is thought to drive the overactive IFN-α signal seen in SLE. Much attention has therefore been focused on the development of more potent TLR inhibitors. Oligonucleotides with nonstimulatory DNA sequences have been used successfully in both *in vitro* assays to block TLR7 and TLR9 activation, as well as improve manifestations of autoimmune disease in lupus-prone mice.[132] A phase I trial of DV1179, an oligonucleotide TLR inhibitor, is expected to begin later this year.

## Conclusion

The approval of belimumab heralds a new era for the treatment of SLE. Cumulative research over the past few decades has yielded many insights into specific perturbations in the immune systems of lupus patients. It is often emphasized among clinicians that SLE is a heterogeneous disease. By necessity in SLE research, individual variations that are discovered more frequently in SLE patients are often generalized to embody a "lupus phenotype." In reality, each

individual patient likely has a distinct set of immune abnormalities that have culminated in the presentation of SLE. With better understanding of these abnormalities, and the development of biomarkers to predict clinical correlations, targeted therapies such as those described here (Table 1) will hopefully allow for individualized treatment regimens tailored to each patient's immune system. And thus the toxicities associated with current broad-based immunosuppression may some day be avoidable.

## Conflicts of interest

The authors declare no conflicts of interest.

## References

1. Mitka, M. 2011. Treatment for lupus, first in 50 years, offers modest benefits, hope to patients. *JAMA* **305:** 1754–1755.
2. Goodwin, J.S. *et al.* 1986. Mechanism of action of glucocorticosteroids: inhibition of T cell proliferation and interleukin 2 production by hydrocortisone is reversed by leukotriene B4. *J. Clin. Invest.* **77:** 1244–1250.
3. Newton, R. 2000. Molecular mechanisms of glucocorticoid action: what is important? *Thorax* **55:** 603–613.
4. Barnes, P.J. & M. Karin. 1997. Nuclear factor-kappaB: a pivotal transcription factor in chronic inflammatory diseases. *N. Engl. J. Med.* **336:** 1066–1071.
5. Albert, D.A., N.M. Hadler & M.W. Ropes. 1979. Does corticosteroid therapy affect the survival of patients with systemic lupus erythematosus? *Arthritis Rheum.* **22:** 945–953.
6. Huscher, D. *et al.* 2009. Dose-related patterns of glucocorticoid-induced side effects. *Ann. Rheum. Dis.* **68:** 1119–1124.
7. Ziegler, H.K. & E.R. Unanue. 1982. Decrease in macrophage antigen catabolism caused by ammonia and chloroquine is associated with inhibition of antigen presentation to T cells. *Proc. Natl. Acad. Sci. USA* **79:** 175–178.
8. Kuznik, A. *et al.* 2011. Mechanism of endosomal TLR inhibition by antimalarial drugs and imidazoquinolines. *J. Immunol.* **186:** 4794–4804.
9. Group, T.C.H.S. 1991. A randomized study of the effect of withdrawing hydroxychloroquine sulfate in systemic lupus erythematosus. *N. Engl. J. Med.* **324:** 150–154.
10. James, J.A. *et al.* 2007. Hydroxychloroquine sulfate treatment is associated with later onset of systemic lupus erythematosus. *Lupus* **16:** 401–409.
11. Petri, M. 2011. Use of hydroxychloroquine to prevent thrombosis in systemic lupus erythematosus and in antiphospholipid antibody-positive patients. *Curr. Rheumatol. Rep.* **13:** 77–80.
12. Izmirly, P.M. *et al.* 2010. Evaluation of the risk of anti-SSA/Ro-SSB/La antibody-associated cardiac manifestations of neonatal lupus in fetuses of mothers with systemic lupus erythematosus exposed to hydroxychloroquine. *Ann. Rheum. Dis.* **69:** 1827–1830.
13. Ruiz-Irastorza, G. *et al.* 2010. Clinical efficacy and side effects of antimalarials in systemic lupus erythematosus: a systematic review. *Ann. Rheum. Dis.* **69:** 20–28.

14. Gourley, M.F. *et al.* 1996. Methylprednisolone and cyclophosphamide, alone or in combination, in patients with lupus nephritis: a randomized, controlled trial. *Ann. Intern. Med.* **125:** 549–557.

15. Illei, G.G. *et al.* 2001. Combination therapy with pulse cyclophosphamide plus pulse methylprednisolone improves long-term renal outcome without adding toxicity in patients with lupus nephritis. *Ann. Intern. Med.* **135:** 248–257.

16. Wang, C.L., F. Wang & J.J. Bosco. 1995. Ovarian failure in oral cyclophosphamide treatment for systemic lupus erythematosus. *Lupus* **4:** 11–14.

17. Radis, C.D. *et al.* 1995. Effects of cyclophosphamide on the development of malignancy and on long-term survival of patients with rheumatoid arthritis: a 20-year follow-up study. *Arthritis Rheum.* **38:** 1120–1127.

18. McDermott, E.M. & R.J. Powell. 1996. Incidence of ovarian failure in systemic lupus erythematosus after treatment with pulse cyclophosphamide. *Ann. Rheum. Dis.* **55:** 224–229.

19. Mok, C.C., C.S. Lau & R.W. Wong. 1998. Risk factors for ovarian failure in patients with systemic lupus erythematosus receiving cyclophosphamide therapy. *Arthritis Rheum.* **41:** 831–837.

20. Ginzler, E.M. *et al.* 2005. Mycophenolate mofetil or intravenous cyclophosphamide for lupus nephritis. *N. Engl. J. Med.* **353:** 2219–2228.

21. Contreras, G. *et al.* 2004. Sequential therapies for proliferative lupus nephritis. *N. Engl. J. Med.* **350:** 971–980.

22. Appel, G.B. *et al.* 2009. Mycophenolate mofetil versus cyclophosphamide for induction treatment of lupus nephritis. *J. Am. Soc. Nephrol.* **20:** 1103–1112.

23. Sinclair, A. *et al.* 2007. Mycophenolate mofetil as induction and maintenance therapy for lupus nephritis: rationale and protocol for the randomized, controlled Aspreva Lupus Management Study (ALMS). *Lupus* **16:** 972–980.

24. Isenberg, D. *et al.* 2010. Influence of race/ethnicity on response to lupus nephritis treatment: the ALMS study. *Rheumatology (Oxford)* **49:** 128–140.

25. Jorge, S. *et al.* 2008. Mycophenolate mofetil: ten years' experience of a renal transplant unit. *Transplant. Proc.* **40:** 700–704.

26. Sahasranaman, S., D. Howard & S. Roy. 2008. Clinical pharmacology and pharmacogenetics of thiopurines. *Eur. J. Clin. Pharmacol.* **64:** 753–767.

27. Grootscholten, C. *et al.* 2006. Azathioprine/methylprednisolone versus cyclophosphamide in proliferative lupus nephritis: a randomized controlled trial. *Kidney Int.* **70:** 732–742.

28. Mok, C.C. *et al.* 2009. Very long-term outcome of pure lupus membranous nephropathy treated with glucocorticoid and azathioprine. *Lupus* **18:** 1091–1095.

29. Skopouli, F.N. *et al.* 1996. Methotrexate in primary Sjogren's syndrome. *Clin. Exp. Rheumatol.* **14:** 555–558.

30. Fortin, P.R. *et al.* 2008. Steroid-sparing effects of methotrexate in systemic lupus erythematosus: a double-blind, randomized, placebo-controlled trial. *Arthritis Rheum.* **59:** 1796–1804.

31. Neiman, R.A. & K.H. Fye. 1985. Methotrexate induced false photosensitivity reaction. *J. Rheumatol.* **12:** 354–355.

32. Farge, D. *et al.* 2010. Autologous hematopoietic stem cell transplantation for autoimmune diseases: an observational study on 12 years' experience from the European Group for Blood and Marrow Transplantation Working Party on Autoimmune Diseases. *Haematologica* **95:** 284–292.

33. Illei, G.G. *et al.* 2011. Current state and future directions of autologous hematopoietic stem cell transplantation in systemic lupus erythematosus. *Ann. Rheum. Dis.* [epub ahead of print].

34. Arbuckle, M.R. *et al.* 2001. Development of anti-dsDNA autoantibodies prior to clinical diagnosis of systemic lupus erythematosus. *Scand. J. Immunol.* **54:** 211–219.

35. Arbuckle, M.R. *et al.* 2003. Development of autoantibodies before the clinical onset of systemic lupus erythematosus. *N. Engl. J. Med.* **349:** 1526–1533.

36. Murawski, N. & M. Pfreundschuh. 2010. New drugs for aggressive B-cell and T-cell lymphomas. *Lancet Oncol.* **11:** 1074–1085.

37. Taylor, R.P. & M.A. Lindorfer. 2007. Drug insight: the mechanism of action of rituximab in autoimmune disease—the immune complex decoy hypothesis. *Nat. Clin. Pract. Rheumatol.* **3:** 86–95.

38. Anolik, J.H. *et al.* 2004. Rituximab improves peripheral B cell abnormalities in human systemic lupus erythematosus. *Arthritis Rheum.* **50:** 3580–3590.

39. Leandro, M.J. *et al.* 2002. An open study of B lymphocyte depletion in systemic lupus erythematosus. *Arthritis Rheum.* **46:** 2673–2677.

40. Ramos-Casals, M. *et al.* 2009. Rituximab in systemic lupus erythematosus: a systematic review of off-label use in 188 cases. *Lupus* **18:** 767–776.

41. Merrill, J.T. *et al.* 2010. Efficacy and safety of rituximab in moderately-to-severely active systemic lupus erythematosus: the randomized, double-blind, phase II/III systemic lupus erythematosus evaluation of rituximab trial. *Arthritis Rheum.* **62:** 222–233.

42. Furie, R. *et al.* 2009. Efficacy and safety of rituximab in subjects with active proliferative lupus nephritis (LN): results from the randomized, double-blind phase III LUNAR study. In ACR/ARHP Scientific Meeting. Philadelphia, PA.

43. Merrill, J. *et al.* 2011. Assessment of flares in lupus patients enrolled in a phase II/III study of rituximab (EXPLORER). *Lupus* **20:** 709–716.

44. Ramos-Casals, M., C. Diaz-Lagares & M.A. Khamashta. 2009. Rituximab and lupus: good in real life, bad in controlled trials—comment on the article by Lu *et al. Arthritis Rheum.* **61:** 1281–1282.

45. Lu, T.Y. *et al.* 2009. A retrospective seven-year analysis of the use of B cell depletion therapy in systemic lupus erythematosus at University College London Hospital: the first fifty patients. *Arthritis Rheum.* **61:** 482–487.

46. Clifford, D.B. *et al.* 2011. Rituximab-associated progressive multifocal leukoencephalopathy in rheumatoid arthritis. *Arch Neurol* **68:** 1156–1164.

47. Daridon, C. *et al.* 2010. Epratuzumab targeting of CD22 affects adhesion molecule expression and migration of B-cells in systemic lupus erythematosus. *Arthritis Res. Ther.* **12:** R204.

48. Mackay, F. & P. Schneider. 2009. Cracking the BAFF code. *Nat. Rev. Immunol.* **9:** 491–502.

49. Castigli, E. *et al.* 2005. TACI is mutant in common variable immunodeficiency and IgA deficiency. *Nat. Genet.* **37:** 829–834.

50. Zhang, L. *et al.* 2007. Transmembrane activator and calcium-modulating cyclophilin ligand interactor mutations in common variable immunodeficiency: clinical and immunologic outcomes in heterozygotes. *J. Allergy Clin. Immunol.* **120:** 1178–1185.

51. Cheema, G.S. *et al.* 2001. Elevated serum B lymphocyte stimulator levels in patients with systemic immune-based rheumatic diseases. *Arthritis Rheum.* **44:** 1313–1319.

52. Navarra, S.V. *et al.* 2011. Efficacy and safety of belimumab in patients with active systemic lupus erythematosus: a randomised, placebo-controlled, phase 3 trial. *Lancet* **377:** 721–731.

53. von Vollenhoven, R.F. *et al.* 2010. Belimumab, a BLyS-specific inhibitor, reduces disease activity and severe flares in seropositive SLE patients—BLISS-76 study [Abstract]. *Ann. Rheum. Dis.* **69**(Suppl. 3): 74.

54. Dall'Era, M. *et al.* 2007. Reduced B lymphocyte and immunoglobulin levels after atacicept treatment in patients with systemic lupus erythematosus: results of a multi-center, phase Ib, double-blind, placebo-controlled, dose-escalating trial. *Arthritis Rheum.* **56:** 4142–4150.

55. Pena-Rossi, C. *et al.* 2009. An exploratory dose-escalating study investigating the safety, tolerability, pharmacokinetics and pharmacodynamics of intravenous atacicept in patients with systemic lupus erythematosus. *Lupus* **18:** 547–555.

56. Waisman, A. *et al.* 1997. Modulation of murine systemic lupus erythematosus with peptides based on complementarity determining regions of a pathogenic anti-DNA monoclonal antibody. *Proc. Natl. Acad. Sci. USA* **94:** 4620–4625.

57. Elmann, A. *et al.* 2007. Altered gene expression in mice with lupus treated with edratide, a peptide that ameliorates the disease manifestations. *Arthritis Rheum.* **56:** 2371–2381.

58. Sthoeger, Z.M. *et al.* 2009. Treatment of lupus patients with a tolerogenic peptide, hCDR1 (Edratide): immunomodulation of gene expression. *J. Autoimmun.* **33:** 77–82.

59. Jones, D.S. *et al.* 1995. Immunospecific reduction of antioligonucleotide antibody-forming cells with a tetrakis-oligonucleotide conjugate (LJP 394), a therapeutic candidate for the treatment of lupus nephritis. *J. Med. Chem.* **38:** 2138–2144.

60. Furie, R.A. *et al.* 2001. Treatment of systemic lupus erythematosus with LJP 394. *J. Rheumatol.* **28:** 257–265.

61. Weisman, M.H. *et al.* 1997. Reduction in circulating dsDNA antibody titer after administration of LJP 394. *J. Rheumatol.* **24:** 314–318.

62. Alarcon-Segovia, D. *et al.* 2003. LJP 394 for the prevention of renal flare in patients with systemic lupus erythematosus: results from a randomized, double-blind, placebo-controlled study. *Arthritis Rheum.* **48:** 442–454.

63. Cardiel, M.H. *et al.* 2008. Abetimus sodium for renal flare in systemic lupus erythematosus: results of a randomized, controlled phase III trial. *Arthritis Rheum.* **58:** 2470–2480.

64. Kyogoku, C. *et al.* 2002. Fcgamma receptor gene polymorphisms in Japanese patients with systemic lupus erythematosus: contribution of FCGR2B to genetic susceptibility. *Arthritis Rheum.* **46:** 1242–1254.

65. Su, K. *et al.* 2004. A promoter haplotype of the immunoreceptor tyrosine-based inhibitory motif-bearing FcgammaRIIb alters receptor expression and associates with autoimmunity. II. Differential binding of GATA4 and Yin-Yang1 transcription factors and correlated receptor expression and function. *J. Immunol.* **172:** 7192–7199.

66. Kaneko, Y., F. Nimmerjahn & J.V. Ravetch. 2006. Anti-inflammatory activity of immunoglobulin G resulting from Fc sialylation. *Science* **313:** 670–673.

67. Smith, K.G. & M.R. Clatworthy. 2010. FcgammaRIIB in autoimmunity and infection: evolutionary and therapeutic implications. *Nat. Rev. Immunol.* **10:** 328–343.

68. Linker-Israeli, M. *et al.* 1991. Elevated levels of endogenous IL-6 in systemic lupus erythematosus: a putative role in pathogenesis. *J. Immunol.* **147:** 117–123.

69. Jeon, J.Y. *et al.* 2010. Interleukin 6 gene polymorphisms are associated with systemic lupus erythematosus in Koreans. *J. Rheumatol.* **37:** 2251–2258.

70. Santos, M.J. *et al.* 2011. Interleukin-6 promoter polymorphism −174 G/C is associated with nephritis in Portuguese Caucasian systemic lupus erythematosus patients. *Clin. Rheumatol.* **30:** 409–413.

71. Illei, G.G. *et al.* 2010. Tocilizumab in systemic lupus erythematosus: data on safety, preliminary efficacy, and impact on circulating plasma cells from an open-label phase I dosage-escalation study. *Arthritis Rheum.* **62:** 542–552.

72. Aringer, M. *et al.* 2004. Safety and efficacy of tumor necrosis factor alpha blockade in systemic lupus erythematosus: an open-label study. *Arthritis Rheum.* **50:** 3161–3169.

73. Ali, Y. & S. Shah. 2002. Infliximab-induced systemic lupus erythematosus. *Ann. Intern. Med.* **137:** 625–626.

74. Favalli, E.G. *et al.* 2002. Drug-induced lupus following treatment with infliximab in rheumatoid arthritis. *Lupus* **11:** 753–755.

75. Llorente, L. *et al.* 2000. Clinical and biologic effects of anti-interleukin-10 monoclonal antibody administration in systemic lupus erythematosus. *Arthritis Rheum.* **43:** 1790–1800.

76. Crispin, J.C. *et al.* 2008. Expanded double negative T cells in patients with systemic lupus erythematosus produce IL-17 and infiltrate the kidneys. *J. Immunol.* **181:** 8761–8766.

77. Wong, C.K. *et al.* 2008. Hyperproduction of IL-23 and IL-17 in patients with systemic lupus erythematosus: implications for Th17-mediated inflammation in auto-immunity. *Clin. Immunol.* **127:** 385–393.

78. Zhang, Z., V.C. Kyttaris & G.C. Tsokos. 2009. The role of IL-23/IL-17 axis in lupus nephritis. *J. Immunol.* **183:** 3160–3169.

79. Kang, H.K., M. Liu & S.K. Datta. 2007. Low-dose peptide tolerance therapy of lupus generates plasmacytoid dendritic cells that cause expansion of autoantigen-specific regulatory T cells and contraction of inflammatory Th17 cells. *J. Immunol.* **178:** 7849–7858.

80. Hueber, W. *et al.* 2010. Effects of AIN457, a fully human antibody to interleukin-17A, on psoriasis, rheumatoid arthritis, and uveitis. *Sci. Transl. Med.* **2:** 52ra72.

81. Griffiths, C.E. *et al.* 2010. Comparison of ustekinumab and etanercept for moderate-to-severe psoriasis. *N. Engl. J. Med.* **362:** 118–128.

82. Chaussabel, D. *et al.* 2008. A modular analysis framework for blood genomics studies: application to systemic lupus erythematosus. *Immunity* **29:** 150–164.

83. Preble, O.T. *et al.* 1982. Systemic lupus erythematosus: presence in human serum of an unusual acid-labile leukocyte interferon. *Science* **216:** 429–431.

84. Ytterberg, S.R. & T.J. Schnitzer. 1982. Serum interferon levels in patients with systemic lupus erythematosus. *Arthritis Rheum.* **25:** 401–406.

85. Garcia-Romo, G.S. *et al.* 2011. Netting neutrophils are major inducers of type I IFN production in pediatric systemic lupus erythematosus. *Sci. Transl. Med.* **3:** 73ra20.

86. Yao, Y. *et al.* 2009. Neutralization of interferon-alpha/beta-inducible genes and downstream effect in a phase I trial of an anti-interferon-alpha monoclonal antibody in systemic lupus erythematosus. *Arthritis Rheum.* **60:** 1785–1796.

87. Desai-Mehta, A. *et al.* 1996. Hyperexpression of CD40 ligand by B and T cells in human lupus and its role in pathogenic autoantibody production. *J. Clin. Invest.* **97:** 2063–2073.

88. Harigai, M. *et al.* 1999. Responsiveness of peripheral blood B cells to recombinant CD40 ligand in patients with systemic lupus erythematosus. *Lupus* **8:** 227–233.

89. Huang, W. *et al.* 2002. The effect of anti-CD40 ligand antibody on B cells in human systemic lupus erythematosus. *Arthritis Rheum.* **46:** 1554–1562.

90. Patel, V.L., J. Schwartz & J.B. Bussel. 2008. The effect of anti-CD40 ligand in immune thrombocytopenic purpura. *Br. J. Haematol.* **141:** 545–548.

91. Boumpas, D.T. *et al.* 2003. A short course of BG9588 (anti-CD40 ligand antibody) improves serologic activity and decreases hematuria in patients with proliferative lupus glomerulonephritis. *Arthritis Rheum.* **48:** 719–727.

92. Robles-Carrillo, L. *et al.* 2010. Anti-CD40L immune complexes potently activate platelets in vitro and cause thrombosis in FCGR2A transgenic mice. *J. Immunol.* **185:** 1577–1583.

93. Kalunian, K.C. *et al.* 2002. Treatment of systemic lupus erythematosus by inhibition of T cell costimulation with anti-CD154: a randomized, double-blind, placebo-controlled trial. *Arthritis Rheum.* **46:** 3251–3258.

94. Merrill, J.T. *et al.* 2010. The efficacy and safety of abatacept in patients with non-life-threatening manifestations of systemic lupus erythematosus: results of a twelve-month, multicenter, exploratory, phase IIb, randomized, double-blind, placebo-controlled trial. *Arthritis Rheum.* **62:** 3077–3087.

95. Larsen, C.P. *et al.* 2010. Belatacept-based regimens versus a cyclosporine A-based regimen in kidney transplant recipients: 2-year results from the BENEFIT and BENEFIT-EXT studies. *Transplantation* **90:** 1528–1535.

96. Weber, J. 2009. Ipilimumab: controversies in its development, utility and autoimmune adverse events. *Cancer Immunol. Immunother.* **58:** 823–830.

97. Yang, J.H. *et al.* 2005. Expression and function of inducible costimulator on peripheral blood T cells in patients with systemic lupus erythematosus. *Rheumatology (Oxford)* **44:** 1245–1254.

98. Nurieva, R.I. *et al.* 2003. Inducible costimulator is essential for collagen-induced arthritis. *J. Clin. Invest.* **111:** 701–706.

99. Hu, Y.L. *et al.* 2009. B7RP-1 blockade ameliorates autoimmunity through regulation of follicular helper T cells. *J. Immunol.* **182:** 1421–1428.

100. Solomou, E.E. *et al.* 2001. Molecular basis of deficient IL-2 production in T cells from patients with systemic lupus erythematosus. *J. Immunol.* **166:** 4216–4222.

101. Scheinecker, C., M. Bonelli & J.S. Smolen. 2010. Pathogenetic aspects of systemic lupus erythematosus with an emphasis on regulatory T cells. *J Autoimmun.* **35:** 269–275.

102. Enyedy, E.J. *et al.* 2001. Fc epsilon receptor type I gamma chain replaces the deficient T cell receptor zeta chain in T cells of patients with systemic lupus erythematosus. *Arthritis Rheum.* **44:** 1114–1121.

103. Krishnan, S. *et al.* 2003. The FcR gamma subunit and Syk kinase replace the CD3 zeta-chain and ZAP-70 kinase in the TCR signaling complex of human effector CD4 T cells. *J. Immunol.* **170:** 4189–4195.

104. Deng, G.M. *et al.* 2010. Suppression of skin and kidney disease by inhibition of spleen tyrosine kinase in lupus-prone mice. *Arthritis Rheum.* **62:** 2086–2092.

105. Weinblatt, M.E. *et al.* 2010. An oral spleen tyrosine kinase (Syk) inhibitor for rheumatoid arthritis. *N. Engl. J. Med.* **363:** 1303–1312.

106. Ghoreschi, K. *et al.* 2011. Modulation of innate and adaptive immune responses by tofacitinib (CP-690,550). *J. Immunol.* **186:** 4234–4243.

107. Garber, K. 2011. Pfizer's JAK inhibitor sails through phase 3 in rheumatoid arthritis. *Nat. Biotechnol.* **29:** 467–468.

108. Kremer, J.M. *et al.* 2009. The safety and efficacy of a JAK inhibitor in patients with active rheumatoid arthritis: results of a double-blind, placebo-controlled phase IIa trial of three dosage levels of CP-690,550 versus placebo. *Arthritis Rheum.* **60:** 1895–1905.

109. Humrich, J.Y. *et al.* 2010. Homeostatic imbalance of regulatory and effector T cells due to IL-2 deprivation amplifies murine lupus. *Proc. Natl. Acad. Sci. USA* **107:** 204–209.

110. Juang, Y.T. *et al.* 2005. Systemic lupus erythematosus serum IgG increases CREM binding to the IL-2 promoter and suppresses IL-2 production through CaMKIV. *J. Clin. Invest.* **115:** 996–1005.

111. Ichinose, K. *et al.* 2011. Suppression of autoimmunity and organ pathology in lupus-prone mice upon inhibition of calcium/calmodulin-dependent protein kinase type IV. *Arthritis Rheum.* **63:** 523–529.

112. Moroni, G., A. Doria & C. Ponticelli. 2009. Cyclosporine (CsA) in lupus nephritis: assessing the evidence. *Nephrol. Dial. Transplant.* **24:** 15–20.

113. Kyttaris, V.C. *et al.* 2011. Calcium signaling in systemic lupus erythematosus T cells: a treatment target. *Arthritis Rheum.* **63:** 2058–2066.

114. Crispin, J.C. *et al.* 2010. Expression of CD44 variant isoforms CD44v3 and CD44v6 is increased on T cells from

patients with systemic lupus erythematosus and is correlated with disease activity. *Arthritis Rheum.* **62:** 1431–1437.

115. Li, Y. *et al.* 2007. Phosphorylated ERM is responsible for increased T cell polarization, adhesion, and migration in patients with systemic lupus erythematosus. *J. Immunol.* **178:** 1938–1947.

116. Biswas, P.S. *et al.* 2010. Phosphorylation of IRF4 by ROCK2 regulates IL-17 and IL-21 production and the development of autoimmunity in mice. *J. Clin. Invest.* **120:** 3280–3295.

117. Wang, G. *et al.* 2010. Markers of oxidative and nitrosative stress in systemic lupus erythematosus: correlation with disease activity. *Arthritis Rheum.* **62:** 2064–2072.

118. Karlson, E.W. *et al.* 2007. Effect of glutathione S-transferase polymorphisms and proximity to hazardous waste sites on time to systemic lupus erythematosus diagnosis: results from the Roxbury lupus project. *Arthritis Rheum.* **56:** 244–254.

119. Suwannaroj, S. *et al.* 2001. Antioxidants suppress mortality in the female NZB x NZW F1 mouse model of systemic lupus erythematosus (SLE). *Lupus* **10:** 258–265.

120. Tewthanom, K. *et al.* 2010. The effect of high dose of N-acetylcysteine in lupus nephritis: a case report and literature review. *J. Clin. Pharm. Ther.* **35:** 483–485.

121. Gergely, P., Jr. *et al.* 2002. Mitochondrial hyperpolarization and ATP depletion in patients with systemic lupus erythematosus. *Arthritis Rheum.* **46:** 175–190.

122. Fernandez, D.R. *et al.* 2009. Activation of mammalian target of rapamycin controls the loss of TCRzeta in lupus T cells through HRES-1/Rab4-regulated lysosomal degradation. *J. Immunol.* **182:** 2063–2073.

123. Lui, S.L. *et al.* 2008. Rapamycin prevents the development of nephritis in lupus-prone NZB/W F1 mice. *Lupus* **17:** 305–313.

124. Fernandez, D. *et al.* 2006. Rapamycin reduces disease activity and normalizes T cell activation-induced calcium fluxing in patients with systemic lupus erythematosus. *Arthritis Rheum.* **54:** 2983–2988.

125. Lu, Q. *et al.* 2007. Demethylation of CD40LG on the inactive X in T cells from women with lupus. *J. Immunol.* **179:** 6352–6358.

126. Zhao, M. *et al.* 2010. Hypomethylation of IL10 and IL13 promoters in CD4+ T cells of patients with systemic lupus erythematosus. *J. Biomed. Biotechnol.* **2010:** 931018.

127. Sunahori, K. *et al.* 2011. Promoter hypomethylation results in increased expression of protein phosphatase 2A in T cells from patients with systemic lupus erythematosus. *J. Immunol.* **186:** 4508–4517.

128. Tenbrock, K. *et al.* 2005. The cyclic AMP response element modulator regulates transcription of the TCR zeta-chain. *J. Immunol.* **175:** 5975–5980.

129. Reilly, C.M. *et al.* 2008. The histone deacetylase inhibitor trichostatin A upregulates regulatory T cells and modulates autoimmunity in NZB/W F1 mice. *J. Autoimmun.* **31:** 123–130.

130. Wang, Y. *et al.* 1996. Amelioration of lupus-like autoimmune disease in NZB/WF1 mice after treatment with a blocking monoclonal antibody specific for complement component C5. *Proc. Natl. Acad. Sci. USA* **93:** 8563–8568.

131. Bao, L. & R.J. Quigg. 2007. Complement in lupus nephritis: the good, the bad, and the unknown. *Semin. Nephrol.* **27:** 69–80.

132. Barrat, F.J. *et al.* 2007. Treatment of lupus-prone mice with a dual inhibitor of TLR7 and TLR9 leads to reduction of autoantibody production and amelioration of disease symptoms. *Eur. J. Immunol.* **37:** 3582–3586.

Ann. N.Y. Acad. Sci. ISSN 0077-8923

# Corrigendum for Ann. N.Y. Acad. Sci. 1242: 26–39

Liu, J.M., J.M. Lipton & S. Mani. 2011. Sixth International Congress on Shwachman-Diamond syndrome: from patients to genes and back. *Ann. N.Y. Acad. Sci.* **1242:** 26–39.

The sentence that begins at the bottom of the left column on page 35 should read as follows:

The most common clonal marrow cytogenetic abnormalities in SDS are i(7q) and del(20q).

doi: 10.1111/j.1749-6632.2012.06459.x